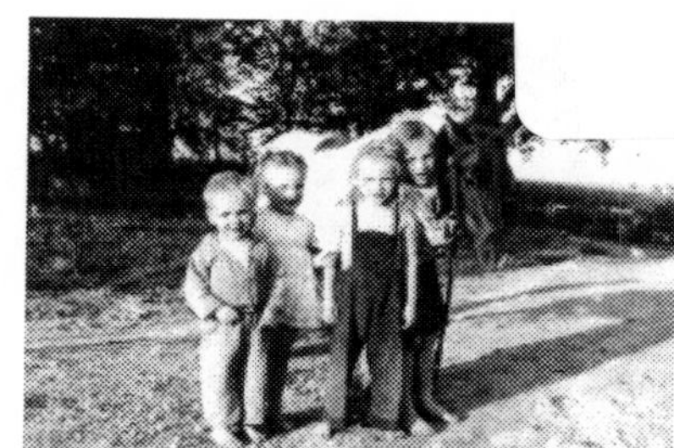

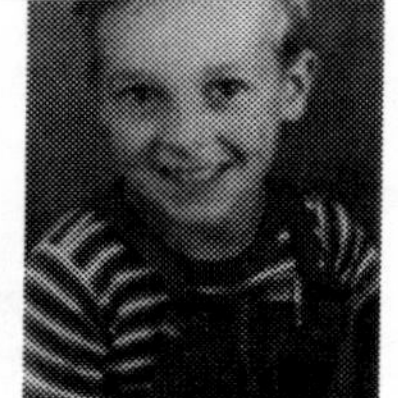

The Upside of the Downside

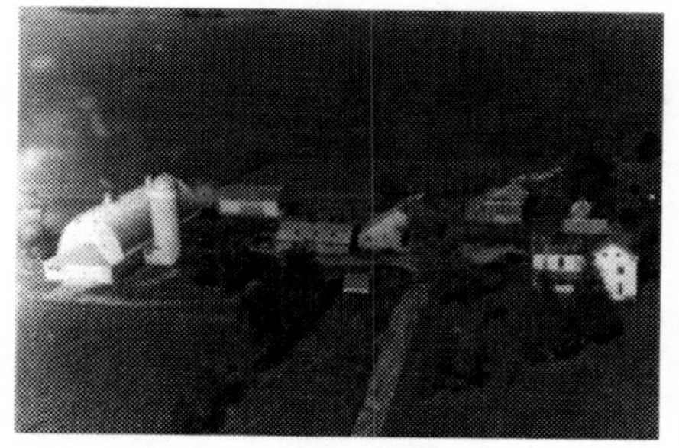

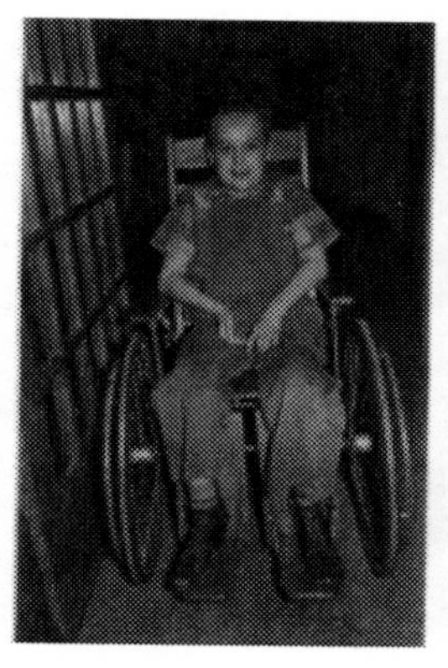

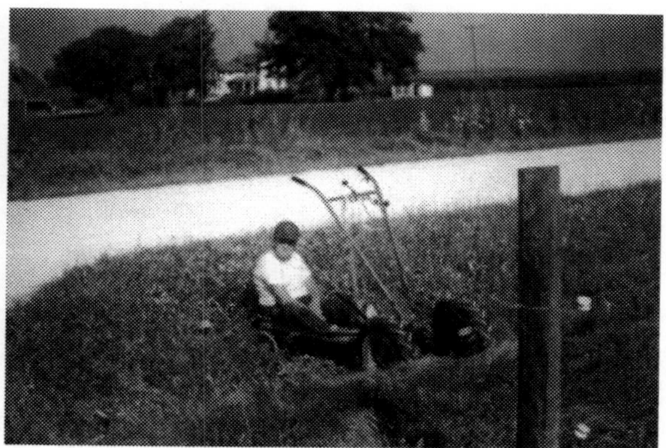

The Upside of the Downside

Journeys with a Companion Called Polio

KENT KLOEPPING

The Upside of the Downside: Journeys with a Companion Called Polio

Published by Wheatmark®
610 East Delano Street, Suite 104
Tucson, Arizona 85705 U.S.A.
www.wheatmark.com

International Standard Book Number: 978-1-58736-641-3
International Standard Book Number: 1-58736-641-X
Library of Congress Control Number: 2006929000

Contents

FOR

My mother, father, family, and countless others
Who made me realize that life is indeed not fair.
I gave only my legs, but in return I received more
Than any one person should expect. There was
Unconditional love, much kindness, continuing
Encouragement, patience in my frustrations, great
Friendships, and limitless opportunities; and because
Of them and what they gave me, I found my way.

Acknowledgements

In drafting this section, I was surprised at the number of people who had made helpful and significant contributions toward the completion of this endeavor. I sincerely hope and trust that I have not overlooked any individuals or failed to mention their name. If I did, please let me know and I will diligently attempt to make amends. In no particular order or priority, I want to acknowledge the following individuals:

Sue Poppaw, a great buddy and college classmate (Southern Illinois University days) comes to mind initially, as she did the major share of typing and retyping of the manuscript. I have terrible handwriting, but she persevered. She also contributed innumerable editorial suggestions, and was willing to point out sections that were poorly written.

My wife, Marlys, lent her excellent language and great proof reading skills, made numerous suggestions on readability and also made certain I didn't "embroider on the truth." Without her tenacity the last several months, I'm not sure that I would have completed the project.

Dr. Murray DeArmond, my former boss at the University of Arizona and a talented writer himself, read the entire work and, along with my Aunt Esther and friend Sue, agreed to help write comments about the book.

Dr. Paul Leung of the University of North Texas was especially helpful with the chapters Illinois Research, Travels, and most importantly, the Epilogue, On Being a Gimp: Differently Abled.

Two special friends, Tom and Tina Bush, provided excellent feedback from the perspective of the reading audience.

Dr. Devon Mihesuah, a gifted writer who has authored ten books herself, advised major structural recommendations, pointed to gaps in the story, and made critically important editorial comments relevant to the potential for publication of the manuscript. She and her husband Josh are good friends.

My mother, her sister Esther, my two sisters Carol and Jolene, my brother Larry, childhood and life-long friend, Dick Rockey, and family friends, Kenny Nott and Fritz Kolb patiently sat through interviews with me. I interviewed Mom on several occasions, and Aunt Esther at least twice. Their thoughts, suggestions, and corrections were helpful in not only shaping topics, but in personalizing material, helping me develop timelines of events, and providing a cohesiveness to the overall story line. There were other family members and friends who continued to inquire about progress, which served to keep me motivated to finish the manuscript.

Somewhere late in the process, Sue Poppaw mentioned the book to her daughter, Lisa Poppaw-Schinerer, a bright, not shy, assertive young woman. Lisa quickly suggested that I needed a real editor, someone like her! I took her up on her offer and discovered that, in fact, she was a talented, up and coming editorial consultant. She made major organizational, structural and editorial contributions to the manuscript.

I also interviewed Linda Scheider, a fellow polio patient in 1948 at the (then) Deaconess Hospital in Freeport, Illinois. Other polio survivors I interviewed were Russell Zimmerman in Illinois, Gloria Schawke in Minnesota, and Madean Perrin from Tucson, Arizona.

Finally, I must mention two fellows, one of whom I know, and the other I wish I had. The first guy is Matthew, my son, who extricated me innumerable times from my Word Perfect foul-ups on our home computer (which he most likely considered hazardous duty). He scanned all the pictures for me and provided candid observations that ultimately helped shape the final organization of the book. He threatened on more than one occasion to stop providing any further assistance, but invariably came to my rescue. I am, without a doubt, a "techno-peasant" who can wreak havoc simply by turning on the machine.

The other guy, Mark Twain, whom I obviously didn't know but greatly admire for his cynical and incisive commentaries on a wide range of social, religious, and political matters, is one of my all-time favorite debunkers of sanctimonious snobs. He had a marvelous command of language, and fittingly, one of his better lines was,"The difference between the right word and the just about right word is like the difference between lightning and a lightning bug."(1)

I often tell Matthew that he too should be a writer. He has a knack for the right word and a wonderful command of language. At times, I see striking similarities between his commentary on issues of today and those of the old curmudgeon Twain.

The Upside of the Downside

I. Foreword.

In 1945, when I was seven years old, I, along with thousands of other Americans, contracted the deadly poliovirus. It would leave me with significant paralysis and render me a lifetime wheelchair user. It would, of course, dramatically alter the course of my life and usher in profound changes for my family as well.

When I retired from the University of Arizona in 1998, I began taking classes in writing. One particular teacher was not only a first rate instructor, but was also very supportive of all the class members efforts. One of her most helpful suggestions was for each of us to write a memoir. So I did.

This is not a very complicated story. Hopefully, however, there are some issues and experiences I've related that will cause you, the reader, to pause and ponder a bit; but nothing so complex as to tax the brain. What I have attempted to communicate is how my life was different from that of an individual who did not have a significant disability. Throughout my life there have been many barriers. Some have been obvious, but more often they've been less visible and quite insidious—things most people may not realize exist.

This story is also about how my family, great friends, and the entire community where I grew up helped me become a "whole" person again. I was rarely—if ever—treated or made to feel like I was a victim. Early on my parents encouraged me take charge of my life, assert my independence, see beyond my physical limitations and confront the obstacles in life that lay ahead for me. Along the way, I had to fight a lot of battles against ignorance and fear of disability. My colleagues and I pissed off a lot of people with our disability advocacy, but we were successful in changing some attitudes.

I was fortunate to find a partner who had learned early on to use her head to overcome problems, as she too was unable to use her legs to run away from the challenges of life. Together we accomplished a lot of good things, with perhaps our best collaborative effort being our son.

Being disabled isn't really funny, in and of itself. But precisely because of the disability, I have experienced, observed or been told of amusing—even hilarious—situations. In this tome, I've included some of my favorites.

What follows are many experiences and events that I and a few other people could recall related to growing up and living with a disability. Looking back, I'd say it has been a good journey, and at 67 years of age, I can honestly say that I am a lucky fellow.

II. Childhood-Changes

When I was a patient at the Kent Cottage in the spring of 1946, our nurses lifted our spirits by teaching us silly songs, including:

Chickory Chick.

"Once there lived a chicken who would say 'chick-chick,'
'Chick-chick' all day
Soon that chick got sick and tired of just 'chick-chick'
So one morning he started to say:

Chickery chick, cha-la, cha-la
Check-a-la romey in a bananika
Bollika, wollika, can't you see
Chickery chick is me?"

Every time you're sick and tired of just the same
old thing
Sayin' just the same old words all day
Be just like the chicken who found something
new to sing
Open up your mouth and start to say

Oh!

Chickery chick, cha-la, cha-la
Check-a-la romey in a bananika
Bollika, wollika, can't you see
Chickery chick is me?" (1)

Autumn in the Midwest is a wondrous time. There is a sense of fulfillment that pervades the rural communities in this heartland of America. The harvest is mostly complete, and the bounty of a summer's labor for these God-fearing people has been stored away. The brilliantly colored leaves gently cascade to earth and are raked into piles to the delight of children. In the cool evenings, the aromatic haze from burning leaves hangs in the air and delights the senses. It is a time of joy and thanksgiving. But in the late summer of 1945, an insidious terror pervaded this bucolic scene. An ancient and stealthy killer was again on the prowl. In the festering, stagnant heat of July, polio had struck in epidemic proportions in northern Illinois. The nation's most severe epidemic of the year had centered in Rockford, Illinois, and Winnebago County. Through the end of that October, the Winnebago County chapter of the National Foundation for Infantile Paralysis reported three hundred and eighty-two cases in the community. I lived there, five miles from Winnebago County. Silent fear gripped every family. I remember my mother speaking in hushed tones on the telephone, and we knew another victim had been claimed. Who would be next? Public prayers pleaded for divine protection, and private supplications asked that others be chosen. My two sisters became quite ill, and unspoken to the four children, were our parents' worst fears. Fortunately, they both recovered quickly without a diagnosis of the dreaded disease. But as the cataclysmic events at Hiroshima were to forever alter the course of human history in the summer of 1945, I, too, was rapidly approaching a catastrophic turning point that fateful year.

In the 1940's, my family, which consisted of my parents, Dale and Christine, my brother Larry who is four years my senior, my sister Carol who is nine days shy of a year older than me, and my sister Jolene who is three years my junior, lived on what had originally been great grandfather Jacob Rodenbough's farm in southern Wisconsin. The land, best suited for dairy farming, was mostly rolling limestone hills with a portion of the land bordering the Illinois state line and an additional eighteen acre plot in Illinois that we called the lot. Old Jacob Rodenbough was from Pennsylvania, and came to Wisconsin in 1872, moving west to buy land and find a new home. The land he chose included ten acres of timber known as the Oakley Woods, which is still in the family.

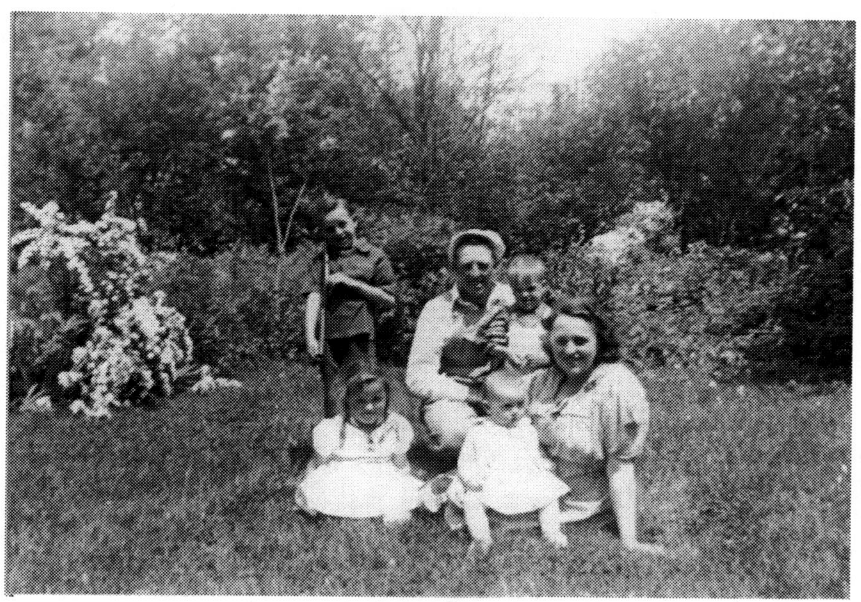

My family in Wisconsin (spring, 1942)

Farm life in the rural Midwest in the 1940's was characterized by long hours of hard, manual labor. There was an abundance of good food, family and friends, but pleasures were simple, as most families did not have money to spend on frills. Even mundane events could be sources of excitement and highly anticipated. Such was the case with a weekly visitor to our farm.

Racing out of the house, letting the screen door bang shut behind me, I always wanted to be the first one to greet him. It was thrilling for a four year old to once again see that huge box shaped truck with the vividly painted advertising on the sides. He drove with the doors open and when he stopped the vehicle, he had to come down two steps to the ground. It wasn't like our truck and it surely wasn't a car. No, it was a special vehicle with a unique mission. When we saw the clouds of billowing dust from the north trailing the speeding vehicle, we knew he was about to make his weekly visit. As near as I can recall, his uniform was dark, maybe brown, and had his name emblazoned on the pocket of his neatly pressed shirt. Sometimes he left the engine running as he leaped off his high stool-like seat, grabbing the large metal carrying case full of those mouth-watering samples, and quickly descended the steps. Always with a big smile and a cheerful, "Hey how are you today?" he headed for the house. As he disappeared through the front door, I'd quickly sneak into the truck, grasping the rail only because it was there. Inside, the truck was lined with shelves, racks, and metal drawers. Deftly sliding out a drawer, I'd marvel at the unimaginable, breathtaking delights. The smell was intoxicating. When I saw him returning, I'd quietly slip out the driver's side door, move away, and wait to bid him good-bye. With a quick salute, he was gone south, dust flying. I stood watching him go, still savoring the heavenly aromas and delectable looking treats that were packed in that marvelous vehicle. Oh, how I wished they weren't so expensive. Maybe, I reasoned, maybe next week we'd partake of his wares. It was one of my favorite childhood memories, the times when the Bread Man came.

Thinking back to that time, I have a strong sense of my parents at work doing chores, especially during the spring and summer months. We never had indoor plumbing, and didn't have electricity until 1941. Our large kitchen, with its massive iron wood-burning cook stove, was the hub of activity in our home. We ate in the kitchen year round, and beginning in late fall and through the winter months, we essentially lived in the kitchen as well, for it was the only heated room in the house. On special occasions—Sunday visitors, for example—we opened the parlor and had a fire in our ornate potbelly heating stove. Our home, without electricity, had almost no conveniences of a modern kitchen. Everything was labored by hand; cooking, baking, cleaning, laundry, and countless other tasks that we, in the twenty-first century, rely on machines to accomplish. Because of the workloads, most families employed additional workers. We called them "hired men" and "hired girls." My parents had numerous of both categories, and some lived with us while others worked by the day. One of them, a lanky seventeen year old soft-spoken Swiss lad from the rolling hills of Argyle, Wisconsin, Frederick "Fritz" Kolb, came to work for us in 1941, and stayed with us for over three years. We would all come to regard him as a member of our family, and although he was the hired man, he was also, to my parents, a combination son, colleague, and friend. During the ensuing years, he became to me not only a big brother but also, at times, a surrogate parent who had no trouble in his role as disciplinarian.

Farmers didn't spend a lot of time going places, as there was always work waiting to be done. Consequently, farm children spent most of their time at home before entering primary school. If there was nothing special happening on the farm like threshing, haymaking, butchering, visits from the Bread Man, or family visiting, we spent our time exploring. By the time I was five years old, I had covered almost every square foot of our two hundred fifty-eight acre farm, including the several miles of old State Line Road that was closed and overgrown with brush and trees. I had explored Grandpa's ten-acre woods and his forty-acre farm, every building on our place and the neighboring Earlywine farm, as well as several other neighboring places that we visited. I was a thin and wiry boy who rarely wore shoes or a shirt during the summer and who, according to my mom, was "brown as an Indian." As a carefree child of the country, the wonders of life had begun to unfold for me—I had found my legs. I was not only swift, but I was also tireless; quite accidentally, I discovered that I was faster than almost anyone, including the eighth-grade boys at our small school of some seventy-five children. I had more endurance than anyone who challenged me. It was an exhilarating feeling for a child of seven to realize that for long distances, I was unequaled. I relished the feeling of winning and being the best. I was very inquisitive and kept myself constantly busy with a vivid and large imagination. I could tell you where every fox den was on the farm, and I had located badger holes and places where pheasants nested. I knew where the best choke cherry trees were, as well as wild strawberry beds, wild plum trees, and even thistle patches. I had the place completely mapped out in my mind.

My mother's parents, Mattie and Luther Rodenbough, lived just a mile north of us on a forty-acre farm. Grandma had a Guernsey cow and made homemade butter, which I didn't like. She was a very talented woman (my mother used to say she was about forty years ahead of her time), who raised a huge garden, was an accomplished artist, played music without reading notes, sewed beautifully, and could get a complete meal in about ten minutes. Mary Martha Rodenbough never fit the mold of the rural midwestern farm wife. She was bright, unpredictable, and often restless, and could pull the wool over the eyes of almost anyone she met if she felt inclined to do so. A short anecdote gives one a glimpse into the mind of this complex woman. As many good rural housewives did in the 1920's, she was attending a local homemaker's meeting, probably sponsored by the University of Wisconsin Extension Service. I could imagine her finding the discussions of domestic issues and gossip boring and a waste of time. I'm told that during those years it had become acceptable, even rather sheik, to have Amer-

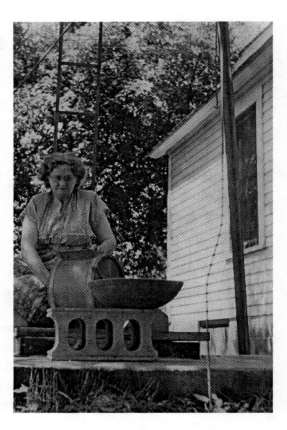

My grandmother "Mattie" Rodenbough churning butter from her Guernsey cow (1950s)

ican Indian blood coursing through one's veins, particularly if the strain was Cherokee, one of the so-called civilized tribes. During the discussion of bloodlines, Grandma took advantage of a pause in the conversation and quipped, "Well you know, I have a little Indian in me also, it's probably about the size of a squirrel." She had informed them that she was pregnant, but had also shocked them enough to end the chatter about Indians. She was a master at squelching the inane.

Grandpa Luther liked to wear a red bandanna around his neck, like a cowboy. Mom told me once he had wanted to go west, but Grandma wouldn't go. He had a team of western horses that carried visible brands. They were half-wild and many farmers were reluctant to drive them. In fact, it seemed Grandpa had lots of wild animals. One day he tried to lead a young heifer from our farm to his place and she attacked him. I still remember him lying in our yard, his face ghostly white, in obvious pain, but he never said he hurt or didn't feel well. He had an old boar hog with huge tusks; it attacked one of his horses, ripping open an artery, killing the horse.

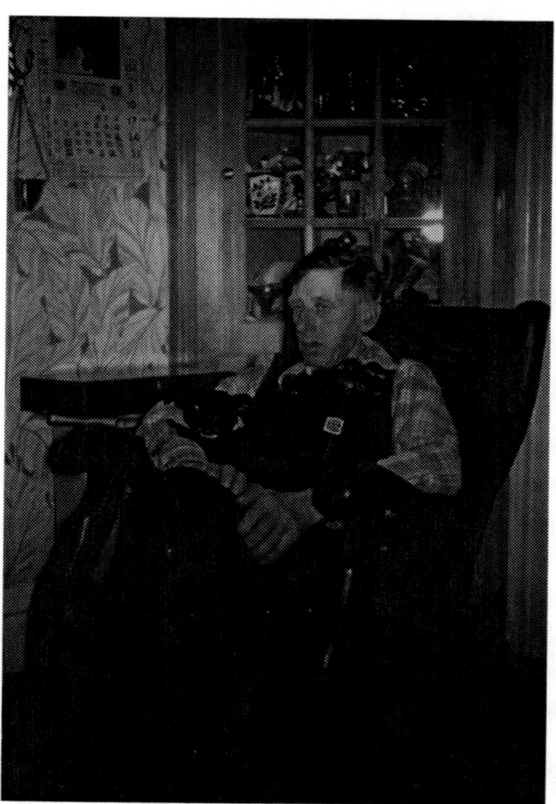

My grandfather Luther Rodenbough and my dog Sparky (January 1954)

He took Larry and I camping

once overnight to the Sugar River, maybe ten miles from our home. It was a fun day, but by nightfall I missed Mom and Dad and wanted to go home. But Grandpa Rodenbough was a fellow who never looked back. Once a task, project, or camping trip was started, it got finished. He had a damn mean dog, Pat, an Irish water spaniel. On our return from the camping trip, Larry went to the car to get Grandpa's shoes and Pat, lying in the car, chewed up and down on both of Larry's arms.

I hated that dog, and secretly rejoiced when a car hit him and he subsequently died. Pat, the dog, had a habit of airing out his penis. He'd sit with fully one-half to two-thirds of it exposed. Just to hear what he would say, we'd ask Grandpa, "Hey, what is that?" Grandpa knew we were fully aware of Pat's exposed anatomy, but he'd chuckle and reply, "Why that's Pat's radish, isn't it?" I thought that was really funny. Grandpa Luther would let us try almost anything we were curious about as long as it wasn't dangerous. He chewed Sweet Burley tobacco, and most of us kids got sick when we tried it. We tasted his brandy, Apple Jack, and homemade wine, which most time we didn't like. Grandma was quite disapproving, but Grandpa would just chuckle and remark, "Well, I'll bet they won't try it again anytime soon."

His mother, who was blind, was still alive in the 1940's. We'd visit her at Mrs. Boyer's home who cared for her in Juda, Wisconsin. She had pure white hair, a wrinkled face with a wonderful smile. I always liked to have her touch me (she said she was looking at me), as her hands were soft and warm. She would feel my arms, face, hair, and then continue talking to me as she held my hands in hers. I didn't really know who she was other than she was my grandmother.

We had another Great-Grandmother, Emma Kloepping, Great-Grandfather Henry's widow. In contrast to the Grandma who was blind, this lady scared the devil out of me. My mother said Great-Grandma had a tendency to spook the kids, and probably did so intentionally. She dressed in long black dresses, had a thin angular, hawkish face and sharp black eyes that my brother Larry said could look right into your soul. He recalls her visits more vividly than I, and he also remarked, "Once she looked at you, you couldn't escape her eyes." My mother told me that she was French/Indian and could not read or write. Her mother died when she was born, and a stepmother who she said was mean to her, raised her. She told my mother that when she was only four years old, she had to wash dishes from a pan sitting on a chair, as she was too small to reach the sink.

She hated housework, and was not a good cook. Mother liked her, despite her direct, outspoken demeanor, as she was honest, witty, and high-spirited. When she visited us, she would have us pick up corncobs that she could use for kindling in her cook stove. A gunny-sack full was worth ten cents, but somehow the dime never materialized, maybe she just forgot. I don't ever remember speaking to her, but I think Larry and Carol did. I mostly stayed out of communication range from her.

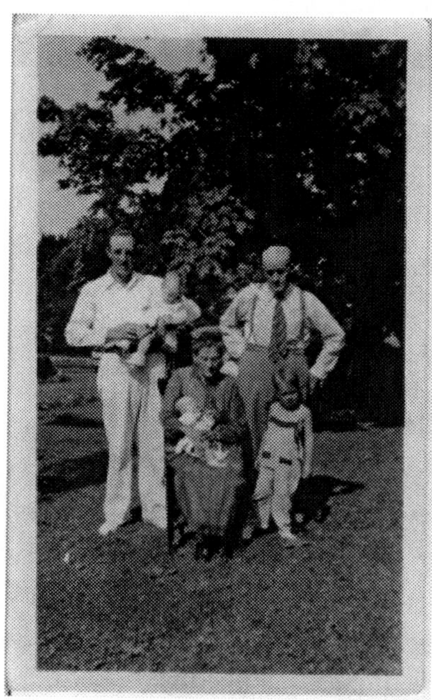

Four generations: my great grandmother Emma Kloepping, Daniel and Dale Kloepping, my brother Larry, sister Carol, and me on Grandmother's lap (summer, 1938)

Occasionally, Larry and I would spend a night or two at Grandpa Dan (old Emma's son) and Grandma Della Kloepping's home. One night I wet the bed; I soaked the sheets, the blankets, the bed and also Larry, as I liked to snuggle up next to him. When I emptied my bladder he got a liberal soaking. Grandma Kloepping always said, "My land," when she was a bit distressed, and it seems she said that several times while changing the bed clothes in the middle of the night. Breakfast was huge at Grandpa Kloepping's household; eggs, toast, jelly or jam, bacon, ham or sausage, oatmeal, and pancakes. Grandma's pancakes were small, two to three inches in diameter and perfectly round. Grandpa Kloepping liked to warm his feet in the oven of the cook stove. When Grandma

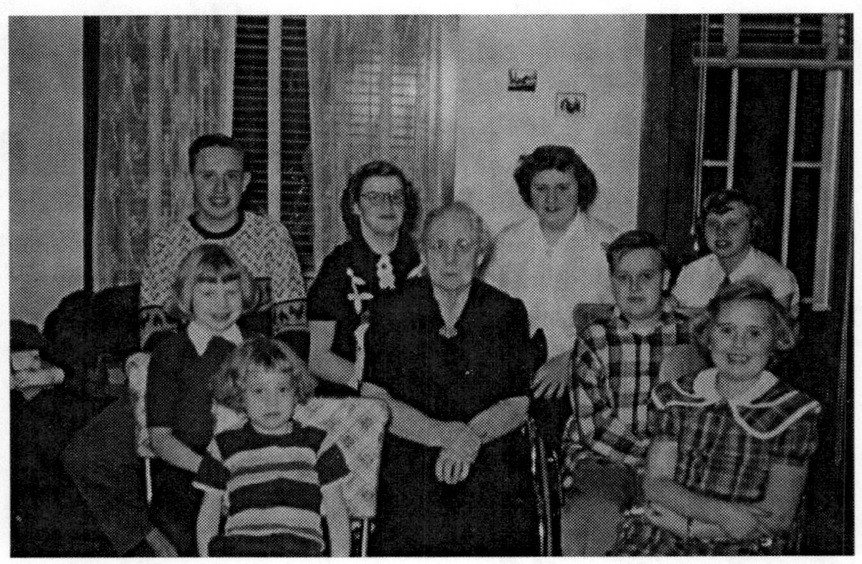

My grandmother Della Kloepping with her grandchildren, and my three siblings and my cousins. Left front: Sylvia and Jody Blunt, Marlene Kloepping behind Grandmother, Sandra Blunt (far right in back). Rock Grove, Illinois, 1950

smelled leather beginning to smolder, she yelled, "My land, Dan, your shoes are on fire!" I don't remember Grandpa Dan being as talkative as Grandpa Luther.

While both old Grandfathers were successful farmers, Grandpa Dan was a true entrepreneur. He was very astute in financial matters, and family folklore is that had he put his money in Sears Roebuck instead of the highly speculative Madison Silo Company, our family might have owned Sears Roebuck. He had asthma, and one of his treatments was Asmador cigarettes. He'd sit on a stool with a metal pan in front of him that had vile smelling yellow smoke billowing up around his face. He'd inhale deeply and when we asked, "What are you doing," he would smile and reply, "curing my asthma?"

Family stories suggest that he was a spirited young man who proved to be a shrewd businessman. His wife, my Grandma Della (Hofmeister), was a genteel, Christian lady, the belle of the Rock Grove, Illinois community. My parents told me that many people were quite surprised at the marriage of such a refined young woman to that rather rough, tough young man. Maybe Grandpa Dan inherited his strong-willed nature from his grandfather Wilhelm Kloepping, who came to America in 1853 from Germany. Later generations of Kloeppings said old Wilhelm had a quick and volatile temper. There is a mill pond story (maybe family folklore) that involves old Wilhelm, suggesting the incident may have led to a quick decision on his part to leave Germany. The story was that the other guy, what was left of him, might still be at the bottom of that pond. There is, to my knowledge, nothing written about the incident, and I had not heard the story until recent years, maybe a rumor, maybe not.

In a successful family farm in the mid-twentieth century, the adults and workers labored methodically to complete the daily chores. Much of the work was repetitive and tedious, thus any variations in daily routines on the farm provided welcome diversions from the daily grind. Seasonal harvesting events, like threshing oats or shredding corn, took on a carnival-like air for the kids. In fact, while holidays and birthdays were occasions for extended family gatherings, it was the summer and fall harvest times, particularly at Grandpa Dan Kloepping's farm, that remain most solidly imprinted on my memory.

On threshing day, the main event was the thrilling appearance of the gigantic steam engine that powered the threshers and shredders. The ground shook and the huge machine clanged, rattled, and banged as if it was about to fly apart as it slowly chugged onto the farm place. Its arrival was a wholly spectacular event. When the local farmers began arriving with their hayracks for hauling oats or corn shocks, it was like a parade. No two teams of horses were alike, and each farmer used a unique set of commands to control his team. The response by the horses to the spoken word was immediate, and most often, unerring. I marveled at the power these men had over these huge animals. There were beautifully matched pairs—bays, blacks, sorrels, huge Clydesdales and Percherons, and the occasional teams of mules. Harness jangled, and sweat and lather flew as the horses strained to haul enormous loads.

Men forked bundles into the machine that threshed the kernels from the straw. A river of yellow-brown oats spewed from the auger into waiting wagons. Fluffy, brilliant, golden straw billowed from a slowly oscillating pipe, cascading down to form a glistening mountain of straw. The rumble of the steam engine was deafening, and the engine whistle shrieked a piercing shrill tone audible for miles, signaling time to eat or break for a brief period of rest.

It was hot, dirty work in the heat and humidity of July and August, but a holiday for the children. It was at these gatherings that we would play with our female cousins, Sandra and Sylvia Blunt and Marlene Kloepping. Marlene was a tough tomboy who was quick to retaliate if we gave her any trouble. But Sandra and Sylvia were gentle, naive, and most important, gullible.

Because I have the advantage of being the writer, I will state unequivocally that Larry was the mastermind of our shenanigans. I must admit to having a pang of guilt thinking back to how we mistreated them. We didn't cause them physical harm; no, our torture was purely psychological. We did things like coax them into Grandpa's large camping tent and then pull up the stakes so it collapsed on them. They were exquisite victims, shrieking and screaming until Grandma Kloepping arrived to rescue them. I suppose our most dastardly deed was getting them to walk down the outside cellar steps and then dropping the heavy horizontal wooden doors. The sheer terror of being trapped in utter darkness was enhanced when we jumped on the doors resulting in a deafening sound in the damp, dank prison we had created for them.

Sandra remained a gentle, ladylike girl into adulthood. Sylvia, however, had no difficulty finding ways to get into mischief. On visits to our farm Dusty Lane, in later years, Sandra usually stayed inside chatting with the moms and my older sister, Carol. Upon arrival, Sylvia's first question was, "Hey, does your dad have any beer in the tank?" And with that, Sylvia, Jolene, and I would head out to the stock tank. During the hot haymaking season in June and July, most all farmers had beer available in their stock tanks, and the easy accessibility seemed an invitation we could not refuse. Sylvia had an impressive number of admirable skills that I longed to emulate. At a very early age, she could chug beer like a fraternity brother and her smoking techniques were unparalleled among the ten-twelve year old crowd. While the rest of us merely puffed on the corncob pipes and cigarettes, she inhaled and blew smoke out of her nose.

Our farm animals fascinated me. We had the basics— pigs, cows, horses, mules, chickens, dogs, cats, but no sheep or goats, ducks or geese. We weren't supposed to tease or torment the animals or try to make them pets, so I mostly just watched them. Abusing farm animals—and potentially hurting or even killing them—could affect the economic well being of the family. While Dad considered the PETA (People for the Ethical Treatment of Animals) folks to be mostly "crackpots," he tended to lend his support to the other PETA (People Eating Tasty Animals) crowd. He was a strong advocate for treating all animals well. With the exception of a few instances, I adhered to his rules about the farm animals. I did, however, chase them to see how fast they could run, and although I tried, there wasn't a single animal on the farm that I could outrun.

Strange as it may seem, with all of the large, imposing and potentially dangerous animals—for instance, we knew to give a sow with baby pigs a wide berth—the animals I feared most were the huge, White Rock roosters. They were fearsome devils that seemed to innately sense your fear. They would give a wicked look, drop a wing, sort of stutter-step sideways, pause, then shift into high gear and race full-tilt at you. They wouldn't follow you very far before they would stop, flap their wings, shake themselves, and crow boisterously as if to say "take that, you scaredy cat!" I never could muster the courage to stand my ground against them.

One sunny day when I was probably three years old, I followed Larry and Carol to a small stream in the East Pasture that, in the spring, had enough water flowing to support a multitude of animals, especially frogs. We were so intent on trying to catch the lightning quick little critters that we failed to notice Dad's Holstein bull rapidly approaching. When he bellowed a warning, we were lucky to be near a scrub willow tree that had grown out of the ditch at about a 45-degree angle. We scrambled up just beyond his head and waited until he vented his rage, butting the tree, bellowing, and pawing the earth. Had we not been in close proximity to that small scrub tree, he would likely have killed one or more of us.

Of all the animals on our farm, it was the horses that most interested me. They all seemed gigantic, and at three or four years old, I was absolutely dwarfed by them. We also had two mules, Jenny and Jumbo. We were warned to steer clear of them because of their nasty dispositions and affinity for kicking people. Unlike our horses, which kicked blindly in the direction of their target, the mules looked at their target, took aim, and usually never missed.

The biggest horse we had was named Goofus. He was a massive animal, a high-spirited, and half Clydesdale crossbreed. At the end of the workday, Fritz would often ride Goofus or another horse for pleasure. In spite of a full day of work, Goofus seemed to have as much energy as when the day started. During the early evening, the entire herd would race full gallop from the field back to the stockyard. We had a fenced lane maybe twenty feet wide and probably a half mile long leading from the field to the buildings. Out in the pasture, they would bunch together and come thundering up the lane, churning up clods of dirt and clouds of dust, whinnying and carrying on. Goofus, in his enthusiasm, would buck and kick exuberantly. Goofus was also the champion farter of all the horses. It was an awesome sight and sound. I mean the dust, the dirt, and fantastic flatus!

Sometimes when I'd see them coming from a distance, I'd lie down and press my ear to the ground. I had heard on the radio that it was an old cowboy and Indian trick—you could hear them coming and feel the rhythmic pounding in the earth. It was thrilling, but also frightening. As the ground began to shudder, I had visions of the herd crashing through the fence. One evening, I was crossing the lane when they began their charge toward home. I panicked and fell several times before scrambling through the wooden fence, seemingly only mere seconds before they roared past.

Children in rural America in the 1940's didn't have closets full of toys as kids do today. We had a few toys, and I fondly recall a scooter with hard rubber tires that wasn't very effective on gravel roads. We had cowboys, Indians, and military figures made of lead, and maybe a toy truck, tractor, or car. When he wasn't working, Dad fashioned toys and games for us out of scrap material. Kites were a favorite project, created from brown paper, sticks, a rag tail, and lots of homemade glue. He also made the original version of lawn darts out of wooden roofing shingles. The object was not to lob them accurately into a circle in the lawn; rather, our goal was to launch them skyward with a twine string sling and achieve maximum height.

However, much of our entertainment was self-generated and not directed or supervised by adults. We had a great deal of freedom during the daytime to think up all manner of mischief. Every day we invented new games, only to have them quickly forgotten by the next morning and replaced with the latest contrivance of our young, creative minds. TV wasn't around, but the radio (after electricity) was often a source from which we derived ideas for things to do, some of which got us into big trouble. I don't know that I misbehaved anymore than the average child, but I recall thinking other children my age seemed more compliant and actively worked to be good. My older sister Carol, for example, always tried to behave and please our parents, her teachers, and adults in general. Maybe like Grandpa Dan, I carried a dose of rogue genes from old Wilhelm. I don't know. What I do know is that I'm not proud of some of the things I did back then, and others I simply won't discuss.

Larry, being older, usually came up with the most creative ideas to pass the time. I was his more-than-willing accomplice. One time he heard on the radio, probably on a cowboy program, that by laying a snare on the ground and stampeding animals over the snare, a quick tug was likely to snag the critter. Using bailing wire, Larry made a loop on one end of twenty-five feet of wire and carefully placed it just outside a loafing shed where the hogs slept. Now the hogs wouldn't know the difference, but we took great care to cover the wire with the mixture of dirt and manure that was in the yard. After all, we knew that the precision and skill involved in concealing the wire in the muck was the key to outfoxing those wily hogs. I was designated to stampede the hogs and Larry was to snag the animal. To our sheer amazement, it worked. Unfortunately, we hadn't thought about how a fifty-pound kid would hold a terrified hundred pound hog, let alone get close enough to remove the snare. By evening, the hog's left front leg was swollen with the wire still wrapped tightly around it. When we heard Fritz yell to our dad, "Dale, what the devil is wrong with that hog?" we quickly vanished from the area. After a bit of encouragement, Larry finally admitted he'd heard of the technique on *The*

Lone Ranger or another cowboy show. Saying Dad was angry was an understatement.

Fritz seemed to have a knack for anticipating our next moves. That's probably because he was no saint himself. He worked hard, played hard, and no matter how late or early he arrived home after a night out, Dad said he never had to call him more than one time to get up for the 4:30 A.M. milking. On one occasion, Fritz caught Carol and I throwing eggs against the cement henhouse wall. We had accidentally dropped an egg one afternoon, and as we watched the chickens erupt in a frenzy of activity, gobbling up the yolk and shell, an idea was hatched. I'm not sure which one of us threw the first egg, but the result was bedlam. Chickens were squawking, wings were flapping, feathers were flying, and we were giggling hysterically. What a scene! We were bent double with laughter when suddenly we heard a voice boom.

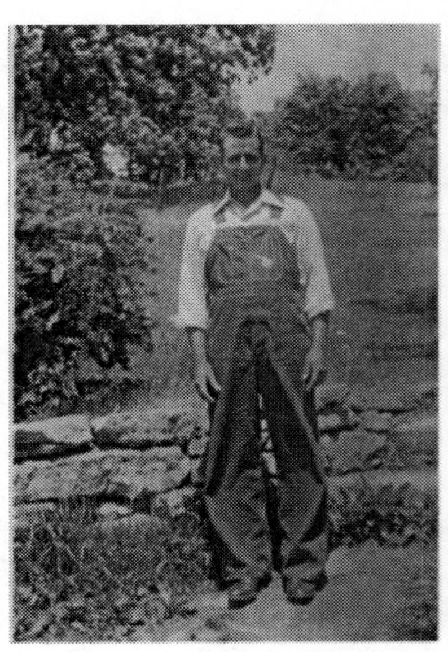

Frederick "Fritz" Kolb, our hired man (1946)

"Well, by God, now I know why your mother is suddenly getting 50 % less eggs. I ought to tan your butts." Fritz had happened upon our little game.

Indignantly we retorted, "You can't spank us, you're not our dad."

With a sly look, he replied, "Oh you don't think so?" and we both got a swat on the butt.

It was probably also Fritz who discovered that we had pushed chickens down through the seats of the outdoor privy. I still remember Dad spending considerable time with a bailing wire snare fishing them out. He wasn't a bit amused, and although I don't recall a spanking, the tongue-lashing was ferocious enough to ensure a non-repeat.

One of my favorite early pastimes was quietly sneaking up on our sleeping farm animals and then shouting as loudly as I could to watch them freak out. Hogs had the most impressive response, with the entire herd racing off in every direction, snorting and squealing. With all the noise and flying dust, it was complete, delicious chaos. Partly as a result of the pig-snaring incident, but primarily from the subsequent tongue-lashing we received, we were again reminded that our farm animals were NOT to be abused.

My brother had a BB gun that I would sometimes borrow without asking permission, and when no one was around I'd shoot everything in sight. A year or two before, I shot all the windows out of Grandpa Luther's old chicken house. That earned me a severe reprimand and a spanking. I shot at dogs, hogs, cows, cats, bees, trees, chickens, and though I never hit one, birds. One day I pinned down my sisters behind a large tractor tire; I was mostly curious to see what they would do. When my parents discovered what I'd done, they were not only angry, but upset imagining how seriously I could have injured the girls. I immediately got a good spanking, and longer term never got my own BB gun.

It seemed that we rarely went to neighboring farms to play, but on occasion, we would visit the Earlywine place about a half a mile away, just over the Illinois state line. Mattie Earlywine was Mom's cousin, and she had a son, Loren "Pete" Earlywine, a rather indulged caboose to three, much older siblings. When I was four or five years old, Larry and I went to play with him at his house. Unlike the majority of rural kids in those days, Pete seemed to have every toy imaginable; a beautiful electric train display, shelves and shelves of toys, and a scooter with inflatable rubber tires. That scooter would coast for almost a mile if you started on a hill. Larry was older than Pete, so Pete greatly admired him. I, on the other hand, was an unwelcome, younger third wheel who was never allowed to touch any of his possessions.

One day, probably in a bid to impress Larry, he picked up a heavy steel rod and said, "This is how we kill pigs," and brought the rod down on my head with a resounding thud. I went down like a dead hog. I saw lots of stars, was briefly disoriented, but staggered to my feet and raced home. As an adult, you couldn't find a nicer person or more solid citizen than Pete. Maybe he wasn't as bad a kid as I thought he was. Several years later, when I contracted polio, he cried all day and stayed home from school, because he felt so sorry for me—but after the incident with the steel bar, I was a bit more cautious and usually didn't turn my back to him.

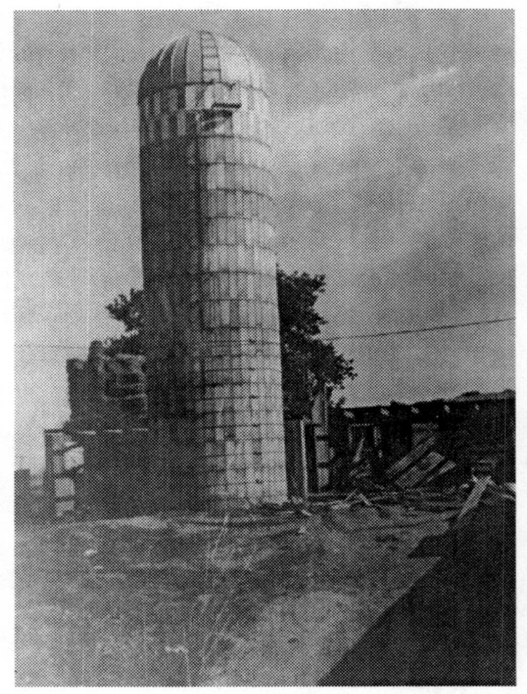

The silo I liked to climb at our Dusty Lane farm (the roof was added)

I also had a tendency to court disaster, and as a result, engaged in some rather reckless and dangerous activities. Dad had a new silo built for corn silage, and we were warned to stay away during the construction due to the risk of falling blocks, steel, and tools. The outside ladder to the forty-foot top ended about ten feet from the ground to prevent children from accessing it. I was intrigued by what I imagined one might see from the top of that silo.

One day, as I sat contemplating how to reach the bottom rung of the ladder, it occurred to me that by grasping the end of the bolts in the metal plates that held the steel rings encircling the silo and climbing up, I could reach the lowest rung. I immediately proceeded up to the top and over into the silo which had been filled earlier in the day by my dad and the hired men. It was indeed a spectacular view, and I experienced a feeling of exhilaration and power. The next day, still filled with excitement, I again climbed the silo. Up and over the top I went, but this time, instead of landing on silage, I dropped down some six to eight feet. The silage had settled. I realized immediately that I was trapped. I screamed, yelled, cried, and cursed to no avail.

After what seemed like being trapped for an eternity, I finally figured out that if I piled enough silage against the wall in one spot, I might be able to reach the top edge of the silo. It worked, and I made it safely down. In hindsight, the thought that I could've fallen forty feet to the bottom of the silo still makes me shudder.

Another time, at about age five, I recall riding in the backseat of our 1935 Chrysler sedan and noticing that the back window had been broken out. Suddenly I got the urge to crawl through the opening out onto the attached rectangular trunk and perch on the top, a 2x2 foot square. I had a great view of the road whizzing by beneath me, and although the gravel road was dusty and bumpy, I hung on. The closest I came to falling off was when Mom realized where I was and slammed on the brakes.

I suppose like many little boys I was fascinated with my penis, not the least of which was its function as a portable water gun. I whizzed on everything; trees, fence posts, bees, buildings, weeds and thistles and in the creek. I also launched streams of urine from things; trees, buildings, bridges, fence posts, and large rocks. But only once did I pee on the electric fence. The terrible shock significantly dampened my enthusiasm for urination experiments.

I don't know if I was a bad or good kid, but I do recall resenting and resisting authority. A combination of extreme curiosity, wanting to experience things for myself, and a deep-seated desire to be independent seemed to drive much of my unorthodox behavior. I didn't have the wisdom to foresee the consequences of my behavior, and Flip Wilson's rationalization, "the devil made me do it," was many years down the road. When I did get caught being naughty, I had to suffer the consequences. Most of my antics were fairly innocuous and usually solitary, although at times I did engage in mischief making as a willing and eager accomplice to others. I learned early on, however, that the downside of group mischief was the increased likelihood that someone would tell on you.

In the fall of 1945, my world abruptly came crashing down. It was October and I had entered the second grade in Mrs. Marie Patterson's primary school room. The Rock City Grade School was the classic two room school house; grades one through four in one room, and grades five through eight in the big room. I was a little fellow who was seemingly always in motion. I liked pushing the limits and one afternoon, going down the slippery slide while sitting on wax paper from my lunch pail to increase speed, the older boys raised the end of the slide three to four feet off the ground and I was catapulted into the air. I landed with a thud on my tailbone. It hurt something awful, but I bit my lip and did not cry. I did not want to be thought a sissy. I didn't feel good for the next several days, and Mom later told me that because I seemed so lethargic, she kept me home from school for a full week.

I returned to school on Monday, but continued to feel bad. By Friday I was very ill. Saturday I continued to worsen, and by Sunday morning, I had developed a blinding headache, was having muscle cramps, and had become extremely sensitive to touch. My parents tried to comfort me, reassuring me that I'd be OK, never betraying what must have been in their minds. That morning, Dad gently laid me on pillows in the back seat of our 1935 Chrysler and said, "Let's go for a ride. Maybe that will help." We ended up in Orangeville, a town about ten miles from home, at the office of a local osteopath named Dr. Ransom Dingis. Dad carried me inside. The doctor placed me on an examining table and began to manipulate my arms and legs. Each movement of my limbs caused shocking jolts throughout my system. After pausing for a few moments, I vividly recall him saying, "I'm afraid it's polio." I had contracted the deadly virus that my entire community feared most. Later that evening, at St. Frances Hospital in Freeport, Illinois, I have clear memories of the spinal tap. I recall Dad holding me curled into a fetal position, and of the terrific sting of the needle going into my spine and withdrawing fluid. I began to see double: two Dads, two overhead lights, and two of each of the other people in the room.

St. Francis, only fourteen miles from home, was filled to capacity and would take no more patients. We returned home and I remember lying on a day couch, suffering with a raging headache punctuated by brief episodes of delirium. I hurt all over, the virus now fully assaulting my body and carrying out its deadly work. I was admitted late that evening into the Winnebago County Hospital in Rockford, Illinois, some thirty miles from home. My parents stayed with me late into the night in that small, dimly lit room. I remember the blue nightlight above my bed that cast a surreal glow throughout the room, illuminating my parents, yet never masking the sadness in their faces.

When I awoke in the morning, they were gone. When I tried to get out of bed, I fell to the floor. I could not get back into bed, and I still remember not understanding why parts of my body were not working. Sometime later, an aide or nurse came in and lifted me back into bed. She was a gentle woman who said softly to me, "Now, you must stay in bed. Don't try to get up again." Within two or three days I was totally paralyzed, absolutely unable to move. I could open and close my eyes, which I did repeatedly, harboring an irrational hope that the activity might somehow help get other parts of my body moving. I couldn't urinate, so a nurse came in and turned the water on in a small sink in the room, hoping the sound of trickling water would help. It didn't and eventually I had to be catheterized. That hurt like the devil, but the relief when my bladder emptied overshadowed the discomfort of the procedure.

I recall little of the ensuing days. Once the infectious stage passed, my parents were allowed their first visit. That was two weeks after my initial admission. They came garbed in white gowns, wearing masks that covered their mouths and noses. Years later, they would share with me that the parents waiting to see their children were all silent, fearing the worst upon seeing their child for the first time since the onset of the disease.

An armed guard was present at the hospital to insure that no one entered the ward until clearance had been given. When I asked when I could come home, Mom didn't, or couldn't, answer, and turned her back, presumably to avoid betraying her emotions. Dad put on a brave face and told me he thought I'd be home in not too long a time. He related the story about an operation he had on his sinuses when he was fifteen years old. The cavity above his left eye had ballooned out (had it ruptured into the brain cavity it could have been fatal), and he said that he was in the hospital a whole month after his operation. I'm not sure I thought of thirty days as a benchmark for my stay, and it's a good thing I didn't. I don't recall the sequence of events for the next six months or so after I was out of quarantine; further, much of what transpired on a daily basis has faded from memory after almost sixty years. There do remain, however, some clear and distinct memories.

I remember the hot packs. The packs were wool fabric that was heated to seemingly scalding temperatures in large mobile stainless steel cookers. The nurses would wheel in the machines, open the lids, and with steam pouring out of the openings, proceed to wrap arms, legs, and torso in the hot, steaming wool. They used tongs to remove the packs from those boiling cauldrons, the wool too hot for them to handle out of the machine, and applied them directly to our bodies. What a sickening smell. You have to be around a bunch of sheep after a rain to appreciate how much wet wool stinks. I felt like I was parboiled and that my skin would peel off when they removed the packs. Much as I dreaded the daily ritual, the hot packs did relieve the cramping, pain, and soreness. All of the toys I had, mostly little cars and trucks, were sterilized as a precaution against transmission of the poliovirus. In 1945, it was yet unclear how the virus was transmitted and a high dose of extended heat was used as a precautionary measure to ensure they weren't contaminated.

On Christmas Eve, Santa paid a visit to the hospital and he gave me an apple that was ice cold.

"Are you really Santa?" I asked.

"Yes, I am," he said, "That's why the apple is so cold. It came from the North Pole."

I knew at that moment that he really was Santa.

Before I was moved into a ward of boys, I had a single room in a dark, gloomy annex of the hospital. I was scared all the time. Before I arrived in the hospital, there had been a kidnapping and murder in Chicago that I'd heard about on the radio. The killer had used a ladder to enter the girl's room and steal her (I still remember her name, Susan Degman) from her bedroom. Nightly, I watched my window for the ladder to appear.

The ladder never came, but one evening I did have an unexpected guest. I smelled her before I actually knew she was there. Suddenly, she was standing in the doorway to my room. At first I saw a tiny figure, wrapped from head to toe in layers of white and other pale pastel garments, and enveloped in a cloud of menthol vapors. When she asked, "How you, lil' boy?" I realized my visitor was a very tiny black lady. Awed by her presence, I didn't answer. She came to my bed, took my hand and said, "Are you feelin' ok?" She looked very old, had nut-brown wrinkled skin, and warm, soft hands. She came every night to my room after dark. I began to wait for her and hope she would come. Later I realized her odor was some kind of menthol balm that she rubbed on her chest and not, as I thought in my innocence, how black people smelled. I don't remember her name (maybe she never told me) or much else about her, but she was a great comfort to me, that little lady with that odd, yet delightful smell. My wife believes in angels. Today, as I think back to that time and how terribly lonely, afraid and abandoned I felt, I sometimes wonder if her appearance was divinely orchestrated. Anything is possible, and I'm sure angels come in a variety of colors, not just glistening white as they are most often depicted. I don't recall when she stopped coming, only that she was suddenly gone. I also don't remember asking where she'd gone. Maybe I already knew that her mission was finished, and that I no longer needed her.

Sometime early in 1946, I was moved into a large ward of boys. I had a bed next to a boy named Ronnie. He was a strange kid who always played with himself because he said it helped him go to sleep. He couldn't have been over eight or nine years old. We were all past the contagious stage of the virus, so I was finally allowed to have visitors on a regular basis. I could now sit up if someone helped me, and I recall Dad cutting my hair with his manual clippers. He gave other kids in the ward haircuts also. Among the visitors I remember was our minister Rev. Bob Hartman and Danny, his son, who couldn't come into the ward because he was too young. He waved up to my window from the car below.

Occasionally, Dad would carry me down the hall to see a young man named Ralph Pratt who was confined to an iron lung. He lay motionless in the huge capsule that rhythmically pulsed, "whoosh, whoosh, and whoosh." Then one day he died. I can still see his mother's face, deep sadness mirrored in her eyes for her son.

Time passed slowly in the ward. There was no physical therapy that I can recall, and the doctors came in but spent little time with anyone. There was no television in 1946, just a radio or two. There just wasn't much activity on the ward. People were afraid of polio, so few, besides family and clergy, came to visit.

Just when my life had become tolerable, a new nurse named Miss Hahn arrived and turned my world upside down. When she came into the ward, the atmosphere changed and a chilling silence descended over the ward. There were maybe thirty little boys, each one of us, confined to our beds, pale, anxious and fearful. We all missed our families and were trying desperately to understand what had happened to us. Not long before, we had been lively, inquisitive, carefree children, who had all changed instantly when the dreaded virus struck. Now all of us, each paralyzed to varying degrees, were jammed into a bleak hospital ward, the beds just far enough apart to allow for foot traffic and gurneys.

I remember the daily routine. The lights were turned on in the morning, beaming from the large translucent globes hanging down from the extremely high ceiling. Probably only two nurses or aides came in to get us going; a washcloth swiped, sometimes not very gently, across the face, a urinal or bedpan and an admonishment to "get it over with." There were far too many patients for only two staff. Cranking up the bed a little, they readied us for our breakfast trays. The food was usually cold, didn't taste good, and mealtime was always absent Mom and Dad, and my brother and sisters. Eating was especially depressing and lonesome. Although we lived in close quarters in that drab room, much of the time we were alone in our thoughts. Supper, as my family called the evening meal, was the worst time for me.

Back home, gathered around the round oak table with the entire family, was a time for not only eating, but also sharing. Everyone had the opportunity to share what they had done or accomplished that day. Frequently, time at the table extended well beyond completion of the meal. Around that oak table, my parents taught us important rules for living; responsible behavior was praised and oft times reinforced with homespun anecdotes. We also had our lapses in judgment or behavior pointed out, but never in a destructive or hurtful manner. Gossip was a special treat, a dose of spice to cap off the meal. "Now don't repeat this" was the signal to pay close attention. "This is just for our family to know and discuss, so keep still." Those words were powerful messages that seemed to strengthen the family unit, and they carried the appeal for loyalty among the six of us who shared common blood. Suppertime was a critical time to learn values and clearly affirm what we believed.

But supper in the hospital was solitary. Few of us were hungry; we tried to think of ways to dispose of the food or places to hide it. We dropped some on the floor, stirred it around on the plate, spilled it on the tray, and even threw some as far as we could. Many evenings, grief and despair would begin to well up inside me and my stomach would churn and my throat would constrict; I'd begin to sob silently and then throw up on my food tray. I was feeling bad, feeling sorry for myself, and wishing Mom and Dad were there.

They weren't, but Miss Hahn was, standing over me, unsmiling and angry, speaking harshly and cruelly about how bad I was for not eating, and for getting sick. Unfortunately, I had fallen into a pattern of upchucking every evening. That fact was most likely recorded on my chart and duly noted by Miss Hahn. She had been an Army nurse who someone said had lost a husband in the war. Maybe she had seen the worst horrors of war and that had hardened her. In any case, she had little sympathy or tolerance for a whimpering seven year old.

"You pull this trick every evening. Well, you aren't going to get away with this. You will eat what is on your plate."

"But I threw up," I protested.

"Yes, I know. You will now eat that also," she coldly replied. I began to cry and she took my spoon, scooped vomit and food, ordered me to open my mouth, and force-fed me the vile, stinking mixture. She continued until I began vomiting again.

She grabbed a cloth and clamped it tightly over my mouth, hissing "Swallow, swallow!" I was terrified, choking. I had thoughts of her doing me in. Suddenly she left, warning, "I'll be back." I can still visualize the table and tray, splattered with my regurgitation, green beans swimming in spilled milk. She returned and again attempted to force-feed me the sickening gruel on the tray and plate. I closed my mouth and refused to open my jaws. While she could pull my lips apart she could not force my teeth open.

"OK, if that's the way you want it," she spat at me then stalked off. She returned with two aides, both short black ladies, their eyes wide, silent, visibly shaken by Hahn's wrath. "Get this bed out of here," she barked. My bed and I rolled out of the ward into the dimly lit hall, my roommates watching silently as we moved rapidly down the corridors. I was wheeled around several corners, finally stopping in front of a closed door.

"Open that door!" she ordered. I went, with the bed and the foul-smelling tray, into a tiny, high-ceilinged room that resembled a giant closet with no windows. "Now, we'll give you some time to think about your behavior. A little time alone might do you some good." She slammed the door abruptly, and I was in complete darkness. There was no light from around the doorsill or from under the door, only blackness. Once Miss Hahn left, I began to relax and was no longer fearful.

Alone, with my gown and bed fouled with stomach acid and bile, I became calm. I slowly began to feel what must have been hatred for Nurse Hahn. The emotion filled my consciousness, completely displacing any remaining anxiety instilled by my tormentor. I cursed her silently with the few words of profanity I knew, damning her for her cruelty. When I had exhausted my limited repertoire of curse words, I realized that I had survived her worst. I resolved to not let her destroy me. I would not allow her to win. Resolute, I fell asleep.

I'm not sure how long I was in solitary, probably nine hours or more. Sometime around 300:A.M., perhaps during the shift change, the door opened and two aides quietly moved me back to the ward. They took the tray, cleaned my gown and bed sheets, and washed my face and arms. There was almost no conversation. As one of the colored ladies (the 1940's term for African Americans) turned to go, she looked at me intently, her soft brown eyes illuminated by the small bedside lamp. She didn't speak, but gently patted my arm, smiled, turned off the lamp and left. I again fell asleep almost immediately, warmed and comforted by the lady who, unspoken, had let me know that she understood and that everything would be okay. I told my parents about the incident, and I don't know if they spoke to Miss Hahn or a superior, but from then on, I never looked at, spoke to, or acknowledged her presence. She decided or had been warned to leave me alone. It occurred to me years later that she might have been the prototype for the Nurse Mildred Ratched character from the movie, *One Flew Over the Cuckoo's Nest.*

Thinking back to that night alone in the closet, I probably owe Nurse Hahn a debt of gratitude. I think maybe her wretchedness helped spark in me a determination to succeed, if only to defeat her. It was an early lesson of my father's later advice, that "What you no longer have in your legs, you must have in your head." I couldn't run from her, but I could escape.

Sometime early in 1946, maybe February or March, a group of volunteers began coming to the hospital to take us swimming at a school in Rockford. President Roosevelt had spent many months in Warm Springs, Georgia, and because of the publicity surrounding his visits to that retreat, water became a recognized form of therapy for polio victims. Those trips to that old brownstone school building were welcome respites from the monotony of our daily routine.

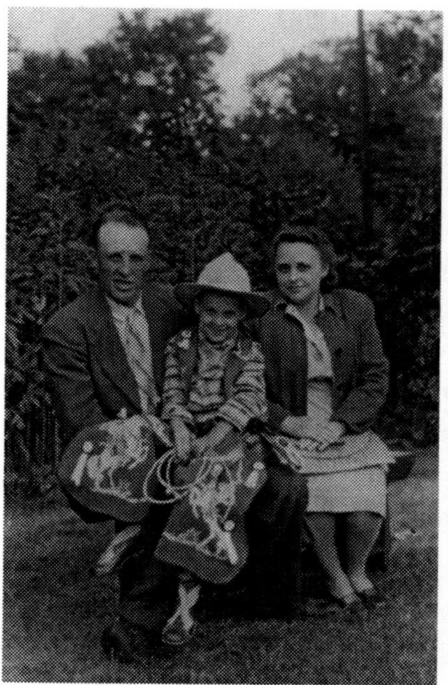

My mother and father and I at the Kent Cottage in Rockford, Illinois. My new cowboy outfit. (Spring, 1946)

Then one day we were told we were moving to a place called the Kent Cottage, at 507 Kent Street, in Rockford across from the Booker T. Washington Center. The Kent Cottage was originally a home and holding center for abandoned and delinquent kids. The facility was like a college dormitory; two stories, very clean, cheery, many windows, and a large beautifully manicured back area with lots of trees, flowers, and green grass. It was late spring, maybe April or May, and although I was not going home, it was as if I had been released from prison. The food was good and the staff mostly cheerful and friendly.

There were many kinds of activities during the week and best of all, we had movies about once a week in the first floor sunroom. There was a primitive little elevator that held one wheelchair, one nurse, and maybe another child standing. It had an accordion-like bottom, which shut off the power when it touched the floor.

After transferring to the Kent Cottage, a lady came in to provide some basic educational tutoring. Many of us had, at that point, been absent from school for a year or more. Although I completely missed second grade, this woman taught me how to spell. I recently discovered a letter I had written to my parents dated March 21,1947, in which I told them I had missed only one word on my spelling test. I had written, "Miss Alm taught me the way." I was obviously very proud of myself, and the letter was one of many from that time that my mother saved.

Ralph, a tough, older boy of maybe fourteen or so, provided another sort of education for groups of younger kids. He held his own unique version of sex education clinics. He'd recruit four or five of us, herd us into his room, and encourage us to expose ourselves. He, of course, was first to bare his genitalia. He managed to convince a dull-witted, post-pubescent girl to provide a little variety. I found the whole thing distasteful, and I escaped in my old wooden-backed wheelchair before it was my turn to exhibit my privates to the group. He also enjoyed extorting money from younger kids, and at one point, had demanded money from me. One Sunday I told my parents I needed money and when they pressed me for a reason, I told them about Ralph. My grandmother Rodenbough had also come along that day to visit, and she immediately provided me with a ready solution. Grandma Mattie had a great imagination and was very creative. She told me to tell the young man to knock it off because our family had Cherokee blood (which is true), and one quick call to Oklahoma would bring several men to "take care of him." It worked. Ralph turned a bit pale when he heard of my fierce relatives from out West, and he never approached me again for money or invited me in to another of his sex clinics.

A primary objective at the Kent Cottage was physical rehabilitation. The goal was to teach skills to compensate for loss of function, as well as prepare the children for returning home. We had daily regimens of therapy, and once the facility had a Hubbard tank installed, sessions in the tub became a daily ritual to loosen and stretch muscles before physical therapy. A Hubbard tank is a large cloverleaf-shaped stainless steel tub with air jets around the perimeter that rumbled, bubbled and foamed. With the regimen of physical therapy I learned to walk—sort of. Hanging heavily on two full-length underarm crutches and heavy leg braces, I could ambulate for short distances on level ground. While I continued to gain strength, and enjoy the return in function of some muscle groups, I began to suffer from institutionalization from having been away from home for over eight months. The doctor felt I needed to go home for a brief period. That week at home resulted in a dramatic change, not only in my mental health, but in my physical condition as well. I didn't have very useful ambulatory skills, we had no wheelchair at home, and Kent Cottage didn't loan me one for the visit home. I had no idea how I would get around in the house from room to room, let alone going in and out of doors.

I wish that I were able to go back to that time and hear the conversation that occurred between my parents when they discussed my homecoming. I would dearly love to know how they arrived at the strategy for the week. Whatever the process that led to the decision, it was a simple solution, and in retrospect, one of great wisdom. They bought me a pair of bib overalls, put me on the floor and said," Go." And go I did. I began to crawl, first from room to room, then out the front door, onto the lawn, around the house, and eventually to every part of our yard. When I got tired, I'd roll, particularly in the grass. Not only was it effective, but also it felt wonderful. In the house, I could also slide on my butt, or "scoot," as we called it.

Upon my return to the Kent Cottage a week later, Ms. Bostrom, the physical therapist, was flabbergasted. My first morning back in therapy she seemed stunned by what I could do.

"Kent, what did you do when you were home for the week?" I started to tell her about friends coming over, going places and playing, but she stopped me and said, "No, no, how did you get around?"

"I crawled," I replied.

Incredulous, Ms. Bostrom called my mother and the next day, there were seventy-five kids of all ages and abilities, on floor mats in the PT gym, rolling, crawling, wiggling, scooting and wrestling with one another. "Floor time," as it was called, became a regular form of therapy and was probably one of the most effective forms of therapy devised. It was born of an uncomplicated, common sense philosophy, characteristic of my parents, "Where there is a will, there is a way."

I spent another year at the Kent Cottage, receiving therapy and continuing to learn ways to care for myself and become independent. Wilma Kurtz, a family friend who was an unmarried schoolteacher in Rockford, began to visit me regularly in the evenings after school. I continued to have difficulty eating (I never did eat very well) and was very thin. Wilma brought me chocolate malts and store-bought hamburgers. They were wonderful, and thanks to Wilma and the store-bought treats, I did gain weight. My parents would later remark, "Well, Wilma probably saved your life." The salvation she provided wasn't literal, but her visits were unquestionably a major factor in improving my physical and mental health. Many of the children had family in or close to Rockford who visited daily. For my parents, frequent visits were not feasible. With the many hours of work each day, in combination with the thirty miles between our dairy farm and the Kent Cottage, it made daily visits impossible. But Wilma came regularly and became a special friend, a confidant, a person I could trust, and a person who bridged the seemingly enormous gap between my community and me.

Richie, a really spoiled kid from Rockford, had parents who showered him with toys, presents and other treats, on a daily basis. His parents brought him fresh blueberries one day, and despite his parents coaxing, he refused to give me or anyone else a single blueberry. He ate them all, a huge bag full, and then proceeded to get sick and splatter himself and his bed with purple-tinted vomit. We called him the "purple puker" after that. When I told Wilma about the incident and his selfishness, she whispered, "Well, we won't share your hamburger or malts with him either." Yes, she was on my side.

While at Kent Cottage, I was fortunate to avoid surgical fusion and joint stabilization as a treatment for polio. These procedures were highly experimental. Hips, knees, shoulders and wrists were favorite targets of overzealous surgeons. For many polio patients, the results proved disastrous. My parents intuitively recognized the problems that would result in my inability to sit, bend knees or wrists, or crawl because the joints on which they operated were permanently locked in position. They refused to allow the surgery, holding fast against the best advice and ultimately the belligerence of an orthopedic surgeon. How lucky I was to have parents with such great horse sense, who recognized the terrible consequences of such surgery and had the courage to hold steadfast in their convictions.

My family came to get me from the Kent Cottage in the late spring or early summer of 1947. They picked me up in a shiny new 1946 Mercury that had wooden bumpers. It was, I thought, maybe the nicest car in which I'd ever ridden. The thirty-some mile ride to my home on that day in 1947 remains one of the best journeys of my life.

III. Polio: The Short Story

> **"Let me tell you a true story about immunization. When I was a little boy in New York City in the 1940's we swam in the Hudson River. And it was filled with raw sewage. Okay? We swam in raw sewage! You know, to cool off. At that time the big fear was polio; thousands of kids died from polio every year. But you know somethin'? In my neighborhood no one ever got polio. NO ONE. Ever! You know why? Because we swam in raw sewage! It strengthened our immune systems. The polio never had a prayer; we were tempered in raw *shit*!" (1)**

Poliomyelitis (polio), also called infantile paralysis, is an acute, and often devastating viral disease caused by the poliovirus. The word, poliomyelitis, comes from the Greek words polios, meaning "gray," and myelos "matter"; "myelitis" refers to an inflammation of the motor neurons of the spinal column.

The poliovirus enters the mouth and initially moves into the spongy tissue of the tonsils, where it begins to multiply. It then travels to the small intestines where it multiplies at an accelerating rate. The virus, released from the tonsils and the intestines, travels to the large lymph nodes under the arms where further multiplication occurs. Approximately ten days to two weeks after being infected, millions and millions of poliovirus dump into the bloodstream and are carried to the neurons in the brain and spinal cord, the key sites of destruction by the virus.

Technically, the term poliomyelitis should not be used to describe everyone who was infected by the poliovirus, as inflammation of the spinal cord motor neurons, or myelitis, did not occur in every case. Dr. Richard Bruno, in his 2002 book *The Polio Paradox*, referring to the work of the pathologist David Bodian, states, "This work revealed that the main event of polio virus infection was not myelitis, an inflammation of spinal cord motor neurons, but an encephalitis, an inflammation of the brain." In every case of polio Bodian studied, paralytic and 'non-paralytic,' he saw consistent patterns of damage to the brain neurons. (2)

There are three different types of poliovirus. Originally they were named "Brunhilde," "Lansing," and "Leon," but became more commonly known as Types I, II, and III. Type I (Brunhilde) was the cause of epidemics and many cases of paralytic polio; Type II (Lansing), sometimes referred to as the "summer grippe," was the least likely to cause paralysis and was responsible for outbreaks of non-paralytic polio. Type III (Leon), the rarest form that is also known as "bulbar," often results in severe damage to the brain stem with resulting difficulties in swallowing, breathing, and blood pressure.

They are all members of the viral family enteroviruses. These viruses infect the gastrointestinal tract, and humans are the only natural host for the viruses. The virus is usually harmless in humans with 80-90% of clinical infections being reported as "minor." Symptoms include fever, fatigue, sore throat, and vomiting, with recovery in twenty-four to seventy-two hours. Only about 1% of individuals infected with poliovirus develop the most severe form.

The poliovirus is spread by direct exposure to an infected person; specifically, when the saliva or intestinal secretions of the infected individual find their way into the mouth of another. Another possible means of transmission, which is the primary mode in countries with poor sanitary conditions, is eating foods contaminated with fecal matter. Despite all the advancements in modern medicine, no one is entirely sure how polio is spread.

Bruno, in his book *The Polio Paradox,* discusses diverse factors that have been associated with susceptibility to polio and states, "You can come up with a kind of equation to help understand why you may have contracted and been damaged by the polio virus." The equation is as follows:

GENES

having more poliovirus receptors, making fewer poliovirus antibodies, or being a fertile ground for poliovirus multiplication

+

RACE

Being white, especially if you're of Germanic or southern European origin

+

BEING MALE

+

COMMUNITY EXPOSURE

Living in a congested city where there was lots of poliovirus, especially if you had moved from a rural area and therefore had fewer antibodies

+

HOUSEHOLD EXPOSURE

Someone in your home had polio

+

POLIO VIRUS VIRULENCE

Being exposed to a powerful poliovirus

+

INJURY

Physical injury or overexertion, receiving an injection, or emotional stress

+

POLIO VIRUS "LOAD"

Being given a large dose of poliovirus

+

YEAR OF BIRTH

Being born later in the century

+

AGE

Having been an infant early in the twentieth century

+

FEMALE HORMONES

Ovulating, just finishing a menstrual period, or being pregnant (3)

In reviewing ten of the eleven factors (excluding female hormones) that may have contributed to my having contracted polio, five of the factors— *race, being male, poliovirus virulence, injury*, and *being born late in the century* —are applicable in my case. Three additional factors— *genes, house exposure*, and *poliovirus load* —were additionally highly probable. Although I did not live in a congested city, the rural locality where I lived had the highest incidence of polio cases reported in America between the months of July to November 1945. (4) I became ill in October of 1945. Thus *community exposure* was the ninth factor that could have played a role in my susceptibility to the virus. That's a 90% probability for me contracting the poliovirus. The odds were stacked solidly against me.

Polio is an ancient virus. The misshapen bones of an Egyptian mummy (circa 3700 BC) may be the oldest known case of polio. (5) A second case of circumstantial evidence is the stone relief of an Egyptian priest named Rom (circa 1580) that depicts an atrophied and shortened leg with a drop foot. (6) Hippocrates, the Father of medicine, mentions cases of "infant paralysis," a rare condition. Roman and Celtic doctors later described polio as, "The pestilence that is called lameness." When Sir Walter Scott, the Scottish poet and novelist, contracted polio in the 18th century, physicians of the day thought it was a new disease. Throughout recorded history, polio had been a mild, infrequent disease of infants with apparently few deaths. Thus for hundreds of years, it was either ignored or misdiagnosed by physicians. In fact, medical documents of most European countries provided no evidence of the existence of the disease to the time of Scott.

The first attempt at a clinical description of polio was by an English physician Dr. Michael Underwood in 1789, who described it as "debility of the lower extremities."

The first authoritative study was published by the German orthopedist, Jacob von Heine in 1840. He was first to correctly describe poliomyelitis as "an affection of the central nervous system, specifically the spinal cord." It was Karl Oskar Medin, a Swedish pioneer, who categorized the disease into three types after an unprecedented outbreak of forty-four cases in 1887. Ivar Wickman, a pupil of Medin, subsequently named the disease "Heine-Medin Disease" after the two. Wickman's experience with a large outbreak of polio in Scandinavia (one thousand cases) in 1905 led him to conclude that Heine-Medin disease was highly contagious, and that both healthy and mildly affected individuals could spread the disease.

Now at this juncture (end of the 19th century and the beginning of the 20th century) in history, bacteria had been discovered as the cause of infectious diseases, and in the medical community there was an explosion of activity in discovering and naming microbes. These microbes were primarily bacteria, and the study and science was called microbiology. Virology, the study of viruses, had yet to be introduced. As far as microbe hunters were concerned, the only difference between bacteria and viruses was one of size. Bacteria were the organisms, which would not pass through a porcelain filter, viruses the ones which would. If the filtration process succeeded in sterilizing cultures of organisms, then they were bacteria. If not, and laboratory animals could be infected after filtration of the culture, it was called a virus. Bacteria became visible under the microscope when stained with certain types of dye; viruses, however, were too small to be seen even through an optical microscope, and it was practically impossible to study them visually before the invention of the electron microscope in 1937.

Despite the virtual invisibility of viruses, the first two human vaccines, (for smallpox and rabies), were virus vaccines. However, as John Rowan Wilson points out, "almost all the really productive developments in this field after the death of Pasteur until 1930 were in connection with bacteria. The reason was because of the technical difficulties in culturing the organisms." In Vienna in 1908, Drs. Karl Landsteiner and Erwin Popper discovered that the infectious agent for poliomyelitis was not a bacterium, but rather a "filterable virus." When Landsteiner and Popper injected filtered fluid taken from the spinal cord of a polio victim into the brains of two monkeys, both animals came down with the disease. Through their experiments, polio not only became a reportable disease, but they established the cause and set the pattern for future research, with monkeys as polio's primary guinea pigs. (7)

The importance of their discovery was widely recognized, not only in America, but in Europe as well. Research into the causes of polio and the search for a vaccine continued for the next forty years. Two men whose work contributed most significantly to the development of a vaccine against polio were Dr. John Enders and Dr. Thomas Wellers. Enders was a Harvard educated bacteriologist and immunologist who, in 1946, established a clinical facility for research in infectious diseases at the Children's Medical Center in Boston. Thomas Weller, also a Harvard graduate, was heavily influenced by Enders, who introduced him to the field of virus research and tissue culture techniques for studying infectious diseases. In 1949, the pair succeeded in growing poliovirus outside the body in laboratory cultures of non-nervous human tissue. (8) Their work won them the Nobel Prize in 1954. With discovery of only three types of polio virus (rather than innumerable strains) and their ability to grow the virus in tissue cultures of human embryonic cells, "the potential to develop a vaccine against paralytic poliomyelitis became a reality." (9)

Dr. Jonas Salk, a medical scientist at the University of Pittsburgh who had been working on a cure for polio, equipped a lab for the latest production techniques. By 1950, he had begun testing his vaccine on children who had had polio. Subsequent blood samples taken from these children showed an increase in antibodies. There was much initial opposition out of concern over the safety of the vaccine, and it wasn't until 1952 that the National Foundation for Infantile Paralysis was convinced that the vaccine was safe. Interestingly, as a national charitable non-governmental organization it had spent ten times as much money in the early 1950's on polio research as the tax-supported National Institutes of Health. Early in 1953, vaccines were given to one hundred sixty children and adults in Pittsburgh, including Salk's three children. Then, in 1954, forty thousand doses of the vaccine were administered in the first large field test. A year later, in 1955, the inactivated Salk poliovirus vaccine was licensed. Dr. Albert Sabin developed an oral poliovirus vaccine the following year, and in the early 1960's, it came into widespread use.

In a time span of only four decades, after the experiments and work of Landsteiner and Popper in Vienna, there emerged a viable vaccine to combat the poliovirus.

The initial major polio epidemic in the United States occurred in Vermont in 1894, with one hundred thirty-two cases reported. The Polio epidemic of 1916 killed seven thousand Americans, with over nine thousand cases in New York alone, and twenty seven thousand total cases reported. The last major outbreak of polio in America was in 1952. It resulted in over three hundred deaths and a total of over fifty-eight thousand cases. Other outbreaks in America were: Los Angeles in 1934; twenty-five hundred cases; twenty thousand cases reported annually between the years 1945-1949; and thirty-five thousand cases in 1953.

Since 1970, there have been only three documented instances of polio outbreaks in America. In 1970, twenty-two cases were reported along the Texas-Mexico border; in 1972, there were eleven cases in a Christian Science School in Connecticut; and in 1979, fifteen cases were reported among the Amish in Pennsylvania, Missouri, Iowa, and Wisconsin. The latter outbreak was the last documented transmission of wild poliovirus in the United States. (10)

(*Note: As this manuscript is in final editing, fall 2005, four new cases of wild poliovirus have been reported again in an Amish community in Minnesota.)

In 2003, polio had essentially been eradicated in the western world. While there are still outbreaks of the disease in third world countries in Africa and India, as well as Mexico, the fearsome epidemics that had struck with increasing frequency in Europe and America in the late 1800's and early twentieth century are now gone.

Worldwide, since 1988 when UNICEF formed the Global Polio Eradication Initiative, dramatic progress has been made in eradicating the disease. "Cases have plummeted by 99% (from 350,000 in 1988 to 784 in 2003). A disease that once crippled children in one hundred twenty-five countries around the world is now endemic in only six—Nigeria, India, Pakistan, Niger, Afghanistan and Egypt. Polio is on course to become the second disease, after smallpox, to be wiped from the face of the earth."(11)

See also ADDENDUM, THE HISTORY OF POLIO: A

HYPERTEXT TIMELINE page 43, for a concise summary timeline of important landmark dates in the history of polio.

While most Americans no longer worry about getting the disease, any discussion these days concerning polio is most likely focused on a topic called post polio syndrome, also called the late effects of polio. Symptoms of the syndrome are varied across individuals but can include increase in muscle weakness (sometimes dramatic and sudden), severe fatigue, pain, intolerance for cold, difficulty in breathing and swallowing, sleep disorders, and other problems. Dr. Richard Bruno has written an authoritative text on post polio syndrome, *The Polio Paradox,* referred to earlier in the text. For any reader who wishes a more in-depth understanding of polio and the late effects of the disease, his book is well written and very readable.

Thinking about the year that I contracted polio, almost sixty-one years ago in 1945, it was not a bad time to catch the virus. In reading about the disease in America, especially in the thirties and forties, I came across the following: "When Roosevelt created the National Foundation for Infantile Paralysis in 1937, it received unprecedented support from the American people. Throughout the Great Depression, World War II, and the postwar years, the fight against polio came to symbolize all that the Americans of the time were most proud of: The response to the great epidemics of the 1930s and 1950s was nationwide and voluntary. Polios were taken care of by their neighbors and communities. The National Foundation and its local chapters provided care to all polios without regard to income or insurance status. The immense cost of care and the search for a vaccine was raised by popular subscription with everyone participating—school children, neighborhood organizations, movie stars such as Mickey Rooney and Judy Garland and, of course, President Roosevelt. The research effort was as complex as building the first atomic bomb or placing a man on the moon, but it was undertaken with absolute confidence that a vaccine could be found. The anti-polio vaccine was, again to quote Basil O'Connor, a "planned miracle." It was all there in the polio effort: Neighbor helping neighbor, American generosity and can-do spirit, America at its very best." (12)

Hollywood has a tendency to overdo, for dramatic effect, things such as cultural clichés and ethnic idiosyncrasies. For example, we've all seen an American Indian movie where the brave warrior, facing imminent death, boldly and courageously intones, "Today is a good day to die."

I didn't die, and although I did face death, given the overwhelming national mobilization to fight the disease, it was a good year to become a "gimp."

ADDENDUM
THE HISTORY OF POLIO: A HYPERTEXT TIMELINE

1789 - British physician Michael Underwood provides the first clinical description of polio, referring to it as a "debility of the lower extremities."

1840 - German physician Jacob von Heine publishes a 78-page monograph in 1840, which not only describes the clinical features of the disease, but also notes that its symptoms suggest the involvement of the spinal cord.

1894 - The first major polio epidemic reported in the United States occurs in Vermont, consisting of 132 total cases, including some adults.

1908 - Polio becomes a reportable disease entity as Austrian physicians Karl Landsteiner and E. Popper identify the poliovirus.

1909 - Massachusetts begins counting polio cases.

1916 - There is a large outbreak of polio in the United States. Though the total number of affected individuals is unknown, over 9000 cases are reported in New York City alone. Attempts at controlling the disease largely involve the use of isolation and quarantine, neither of which is successful.

1921 - Franklin Delano Roosevelt (FDR) contracts polio and is left with severe paralysis.
1924 - FDR travels to Warm Springs, Georgia and checks into a

cottage on the grounds of the dilapidated Meriwether Inn based on reports that the waters there could somehow "cure" paralysis.

1926 - FDR purchases the Meriwether Inn, and the Warm Springs Foundation is formed.

1928 - Philip Drinker and Louis Shaw develop the iron lung, a large metal tank equipped with a pump that assists respiration. The device is field -tested and goes into commercial production three years later.

1932 - FDR is elected president of the United States. The first and only U.S. president to use a wheelchair, he successfully hides the extent of his disability from the American public throughout his presidency.

1934 - There is a major outbreak of polio in Los Angeles. Nearly 2500 polio cases are treated from May through November of that year at Los Angeles County General Hospital alone. The first Birthday Ball is held on FDR's birthday (Jan. 30) to raise money for the Georgia Warm Springs Foundation.

1935 - Physicians Maurice Brodie and John Kollmer compete against each other, with each trying to be the first to develop a successful polio vaccine. Field trials fail with disastrous results as the vaccines are blamed for causing many cases of polio, some of which are fatal.

1937 - FDR announces the creation of the National Foundation for Infantile Paralysis.

1938 - Entertainer Eddie Canter coins the name "March of Dimes" as he urges radio listeners to send their spare change to the White House to be used by the National Foundation for Infantile Paralysis in the fight against polio. The name sticks.

1940 - Sister Elizabeth Kenny, an Australian nurse, travels from her native Australia to California where she is virtually ignored by the medical community. She then travels to Minnesota where she gives the first presentation in the United States to members of the Mayo Clinic staff regarding her procedures for treating polio patients by means of hot-packing and stretching affected limbs.

1942 - The first Sister Kenny Institute opens in Minneapolis.

1943 - The Sister Kenny Foundation is formed, and Kenny's procedures become the standard treatment for polio patients in the United States, replacing the ineffective traditional approaches of *"convalescent serum"* and *immobilization.*

1945 - World War II ends. Large epidemics of polio in the U.S. occur immediately after the war, with an average of more than 20,000 cases a year from 1945 to 1949.

1947 - Jonas Salk accepts a position in Pittsburgh at the new medical laboratory funded by the Sarah Mellon Scientific Foundation.

1948 - Salk's laboratory is one of four awarded research grants for the poliovirus-typing project. Salk decides to adopt the new tissue culture method of cultivating and working with the poliovirus that had recently been developed by John Enders at Harvard University. Other researchers, including Albert Sabin, who would later develop the oral polio vaccine, continue to do their work with monkeys infected with the poliovirus—a more difficult and time-consuming process.

1952 - There are 58,000 cases of polio in the United States, the most ever recorded. Early versions of the Salk vaccine, using killed poliovirus, are successful with small samples of patients at the Watson Home for Crippled Children and the Polk State School, a Pennsylvania facility for individuals with mental retardation.

1953 - Amid continued "polio hysteria," there are 35,000 cases of polio in the United States.

1954 - Massive field trials of the Salk vaccine are sponsored by the National Foundation for Infantile Paralysis.

1955 - News of the successful vaccine trials is announced by Dr. Thomas Francis Jr. of the University of Michigan at a formal press conference held April 12 in Ann Arbor (the site where the research data from the field trials had been gathered and analyzed). A nationwide vaccination program is quickly started.

1957 - After a mass immunization campaign promoted by the March of Dimes, there are only about 5600 cases of polio in the United States.

1958 and 1959 - Field trials prove the Sabin oral vaccine, which uses live, attenuated (weakened) virus, to be effective.

1962 - The Salk vaccine is replaced by the Sabin oral vaccine, which is not only superior in terms of ease of administration, but also provides longer-lasting immunity.

1964 - Only 121 cases of polio are reported nationally.

1974 - Dr. Donald Mulder of the Mayo Clinic writes an article describing the "late progression of poliomyelitis."

1977 - The National Health Interview Survey reports that there are 245,000 persons living in the United States who had been paralyzed by polio. Some estimates place the number at more than 600,000.

1979 - The last indigenous transmission of wild poliovirus occurs in the U.S. All future cases are either imported or vaccine-related.

1981 - Time Magazine reports that many polio survivors are experiencing late effects of the disease.

1984 - Researchers, including Dr. Lauro Halstead, organize a conference at Warm Springs Institute for Rehabilitation because of growing concerns about the late effects of polio (post-polio syndrome).

1988 - With approximately 350,000 cases of polio occurring worldwide, the World Health Organization passes a resolution to eradicate polio by the year 2000.

1993 - The total number of reported polio cases worldwide falls to about 100,000. Most of these cases occur in Asia and Africa.

1994 - China launches its first National Immunization Days, immunizing 80 million children. The entire Western Hemisphere is certified as "polio free."

1995 - India follows China's lead and organizes its first National Immunization Days. More than 87 million children are immunized.

1997 - The Franklin Delano Roosevelt Memorial opens on May 2.

1999 - More than 450 million children are vaccinated, including nearly 147 million in India. In the 11 years since the World Health Assembly Initiative, the number of reported cases worldwide has fallen to approximately 7000.

2000 - Wars, natural disasters, and poverty in about 30 Asian and African nations prevent the complete eradication of polio. There is even a polio outbreak in Haiti and the Dominican Republic, which, along with the rest of the western hemisphere had been polio free since the early 1990's. A new target date of 2005 for worldwide eradication is set by the Global Polio Eradication Initiative.

2001 - 575 million children are vaccinated in 94 countries.

2004 - Ministers of Health from the six remaining polio-endemic countries meet and agree to take the final steps toward polio eradication. Polio cases in Asia decline by 50%, and over 80 million children are vaccinated in western and central Africa. In spite of these efforts, there are 1170 cases of polio in 2004, 760 of which occur in Nigeria.

2005 - Polio spreads from Nigeria to the Sudan, with 105 confirmed cases. This latest outbreak illustrates "the high risk posed to polio-free areas by the continuing epidemic in west and central Africa" (WER, 80 (1), 2005, p. 2).

IV. Dusty Lane Days

"There is no use crying about what you can't do. Now what you no longer have in your legs, you must have in your head." (1)

In that glorious late spring of 1947, when I returned home for good, I was a frail, thin, eight year old, who weighed less than sixty pounds. I could walk, sort of, leaning heavily on two underarm crutches, a long, steel brace on my right leg, toe to hip, and a short brace on my left leg, toe to knee. Trying to walk was tiring, and as I became fatigued I would frequently fall. With gimpy hands, no triceps muscle in my right arm, and my awkward crab-like walking gait, I could easily get out of sync and down I would go. I was especially vulnerable when on uneven ground, trying to negotiate a single step, and on slippery floors and rugs.

Thus, when we went out most often I left my braces and crutches at home, and my father carried me. Dad was a strapping German fellow who, at 6-2 and two hundred-ten pounds had amazing stamina. He would simply carry me to and from the car and deposit me in a chair; or, in warm weather, he would put me outside on the ground in a grassy yard. With relatives, I was comfortable crawling or scooting on my butt around the house or yard. For an all-day outing, like the Violas Park Zoo in Madison, the Green County Fair, or a Saturday night in Monroe, Dad carried me the entire time. I could tell when he was becoming tired, as he would find a place to sit or lean to relieve the excess weight on his legs and back.

Realizing that I was a burden to him, I'd sometimes ask, "Are you OK, Dad?"

His reply was always the same, "Oh, I'm OK."

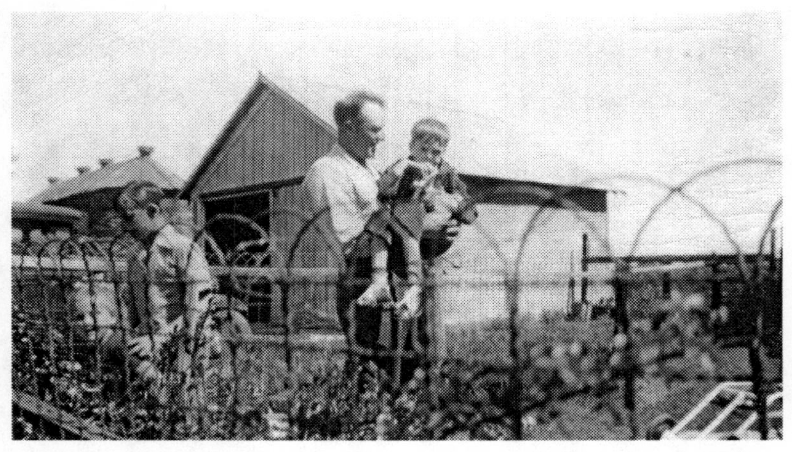

My father carrying me, after I came home (summer, 1947)

Around home, my braces and crutches quickly became a nuisance. I discovered that I was far more mobile when I simply got down on the floor and crawled. My brother told me that when I first returned home, he remembers that our mother would repeatedly warn my siblings and other neighborhood kids, "Be careful, don't step on Kent!" I was literally underfoot the majority of time.

June through August of 1947 was truly a summer of serendipity for me. Many mornings I would awaken to the familiar and comforting sound of my father's voice calling his dairy herd to come in for the morning milking. During the night, I could clearly hear the melody of bells as the herd grazed contentedly in the cool dampness of the Illinois summer night. Neighborhood dogs barked and howled into the early morning hours, disturbing sleep, and roosters that were up

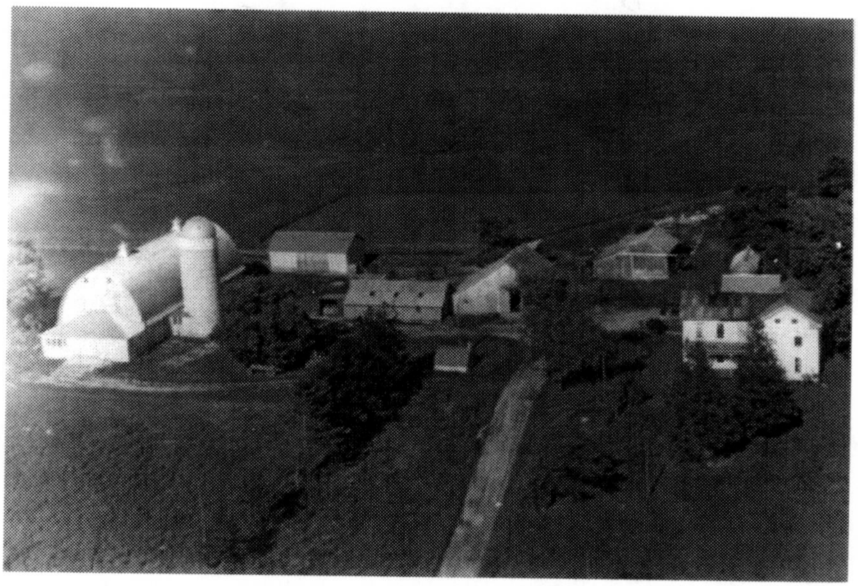

Dusty Lane: a time and place that healed me physically and spiritually

much too early began to crow. These were the sounds of home, and all reassured me that I was back with my family where I belonged. Every day someone came to our farm to visit—relatives, neighbors, and friends of all ages. My family was welcoming to all.

While all of these folks came to visit our entire family, it became clear to me that their specific mission was to deliver good wishes, hopes and prayers for my continued recovery. The community showered our family with love and affection. Home had not only become the place where I lived and felt safe and secure, it was an environment filled with fun, laughter, excitement and people, many people, whose presence nourished our family's spirits. I flourished physically and emotionally at this place called Dusty Lane.

My Aunt Esther, commenting (in 2003) on that period and the ensuing years observed, "Your parents had a great attitude about your situation; they took a very practical approach to each new challenge, confident that they could handle the situation. Your parents gave all of you children tremendous freedom growing up on the Rock City farm. My own children Audrey and Elaine loved coming to the farm; it was their destination of choice."

Cousin Audrey was the game girl; she learned every new game that came out, and taught us how to play by the rules. I especially remember canasta. The biggest obstacle was learning how to hold all those darn cards. Elaine, her sister, nine years younger, also spent much time at our farm, Dusty Lane. She wore orthopedic shoes with steel inlaid toes, and she was very adept at hitting shinbones with a well-placed kick. She loved horses and riding them, until one day our dogs spooked a huge white gelding, and he threw her. It was early spring, very crisp outside, and Elaine, maybe seven, was bundled up in heavy clothes, stocking cap, scarf, and boots. That old horse launched her like a rock out of a catapult. She sailed through the air like in slow motion, and then hit the ground with a thud. I thought she was dead as there was no sound. Then she let out a blood-curdling yell, jumped up and raced to the house. I don't think she was even bruised.

Another little girl who loved animals was the youngest sister of my cousins Sandra and Sylvia Blunt. Her name was Joann, but everyone called her Jody. She loved cats and had a huge old tomcat named Mickey. Because her mother, my Aunt Corrine, had terrible allergy problems, they decided that Mickey should live at our farm. Jody was terrified that our dogs might hurt the cat, as he was a stranger. Upon the cat's arrival, my Boston terrier, Grumpy, began to bark at Mickey, and continued for what seemed an hour. He yapped and lunged, towards and then back, dancing ever closer to the seemingly unconcerned feline, Mickey lay motionless except for a rather violent switching of his tail. Eventually Grump got within striking distance, and with a lightning-quick slash old Mickey buried his claws deep into the top of Grump's head. Well, that ended any further harassment towards Mickey. As I recall, he lived a peaceful, uneventful life the rest of his days on our farm.

My parents were always very supportive, but at the same time recognized that learning to overcome my physical limitations was primarily my responsibility. Their attitude was simply that I needed to address each situation as it arose and figure out how to cope with or solve the problem. When I initially returned home that spring, I was given a downstairs bedroom while the rest of the family slept upstairs.

As the only one sleeping downstairs, I was frightened. I could trace the origin of my fears to the kidnapping and murder of that young girl in Chicago. Just as I had watched the window in my hospital room, I now watched, at times absolutely terrified, for a strange face to appear leering in at me from outside the window of my home. They tried to allay my fears, but to no avail. Exasperated, Mom finally said, "Well, there is room for you to sleep upstairs, but we can't carry you up and down each day. How will you get up and down?" Relieved at not having to be downstairs alone any longer, I learned to crawl up those eighteen-twenty stairs on my first attempt. Coming down I simply bumped down one step at a time on my butt.

Almost daily, I increased the range of my crawling or scooting, and by the end of the summer I could negotiate my way, even over gravel, to our dairy barn, a distance of probably fifty yards. Fritz Kolb, our former hired man, came for a visit one Sunday and I happened to drag myself to the barn where he was chatting with my father and a few other men. Fritz later recalled wondering, "What kind of life will that kid have?" Each small feat I accomplished—crawling to the barn, crawling up the stairs each night, discovering that I could get up on a chair from the floor and then to a counter top to reach a high cupboard—was empowering, and overcoming each new challenge was part of a critical learning process for me. Julian Rotter, a social psychologist, had a theory regarding an individual's "generalized expectancy for reinforcement in life." Simply, the idea is that we either believe we control our lives or we believe that outside forces control us. I was, in his terms, learning that I could control my life by developing an "internal locus of control." And it was true. The more I figured out how to do things for myself, the more confidence I felt in my ability to solve the challenges that I faced. By contrast, people with an "external locus of control" see life contingent on luck, fate, or chance, but always on circumstances beyond their control.

Notwithstanding my growing confidence, I knew that fall was approaching, which would bring the start of a new school year. How would I negotiate the six steps at the main entrance, and the two steep steps down to the indoor bathroom? What would the kids think of me? Would they tease me? I fretted daily as the first day of school drew closer. The reception was nothing like I could have imagined.

The entire school turned out to welcome me back. Everyone wanted to do something for me. Although a bit overwhelmed initially, I soon was basking in the glow of something akin to celebrity status. After overcoming the apprehension about the first day, school was a breeze.

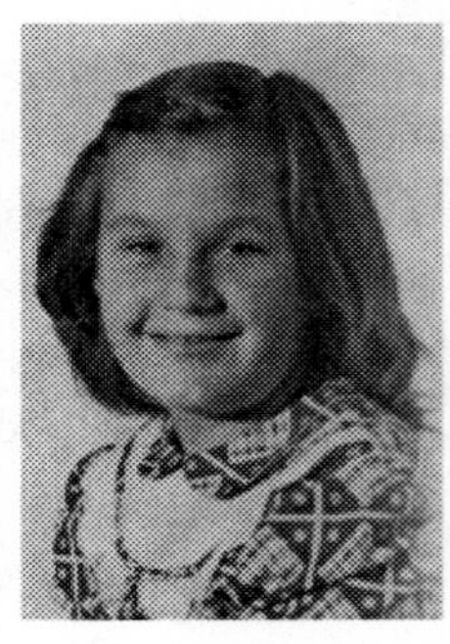

Dorothy, my first girlfriend (third grade, 1947)

Aunt Esther later commented, "You were easy to get along with, and didn't feel sorry for yourself. It's always easy to help someone who is good natured." I clearly remember one little girl who would stay in with me at recess. Her name was Dorothy and she had piercing gray eyes. She would sit next to me and watch me intently, waiting to help if I needed something. She was, no doubt, my first girlfriend, and I still remember her kindness and attention. Later on when our relationship had blossomed a bit more, she told me my first dirty limerick; it went, "I have a girl and you can't beat her, she has a hole to fit my peter!" I thought that was absolutely wonderful. My relationship with little Dorothy transformed from infatuation to friendship throughout grade school and high school, and I can still see her sitting across the aisle in her desk, a devoted little friend.

The year, 1947, and third grade ended with not only many new milestones in my life, but also for America. A guy named Branch Rickey overturned convention, maybe more accurately the course of history in our nation, by signing a young black man to a major league baseball contract. I doubt that Rickey, as a general manager of the Brooklyn Dodgers, or Jackie Robinson, the talented young athlete from UCLA, had any idea of the significance of Jackie "breaking the color barrier" in baseball for our country. I was yet to become a serious baseball fan and the signing of Robinson was mostly a curiosity for me.

Besides I was living at home, feeling like I was a normal person again, and I knew that 1948 was going to be another great year with the family and my neighborhood friends. Then the bottom dropped out of my world. My parents, trying to ensure that I gained as much physical return as possible, signed me up for a year at Deaconess Hospital in Freeport, Illinois, about fifteen miles from home. I was devastated. There were six or seven young people who were post-polio in what was essentially a mini-rehabilitation center that occupied several rooms at the South end of the first floor of the hospital. Despite initial bouts of homesickness, I adapted readily to my new environment and the daily routines of therapy and school. My zany roommate, Jerry, another ten year old who was an unwitting clown, kept life interesting.

The day I arrived at the hospital, Jerry, as sort of a welcome gesture, demonstrated that the thick lenses of his glasses were unbreakable. He had recently broken an older pair, and he was quite proud of these new, indestructible ones. He ripped them off his face and threw them to the floor. One lens shattered as if a BB had hit it dead center. The nurses and his family were quite pissed at him, but Jerry just squinted through his shattered lens for what seemed like weeks before another new pair arrived. "Oh, I can see okay" he reported, and in fact, it didn't seem to bother him. Jerry and I spent the year at Deaconess Hospital getting into all sorts of mischief, especially on weekends. He was ambulatory, and I got around pretty rapidly in an ancient, wooden, hard-rimmed front wheel drive wheelchair. We played hide and seek throughout the hospital; snuck up to the surgery suites, downstairs to the kitchen and laundry, and in the subbasement that was jammed full of beds, chairs, obsolete equipment, boxes, containers, and all manner of junk. Only once did we go into the morgue. The door was not locked and we went in, but it didn't take long for both of us to get the creeps and abandon that adventure.

We frequently visited the firehouse station about two blocks from the hospital, enjoying the company of the firemen who usually had a sweet treat for us. On more than one occasion the nurses had to come to the station to retrieve us. The consequence of being AWOL was being grounded for a couple of weeks. Ed Yde, a huge Freeport police officer, was a favorite visitor to the ward, although the hospital staff wasn't always pleased when he brought us fattening treats. He would treat us to ice cream by the gallon, candy, snacks, movies, tickets to the Golden Gloves boxing matches, and toys. It was always something special. As the city's only polio ward, we got quite a lot of attention from the community.

Anyone who was a quart low on doing good deeds would visit us. There were singing groups, dancers, comedians, clowns, storytellers, and puppeteers who came to the ward to cheer us up. Some of the entertainment wasn't too bad, but regardless of the quality, we really didn't have a choice about attending. The hospital wasn't going to risk damaging their image by making the do-gooders play to an empty house. We learned to put on our plastic smiles for our benefactors and the press, who always showed up for the photo ops. Jerry and I had our mugs in the paper on a number of occasions, once with a caption that stated, "Young Dancers Entertain Polio Ward."

There we sat with our hair slicked back, nicely posed with stupid

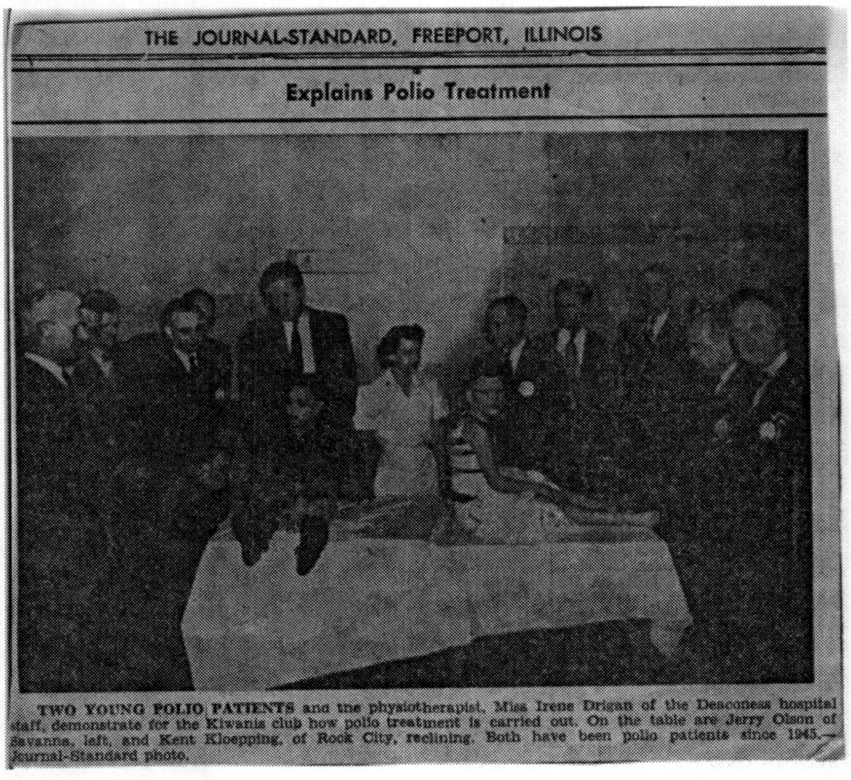
THE JOURNAL-STANDARD, FREEPORT, ILLINOIS

Explains Polio Treatment

TWO YOUNG POLIO PATIENTS and the physiotherapist, Miss Irene Drigan of the Deaconess hospital staff, demonstrate for the Kiwanis club how polio treatment is carried out. On the table are Jerry Olson of Savanna, left, and Kent Kloepping, of Rock City, reclining. Both have been polio patients since 1945.—Journal-Standard photo.

Explains polio treatment

Young Dancers Entertain Polio Ward

July 1945

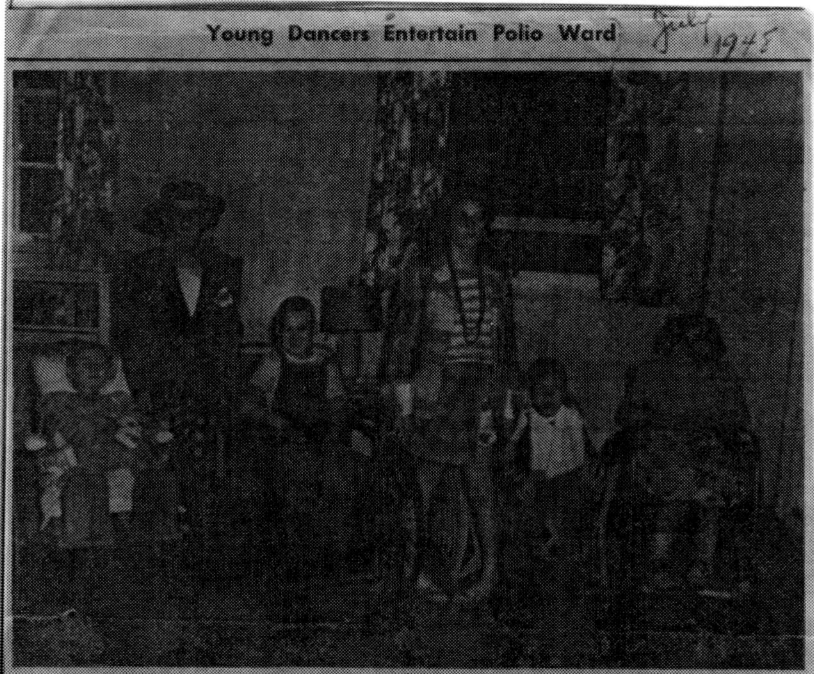

PATIENTS AND ENTERTAINERS are (left to right): Mary Ann Morris, Harry Bird, Kent Kloepping, Harriet Bird, Jerry Olsen and Mary Lou Mienert.—Photo by Dwight Garnhart.

Hospital Ward Is Dance Stage

The polio ward at Deaconess hospital, with the four children who are making progress from paralysis suffered in the epidemic of 1946, had an entertainment to their taste.

A dance program, in costume, was presented by two young entertainers, Harry and Harriet Bird of Huntington, W. Va., children of Mr. and Mrs. Harry F. Bird, formerly of Freeport. They are here visiting their grandmother, Mrs. Emma Hamlyn, 312 North Powell avenue.

Harriet gave a tap characterization of a southern belle, and a toe dance. Harry did a buck-and-wing solo. Together they did a "symphonic" tap dance and a comedy rube dance.

The youngsters of their audience were delighted.

Also Visit Fire Station

Of the four patients, Jerry Olsen is now the most advanced and has been walking since the first of the year. Mary Lou Mienert and Kent Kloepping are still in wheel chairs but making fine progress. Mary Ann Morris, who formerly had to be in an iron lung all the time, still sleeps in an iron lung but does not require it all of the day.

Neighbors of Deaconess hospital enjoy the children's daily tour of the neighborhood when the weather permits the nurses to take them out. Favorite destination is the fire station. The firemen lift their small visitors into the engine cab, and help them make the siren sound.

The four children are cared for by Miss Mabel Hayes, polio nurse supplied by the National Foundation of Infantile Paralysis, and by Miss Irene Drigen, Deaconess hospital physical therapist.

Care Of New Cases

Convalescent cases are cared for at Deaconess hospital. New cases are cared for during the acute and contagious stage at St. Francis hospital.

Wednesday the first 1948 Carroll county case was transferred from St. Francis to a room near the other four children at Deaconess. This was Betty Lou Curbey, Mt. Carroll route 3, who was brought to the hospital 16 days before, and is making fine progress.

The first Stephenson county case was brought to St. Francis hospital at noon Wednesday. Danny Albert Grenoble, 103 West Clark street. He is 13 years old.

Young Dancers Entertain Polio Ward.

grins on our faces, staring with rapt attention to whatever inane entertainment was being foisted upon us that day.

We had some great nurses, like Mrs. Fager and Mrs. Huber, really nice ladies who brightened each day. We also had a few really cute nurses like Allie Nelson a foxy blonde and Miss Irene Dregan, our physical therapist, a petite brunette.

Another nurse, although she was fairly pleasant, gave Jerry and I a good bit of grief for a period of time. That was in the person of a rotund spinster, Miss Kramer. She must have been a frustrated old maid with no prospects for a roll in the hay anytime soon. Well, Miss Kramer liked to spank Jerry and I. At the least provocation or

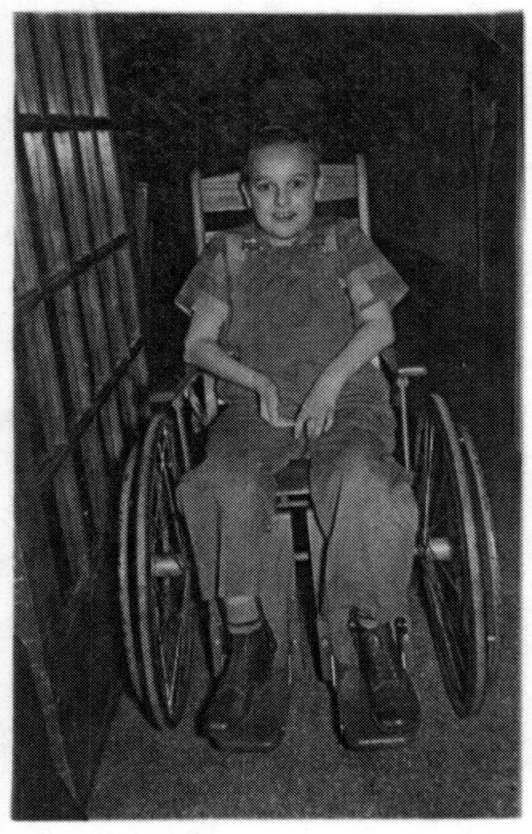

My ancient wheelchair at the Deaconess Hospital in Freeport, Illinois (1948)

rule infraction, she'd grab a yardstick and whale away on us. Never both the same day as I think she saved her strength so she could administer a thorough beating. Frankly her assaults got tiresome, and further they stung like the devil. Jerry and I had to come up with a new strategy to combat her. We had noticed that she would whack us until we began to cry and then stop the assault. We made a pact not to cry, no matter how much the whippings hurt or stung. "Let's laugh, if we can." I was next on her hit list and I didn't whimper once. I began to laugh at her, which caused her to increase the fury of the spanking. The harder she hit me, the more I laughed. Abruptly, she burst into tears and rushed out of the room. Several days later Jerry got her attention, by golly, he hung in there, laughing with a strange high-pitched cackle (I thought he had lost it) with the same result. Miss Kramer again fled in tears and never again threatened us with corporal punishment.

I returned home in the spring of 1949, and began in earnest to try and figure out how to fit in. My desire was to participate fully in a community filled with people who were not disabled. I especially wanted to be included as a member of my peer group. Then I discovered baseball. I had listened to the 1948 World Series between the old Boston Braves and the Cleveland Indians while in the hospital in Freeport. Boston had two great pitchers, Warren Spahn, a big left-hander from Hartshorne, Oklahoma, and a right-hander named Johnny Sain. The byword in Boston was, "Spahn and Sain and pray for rain." I thought that was about the coolest saying I'd ever heard. The game had all kinds of esoteric jargon, superstitions practiced by the players, but best of all, statistics on it seemed everything that happened on and off the diamond. Many players had great nicknames: "Stan The Man," the "Splendid Splinter," the "Yankee Clipper," "Country Slaughter," "Pee Wee," "Yogi," "Preacher," "The Whip," "The Bear," "Moose," "Sal The Barber," and of course, "The Say Hey Kid."

I was hooked. I became a devoted fan and strove to be an expert in baseball trivia and statistics. I decided that my teams would be the Cubs and the Yankees. The Cubs were awful, and the Yankees were, arguably, the best team in baseball during the waning days of the great Joe DiMaggio. Dick Rockey, a new neighbor in 1949 who was my age and would become a life long friend, picked the Dodgers—the real Dodgers, from Brooklyn—as his National League team, and Cleveland as his American League team.

Brooklyn had a fabulous array of stars. There was Jackie Robinson, Pee Wee Reese, Roy Campanella, Gil Hodges, Duke Snider, Billy Cox, Carl Furillo, Preacher Roe, and more. Cleveland had great pitchers in the aging Bob Feller, Mike Garcia, Early Wynn, and Bob Lemon. God, we could argue forever about who was the better player or team. I listened daily to the Cubs or the Yankees (but only if they were playing the White Sox, because we could only get Chicago games on the radio), read baseball magazines, record books, and memorized statistics. I could spew all manner of minutia related to players and teams. My all-time baseball hero, Mickey Mantle, from Commerce, Oklahoma, arrived in the majors in 1950.

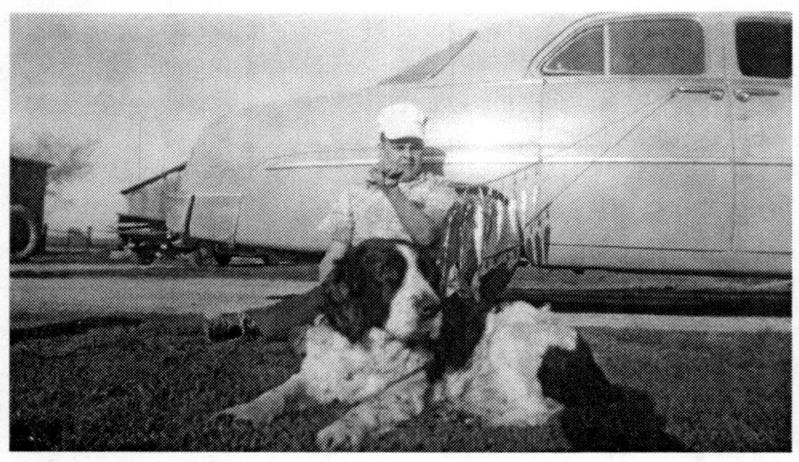

A nice catch from the Rock Run Creek, which ran through our farm. The dog was old Butch. (1953 or 1954)

Baseball wasn't my only interest. I began fishing regularly in the Rock Run Creek that ran through our farm. I also learned to play croquet, a game at which I got quite good. Dick Rockey and I would play with my older sister Carol, and we usually cheated. One afternoon, in a fit of anger, she flung her mallet at us. It whizzed past our heads like a large boomerang, knocking a substantial hunk of siding off the house just below the living room window. Dad never did fix it.

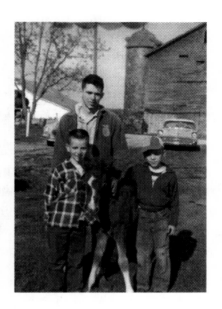

Childhood and lifelong friend Dick Rockey, with his younger twin brothers and colt (1955 or 1956)

I played a version of softball with the neighborhood kids; my bases were shorter and I batted sitting on the ground. If I hit the ball I crawled to first base, second, and so on. I wasn't very mobile in the field defensively, but once I did catch a line drive off the bat of our neighbor girl. It knocked me over, but I hung onto the ball. A person could also be put out by rolling or throwing the ball in front of them before they reached a base. My mother put a lot of patches on the knees and the rear of the bib overalls I wore. They worked best for crawling, as the shoulder straps kept the pants on. I especially remember the Coleman kids from the farm across the road being willing to include me by playing this rather odd game of softball

Wilma Kurtz, the family friend who had been so good to me at the Kent Cottage in Rockford, continued to be supportive and thoughtful even after I returned home. She not only took me on special day-outings like the Brookfield Zoo in Chicago, but also tried to pique my interest in different hobbies. She brought me a pair of hamsters, and presto, I was in the hamster business. Raising the little buggers was okay for a while, but they multiplied so fast, I began to feel like rodents surrounded me. My career as a hamster farmer was short-lived, much to the delight of my parents.

By 1951, the activity at our farm in rural Rock City, Illinois, had reached whirlwind levels. I was thirteen years old and my siblings, ages seventeen, fourteen, and ten, each had a different group of friends whose choice destination, year around, was our farm. We rode horses and ponies, drove old buggies, played all sorts of outdoor games, and swam in the local creek.

My brother and his buddies built rafts and piers, and we spent the day in the brown, mud-filled swimming holes, ignoring the cow turds that regularly floated by. I swam with a life jacket when I first began returning to the creek with the neighborhood kids. It was heavy and cumbersome, and one afternoon, I took it off. I was overjoyed to discover I could stay afloat without it. I practiced holding my breath underwater, and soon became the champion underwater king. Two and a half minutes was my record. Almost invariably each day's swim ended with a mud fight, particularly if the swimmers were an all-male group. The city kids were singled out most often for the pelting with the sticky black goop that stuck like glue to body and hair. Rinsing off, gingerly getting out of the creek, drying off, and getting into your clothes took a good bit of strategy to avoid the barrage of muck

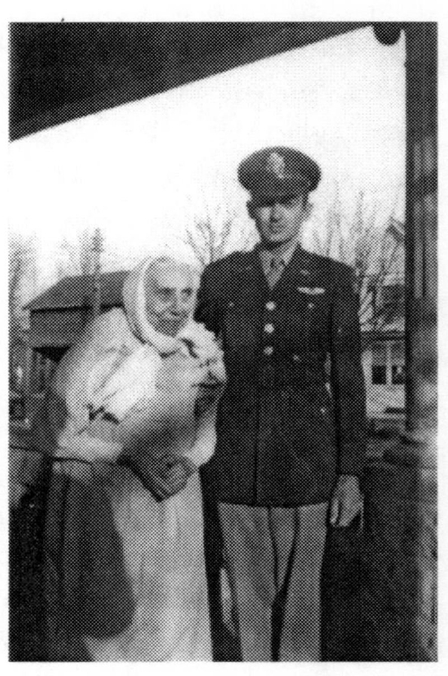

Uncle Jacob Rodenbough, a B-17 pilot, and his grandmother, Mary Rodenbough, whom we called "blind Grandma." Juda, Wisconsin (November or December 1943)

During these memorable carefree days, we always looked forward to visits from our Southern relatives, Uncle Jake Rodenbough, (Mom's brother), his wife, Aunt Ethel, an attractive dark-haired Cajun from Louisiana, and their kids, Martha, Francis, "Bud," and later, Richard. Uncle Jake was a B-17 pilot in World War II, flying thirty plus missions over Germany from his base in Lavenham, England, with the 487th bomber group. My first recollection of him was the

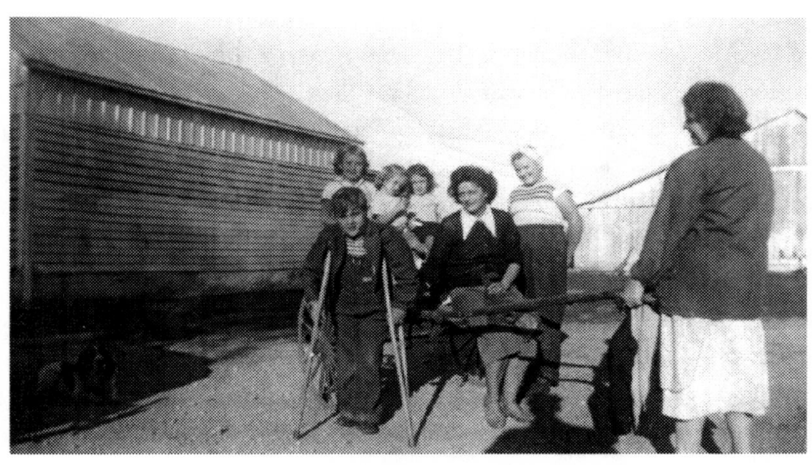

Aunt Ethel Rodenbough and daughters (in the pony cart) at our farm (summer, 1948 or 1949)

Christmas of 1943 when he brought his new wife, Ethel, to Wisconsin to meet the family. The adults said she was from Louisiana. I didn't know where that was, but in my imagination she was from some far away land, like maybe India or Arabia because she was an exotic woman with dark eyes and an alluring laugh. He retired from the Air Force as a Lieutenant Colonel, and only after his passing in January 2000, did the family begin to fully appreciate his exemplary military career. He was one of our family's brightest stars, a quiet, unassuming, gentle man who did his job well without fanfare. He was truly a member of the valiant warriors that Tom Brokaw labeled, *The Greatest Generation,* in his book of that title.

One of the best parts of Jake and Ethel's visits was listening to them talk. Those Southern drawls (Ethel particularly) were new sounds. Their arrival always meant exciting times. There was usually at least one huge extended family gathering with old folks, young folks, (many I didn't really know), but all who were supposedly relatives. They always brought a unique gift of some sort; one I still have is a regulation bomber pilot flight cap with attached flip-down sunglasses.

Life was good, fun and frivolity every day. But again, I was to have my life put on hold as my parents sent me to a private Rehabilitation Center at Oshkosh, Wisconsin. The facility was the former home and estate of a guy named Milton Berry. The Milton Berry School, we later decided, was mostly a dumping ground for individuals that families didn't want to have underfoot. My parents' motivation was quite different, and I'd guess it was as difficult for my parents to have me leave as it was for me. But Eddie Herbert, a local man who had polio in the 1920's, realistically felt I would profit from their brand of therapy and the new braces with a waist-collar that he fabricated. That fact, plus a great sales pitch from a slick-talking representative of the organization convinced my parents that it was worth a try, even though the tuition was quite expensive.

The setting was gorgeous, a lovely wooded estate on Lake Winnebago with beautifully decorated rooms in the main house. My room was formerly Berry's office; mahogany paneling with elegant French doors leading to what had been an open-air sun porch.

There was a young man in his early thirties from New York who had obviously been farmed out by the family. He had a neurological condition that caused him to walk with a lurching, unsteady gait. He was also mentally slow, but he was streetwise and he loved baseball, especially the New York Giants. He was quite knowledgeable about the game, and we spent a good deal of time talking baseball. The National League pennant race in 1951 was the year of an amazing comeback by the Giants, who beat the Dodgers on Bobby Thomson's dramatic three-run homer in the bottom of the ninth inning in the last of a three-game playoff series. Henry was listening to the game in his room on the second floor, and when Thomson hit the ball, he howled at the top of his lungs, leaped out of bed, and fell flat with a thump on the wooden floor. After he righted himself and staggered to the top of the stairs, he screamed almost hysterically, "Ginas win! Ginas win! Ginas win!" He tripped and tumbled head over heels down the long flight of stairs yelling all the way down, "Ginas win! Ginas win!" He had quite a speech impediment, and "Giants win" came out "Ginas win." It was amazing he didn't break his neck celebrating the victory of his favorite team. Later that evening, I brought Henry a Coke from the well-stocked kitchen to celebrate the "Ginas" victory. He sat quietly, chuckling and mumbling to himself as he slurped down his soda. He was a strange, lonesome little man, but during the months I spent at Berry's, Henry and I shared a bit of camaraderie over baseball.

Earlier that fall, Aunt Esther got tickets for the Cubs and Dodgers for a game on September, 16 at Wrigley Field; my first major league game. On leave that weekend, from Oshkosh, Uncle Hub, Dad, Esther and I went to the game. It was a thrill to actually be at the ballpark, but what happened that day in Wrigley Field transcended a mere baseball game. Several years prior to this memoir, I wrote an account of that day for a writing class: I have included the text *A Day at Wrigley* as an addendum to the end of this chapter. Jackie Robinson and the rest of the great Dodger team were there that day, and what a day it was.

I had only been in residence at Milton Berry for six months when, because of the high fees and the fact that I made little progress in becoming more functionally independent, my parents felt that a more normal situation was, after all, the most beneficial situation for me. I returned home from Oshkosh sometime before Christmas, back to the two-room school at Rock City and all my buddies. In 1952, I turned fourteen years old. With each passing year, my mobility was becoming more of an issue for me. My interests had expanded beyond my crawling range, as had my girth, which necessitated a new mode of travel for me. I was a "Kloepping eater," which meant consuming food in large quantities. I had become quite heavy, and although my weight wasn't so excessive that it interfered with my functioning, it was limiting how far I wanted to crawl.

In the early 40's my Grandfather Rodenbough had bought me a wheelchair, but I rarely used it. It had large front wheels and small ones in back, with both sets comprised of hard rubber on steel rims; it folded up, back to seat, and the front wheels would pop off. It reminded me of a folded up lawn chair when not in operation. It was okay, but in those days every building and house had steps. Homes had basements, fifteen to twenty steps down, and the same number upstairs. Front doors, especially in cities, always had a front stoop with half a dozen (sometimes more) steps. Curbs in cities were eight or ten inches high to deflect snow and water. In the face of those substantial physical obstacles, the chair had limited value. On a one hundred-forty acre dairy farm in northern Illinois, it was even less practical. I was beginning to tire of bleeding hands and torn-up knees, and in the dead of summer when I never wore shoes or socks, I also had raw toes and feet.

My temper brought the issue to a head one day when I wanted to go fishing at our creek, which was about a half mile away as the crow flies. A friend was visiting for the day, but we couldn't get anyone to drive us there. I got so pissed I told Danny, "You carry the fishing poles, worms, and pail, and I'll crawl to the damn creek!" Well, I did, but it was the last time. My hands, knees, and feet were shredded. It took several weeks for the cuts and bruises to heal. I had to do something, and soon. I thought of building a cart with a gasoline motor, but the time it would take to do so was daunting. Some catalogs sold small electric cars, really toys, but they were prohibitively expensive. Then one day I saw the answer sitting in our machine shed. It was our garden tractor. This rugged little implement was driven by a five HP Briggs and Stratton gasoline engine, which delivered excellent power. It had two large front wheels with handlebars coming up and back from the engine, mounted at about a 30-degree angle. Different kinds of tilling accessories or a mower could be attached to the draw bar behind the engine. Then the operator walked behind guiding the machine with the handlebars. With the power unit at hand I needed some kind of wagon or cart that I could ride in. I had to figure out a way of attaching the wagon to the machine that would stabilize the handlebars. Without a tilling implement attached, it simply tipped forward resting on the front bumper.

Then Dad came to the rescue. He removed the front wheels and axles from one of our coaster wagons, and mounted a wood 2x4 tongue underneath the wagon that extended about two feet forward beyond the front of the wagon. He drilled a hole in the tongue for a bolt that would drop into a slot on the tractor. When hooked up, the front of the tractor elevated and the handle bars extended straight back at about a 60-degree angle. They were a little over my head and I had to reach up to steer the machine. It was probably the prototype for the Harley "Hogs," the motorcycles with the outlandish high bars. I'll bet some dude saw me motoring down our old county gravel road hanging high on those bars and thought that was a neat style of riding. Maybe I need to write Harley-Davidson and ask for royalties for developing the prototype.

The last major hurdle in using the system independently was being able to start the engine. It didn't have a push button starter, so you had to use a rope, wound around the exposed small crankshaft of the engine, and then give it a rapid pull. If the engine backfired, it would almost tear your arm off. But I was determined to learn to start it, and I did, in rather unconventional fashion. I found that sitting in front of the tractor leaning against the engine and then falling backward to the ground created enough leverage to start the engine. I learned a hard lesson one afternoon having forgotten to put the clutch in neutral. Using my usual procedure, I successfully cranked up the machine, and I was run over by the tractor and wagon. No permanent damage, but a bruised ego. We had an endless supply of twine string, which was strong, light weight, and wrapped easily around the crankshaft. I began to carry an extra starter rope after one broke when I had gone fishing alone at our creek. I was really "up the creek" to

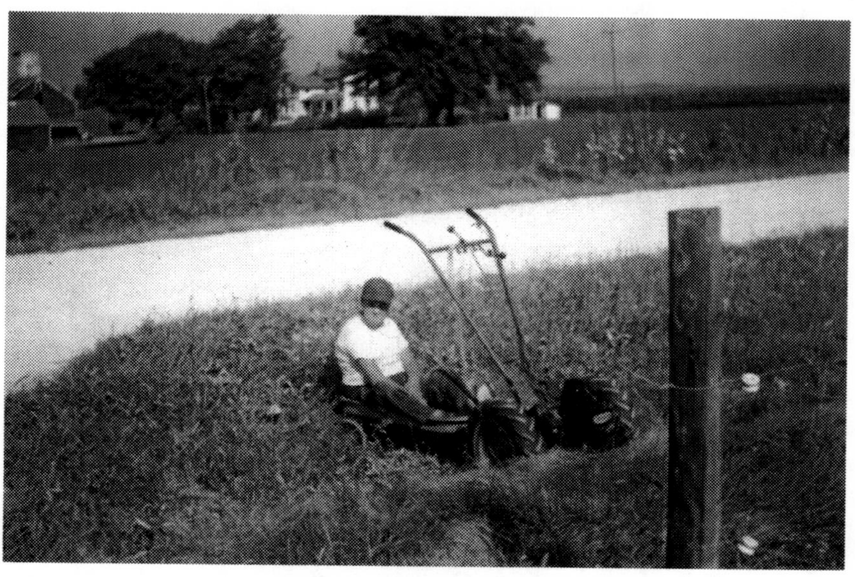

Stuck in a ditch. My tractor couldn't overcome every obstacle. (1952 or 1953)

paraphrase the old adage. I wasn't missing a paddle; I needed a rope. Fortunately, I had given up bib overalls as too juvenile, and now wore slacks with suspenders. Presto, the suspenders worked, I tore them in half, but the engine started.

My new transportation system greatly improved my range of mobility on the farm, and it also gave me a tremendous sense of freedom and independence. I could reach any part of our 140-acre farm. I used the system extensively over the next several years, broke a piston once, went through dozens of hard-rimmed coaster wagon wheels, and had a number of mishaps only one potentially serious. Driving at twilight along our rural dusty gravel road, a beginning driver didn't see me and nearly ran over me before I made it to the ditch. I got stuck on a number of occasions, and had to wait for someone to miss me and come looking. If my father were alive, he would probably tell about an incident that occurred one evening during milking when I rolled the tractor, wagon, and myself over a concrete bridge leading out of our dairy barn yard into a foot of cow yard soup. Once he realized I wasn't hurt, he burst out laughing, and continued to chuckle while he power-washed the tractor, wagon, and me. Aside from a few mishaps, my homemade hog provided countless hours of enjoyment and transportation for the next three or four years.

In addition to fanatically following major league baseball, I began to keep track of college teams; I followed amateur tennis and track, golf, and every sport of the local high schools in the area. And then I developed a passion for fishing. I fished in creeks, lakes, rivers, and ponds. My gear was a cane pole and angleworms. My family, friends, uncles, and neighbors took me fishing. I ought to write a book about my literally hundreds of fishing expeditions. Undoubtedly one of the most entertaining chapters would be those times with my Uncle Hub Andereck.

Hub was a good-natured, kind man, always optimistic about our chances for a big haul. He brought every new fangled lure on the market, fish scents, humming lures, buzz baits, poppers, divers, skippers, fake worms, bugs, frogs, and flys until he had an unbelievable arsenal of bait with which to trick those wily water creatures. Hub had a heart of gold, but on our fishing outings we had the luck of Al Capp's cartoon character, JOE BTFSPLK. Like Joe who walked around with a rain cloud overhead, when Uncle Hub and I went fishing it seemed that we were jinxed. We never had any big tragedies, but that rain cloud seemed to follow us.

Here are a few examples: 1) On an all day fishing trip to Lake Kegonsa where everyone was catching dozens of huge bullheads, I caught one large bullhead and Hub and my brother got none. Despite our poor luck I was thrilled, as the fish was going to be our dinner; Hub put the fish in a pail of cold water on the front stoop to clean it, left it unattended for about one minute and it disappeared. He did return in time to see a large gray cat bounding off into the field, fish in tow. 2) In a rush to get to the river one evening before a summer storm broke (a great time to catch fish), Hub couldn't find his 6-12, the mosquito repellent, so he grabbed a can of Raid and liberally doused his arms. The rain shortened our early evening trip, and by the time we arrived home, his arms were terribly swollen and itching. 3) On the first day of a week long trip to Lake Wisconsin, he insisted I use his brand new, never before used, forty dollar casting reel, which promptly flew out of my hand on my first cast, sinking to the bottom of the swift flowing waters of the river. We broke two more rods trying to retrieve the new reel, which we never found. 4) On that same trip on a particularly hot day, he took off his shirt while in the boat on the lake. He was fair skinned and almost never exposed his body to direct sunlight. He got terrible sunburn; he got the chills and had to go to bed in the middle of the fishing trip. Notwithstanding our lack of success and a few fiascos, I always looked forward to going with him as he was so optimistic about the next time and his attitude was infectious

Between trips with Uncle Hub, Dad's bachelor brother, Lamont, would sometimes stop and ask me if I wanted to go to a local creek or nearby river. He was a quiet, shy man and never called ahead, just showed up. Our conversations were very limited on those trips, and if he or I caught a nice fish he would only smile.

Also some days, Bob Breed a neighbor, would suddenly appear unannounced at our farm. "The bullheads are biting Kent, get your pole." We always got a bunch, and then Leah his wife fried them for supper. Those were fun days.

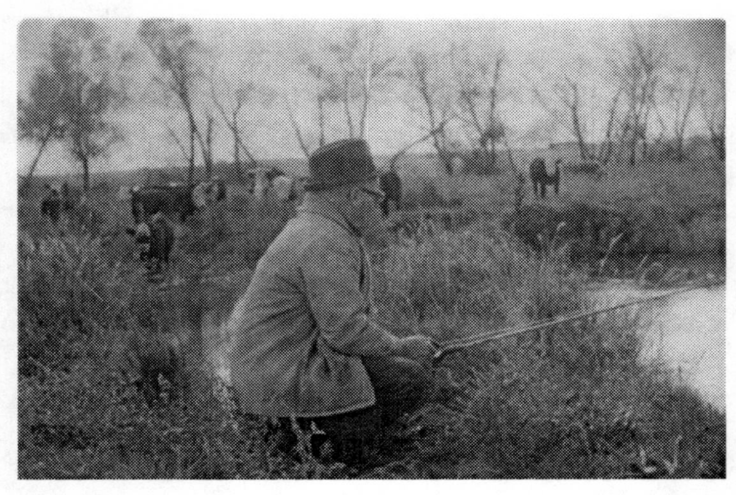

Uncle "Hub"—he'd go fishing anywhere, anytime (1950s)

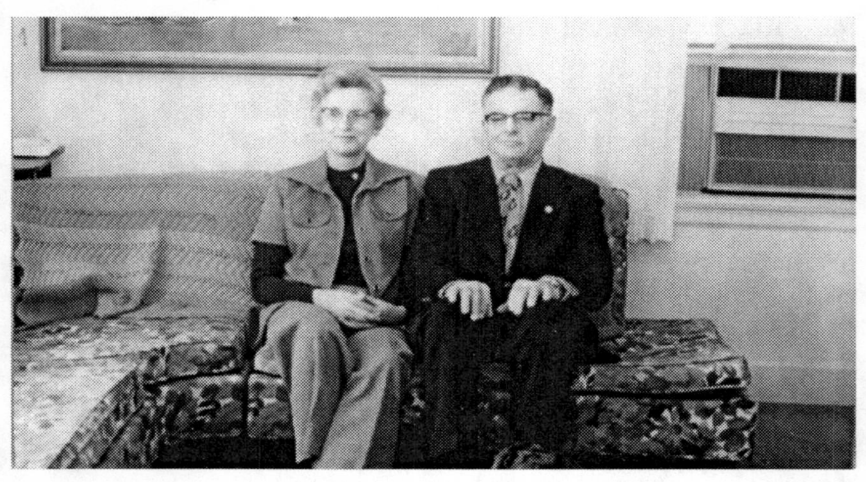

Aunt Esther Andereck and Uncle Herbert "Hub" Andereck,
Juda, Wisconsin (1970s)

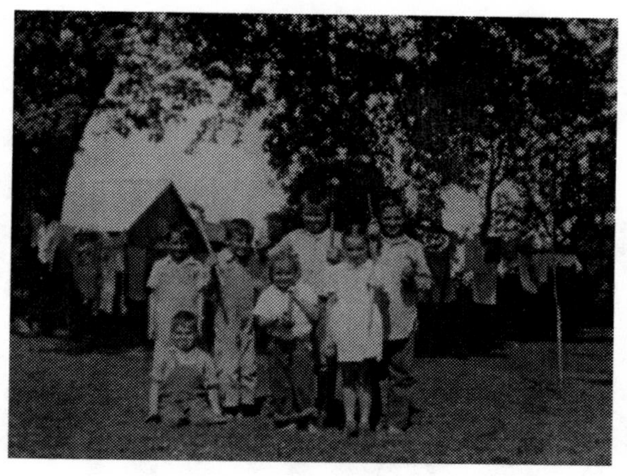

Neighborhood kids in our backyard; I'm on the ground (summer, 1947 or 1948)

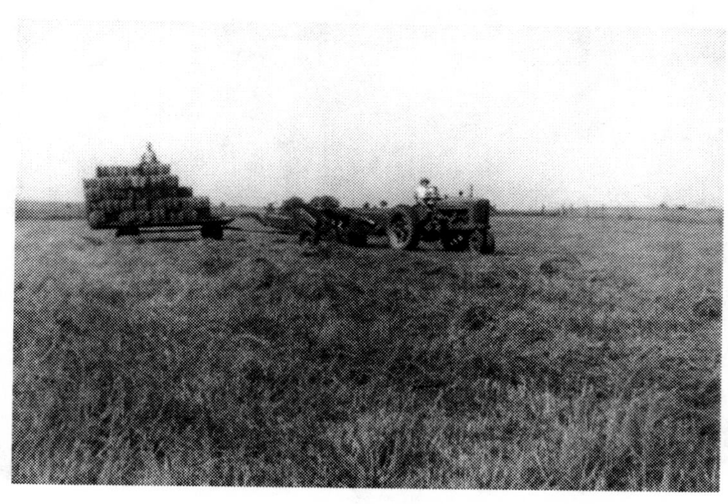

Riding on baled hay. I couldn't help much but I was usually there. (summer 1955 or 1956)

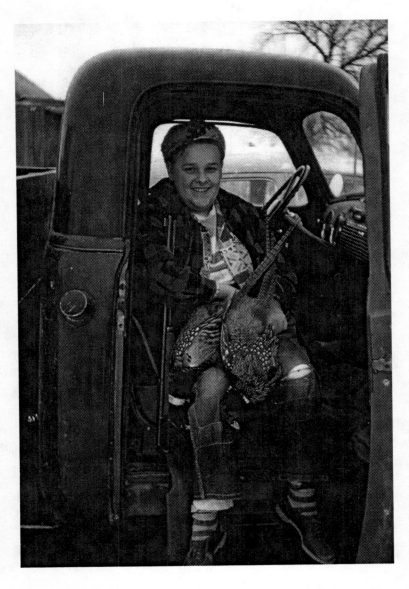

The first two pheasants that I got shooting from the truck (1951 or 1953)

The period 1947-1953, after my initial return home from my hospitalization up to the beginning of high school, was most likely the most important six years of my life from a developmental standpoint. The years of one's life between the ages of around ten to fourteen were for me as for many young persons, a time of transition and awakenings. Childhood through puberty to the threshold of young adulthood is a time of radical change. My disability added a significant variable in the process for me and without the tremendously supportive environment in which I lived, my ability to adapt successfully could have been much more difficult. The attitudes of my parents and also my siblings in accepting me as a normal part of the family unit was key to my integration socially, emotionally, and physically into the mainstream of our community life. The extended family members were also very supportive of me, as well as to our family members.

H.L. Mencken, contrarian and skeptic once remarked, "Don't over estimate the decency of the human race." Maybe taking the entire population as a whole there would be a degree of validity in his view, but in the community where I lived in rural Rock City, Illinois, in the late 1940s and on into the 1950s, that was not true. In an interview with her several years ago, my Aunt Esther remarked, "You know, Kent, you were very fortunate to be living in a rural community when you got sick. Your family was well known and established; and unlike a large urban center, you and your family became a focus of community concern. If you had to get polio, I think your timing was good; there was great attention and resources given over to caring for polio patients in 1945, and subsequently, upon your return home, a continuing continuity of care and concern was provided by your community."

In developing background material for this memoir, I interviewed my siblings, childhood and high school friends, people from our old neighborhood, relatives (chiefly my Aunt Esther), Fritz Kolb, our hired man in the 1940's, a fellow polio patient from the Deaconess Hospital, and my mother, numerous times. In the process of reminiscing, recalling, remembering, hearing new things and then writing, I came to more fully understand and appreciate how fortunate I was to have lived in that place with my family. I can never thank all of the people who helped and supported me. Even though

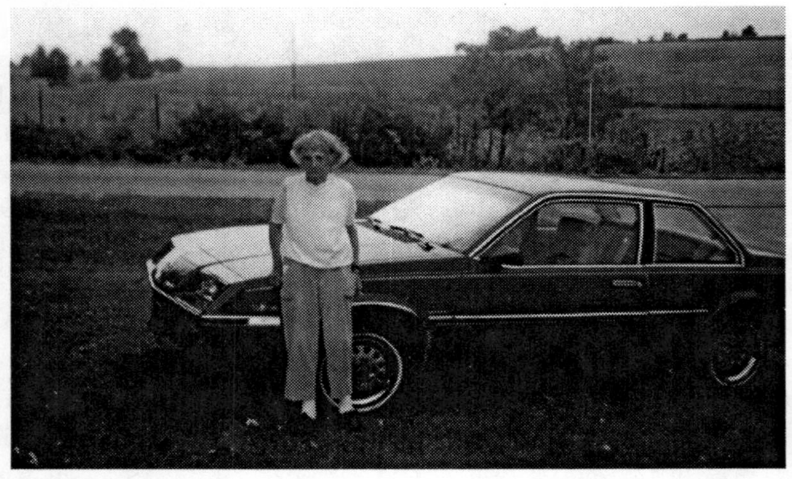

Our family friend and my early mentor, Wilma Kurtz (1991)

most are not named, one lady I feel compelled to again acknowledge was a family friend named Wilma Kurtz.

So as not to end this chapter sounding too maudlin or as my family would say, gushy, I thought about a remembrance that might bring some balance to this previous rhetoric. It also serves to demonstrate that during this time not everyone's motivations were always altruistic.

One day while my family and I were at a local county fair, it occurred to me that at these kind of events (carnivals, and community celebrations,) my younger sister, Jolene, always seemed to be at my side, especially when we were in the midways. That's where all the games of skill or chance were located. Throwing baseballs at milk bottles, pitching pennies into dishes, softballs into bushel baskets, shooting ducks, and throwing darts at balloons were just a few of the games. Many, if not most, of the games were rigged back in those days. However, Jolene, only eleven or twelve years old, had very astutely observed that more often than not I would win at these games.

Our family had gone to a local small town celebration that had all the usual carnival games. There was a game in the midway that required tipping up an empty Coke bottle resting at a 45-degree angle on a block of wood. Using a two-tined long-handled fork, one simply raised the bottle to the upright position. The problem was that when upright the bottle sat on a crack between two boards that were covered with a heavy green felt material. With a well-timed step on a concealed pedal, one of the boards would lift, imperceptibly, but enough to topple the bottle. Enter Kent. With much fanfare, the game operator got everyone's attention shouting with something like, "Come on folks, and let's see if this brave young handicapped fella can do it?" Sure enough, I won. Imagine that. My bright-eyed little rascal of a sister would then plead, "Oh, try it again, just one more time." Wow, two wins in a row and now two big stuffed toys, one for me, one for Jolene.

Yes, the mercenary little cuss had figured out that a crippled kid often wins. Like little Addie (Tatum O'Neal) in the movie *Paper Moon,* my baby sister had a scam of her own. I didn't question her motives then and I wouldn't today. Maybe it's sufficient to share a quote I heard from my son; "In all good people there is probably some bad, and in all bad people there is probably some good."

On balance, I think I must have known mostly good people.

ADDENDUM

A Day at Wrigley

In 1951 major league baseball was no longer the exclusive domain of white men. It was only four years since one of baseball's moguls, a man named Branch Rickey, recognized the huge financial rewards to be reaped by allowing some of the best athletes in the world, African Americans, to join big time baseball. I never believed it was completely a decision of conscience; I'd guess winning and money were equally important issues. It seems the dollar often sends one on towards the path of enlightenment. That year I attended my first major league baseball game, and neither my family nor I were prepared for what was to transpire that day.

As a thirteen-year-old kid, I, like millions of other Americans, religiously followed the fortunes of my favorite major league team. Daily I listened to the radio play-by-play of my heroes, carefully devouring any new statistical data that the announcer slipped in between calling the action. In those days, as fans, we were loyal to our teams and ferociously defended our heroes, those "boys of summer." Being loyal to your team if you lived in Illinois in the '50's was an act of courage, for my team was the Cubs, those lovable losers from the North side of Chicago. The '50's were lean years for the Cubbies and their fans. They would typically start the year quickly, play well, raise our hopes and expectations, but around the middle of June began to wilt like early spring flowers in the summer heat. We tried to remain hopeful, privately praying for miracles, publicly maintaining our bravado in the face of yet another season deteriorating with the dog days of summer.

My Aunt Esther got tickets for a late September game, the 16th, and my father, Uncle Hub, Aunt Esther, and I were off to Wrigley Field for a Sunday afternoon game. Wow, the Dodgers arguably were the most powerful team in all of baseball. Their lineup was sprinkled with future hall-of-famers, names like Pee Wee Reese, Duke Snyder, Gil Hodges, Roy Campanella, Don Newcome, and a spirited fellow, Jackie Robinson.

The Cubs, by contrast, were again a struggling last place team, lots of heart, and lots of losses. But they were my team, and today they could win. I was awe struck by the sights and sounds of the ballpark. The giant stadium with Ivy covered brick walls, dark green grass in the outfield, beer vendors, memorabilia salesmen, smartly dressed Andy Frain ushers, and the buzz of the people. The crowd was fascinatingly diverse, kids, oldsters (men and women) and young folks; but most notably, a large percentage of people in the stadium were not white. Many were African Americans, a different experience for me, having been born and raised in almost a 100 % rural white community. As I looked over the throngs of people, I was struck by the formal dress of many, particularly among the black folks. The majority of the men were in white shirts and ties, some with sport coats, and sharp Sunday hats. Most of the women wore beautiful colorful dresses, long stockings, and lots of jewelry, high heels, and out-of-this-world fall bonnets.

As game time neared, the excitement and noise levels increased in anticipation. Then suddenly it was quiet for the National Anthem. At the final note of the anthem, the thirty thousand plus fans erupted with a single mighty roar. As the din subsided, a strange hush fell over the entire stadium. Almost imperceptibly at first, a faint murmuring sound began. The air seemed charged with a building force of energy. I suddenly felt extremely uneasy.

I gasped for air, "Dad, what's happening, can you feel it?"

"Yes," he replied quietly as he looked down at me.

Trembling, I asked, "What is it?"

"It's Robinson I think, Jackie." I stared at my father in amazement.

"What do you mean, it's Jackie, what's he doing?" What was this silent, yet powerful crescendo surrounding everyone? The loud staccato voice from the P.A. system jolted me, "Attention, attention, now batting for the Brooklyn Dodgers, playing second base, Jackie Robinson." The crowd rose as one; another mighty roar came from thousands of throats. There was a strange dissonance of sounds, chords of adulation, shrieks of joy, his name spoken repeatedly, and almost prayerful supplications, to a master or a Messiah. Everyone was standing, swaying, and I sat unable to stand, shivering, fully engulfed in this unknown force and energy. But the moment passed, Robinson got a hit, and in an instant the stadium was suddenly transformed into a gleeful raucous baseball crowd. Familiar sounds that I understood, the simple joys of the ballpark, the "Cubbies" and "da bums," playing America's game.

The Cubs lost 6-1, and their season record fell to 58-85, good for last place. Clem Labine, a Dodger rookie beat Bob Kelly, a journeyman pitcher. Oh well, maybe next year. Riding home, exhausted, stuffed with hot dogs, candy, peanuts, and soda pop, snug in the back seat of Uncle Hub's Chevy, I dozed dreamily, thinking of the day. I thought about that strange, overwhelming moment, unable to comprehend its meaning. What was clear was the overpowering surge of energy that swirled around us for a brief time, seeming to gently cradle the man, Jackie.

That day, now over fifty years ago, remains indelibly etched in my memory. I'm not sure that I'll ever fully understand or appreciate what happened at Wrigley Field. What I do know is that Jackie Robinson was much more than just the Dodgers second baseman. It was true then for millions of Americans, and it is true today. (7)

V. High School

OK guys—ready? Go!" And on that signal, we did go, up two flights of stairs, one landing in between, me in my wheelchair carried by four burly Midwestern farm boys, racing to beat the time for the fastest trip up to the second floor where all my high school classes met. Dangerous, I suppose, but I recall only a handful of times that one guy tripped sending all five of us and the wheelchair into a tangled heap perched precariously on the stairs. It was much worse having them run down the stairs. That really got my adrenaline flowing. One misstep and, oh, I don't want to think about it.

I graduated from Rock City Grade School in 1953 and was ready for high school. I lived in the Dakota Community High School district #201 in northern Illinois, but it seemed unlikely to me that I would be able to attend that school. The high school was located on the second floor of an old brick building that housed the elementary grades on the first floor. The building had an attached gymnasium on the west end of the building, with the high school study hall over the gym. I could not negotiate steps; I walked, sort of, with underarm crutches and leg braces, but I was quite unsteady on anything but level terrain.

I envisioned all kinds of scenarios that might be implemented to accommodate me—being shipped off to a school for disabled kids; homebound instruction; or being sent to another district with a newer, more accessible school building. While I worried, fussed and stewed, my parents, unknown to me, had met with the high school principal, Mr. Donald Johnson ("DV," we called him), who encouraged them to send me to the local high school. I began school at Dakota High School that fall, 1953, feeling much trepidation. Little could I have imagined that a great bunch of kids and fellow classmates were to make the next four years one of the happiest periods of my life.

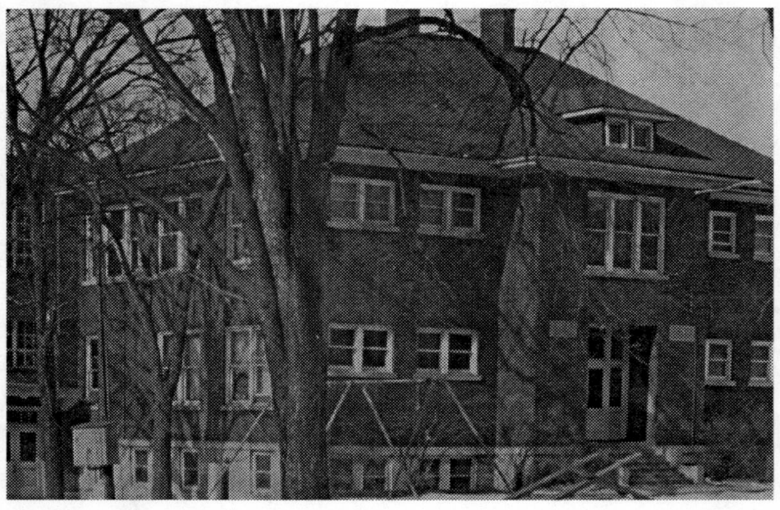

The old Dakota High School building where my fellow students daily carried me up and down two flights of stairs for four years

There was a great sense of optimism in America during my high school years, and the feeling continued for several years after I graduated. It was a time of prosperity for millions of Americans, including our rural community in northern Illinois. There was mostly peace in the world, and most of us had high hopes for the future. On the international scene, the Korean Conflict had been concluded with a cease-fire at the 38th parallel and peace talks were under way. Harry "Give 'Em Hell" Truman had fired Douglas MacArthur for insubordination and acting on his desire to chase the Chinese back across North Korea's border, the Yalu River, and all the way to Manchuria. Getting sacked probably didn't do MacArthur's candidacy for the presidency any good, so instead, we got everyone's World War II hero, Dwight (I Like Ike) Eisenhower, architect of the June 6, 1944, D-day invasion of Europe. Despite the Cold War and communism, we somehow managed to remain insulated from these threats in our daily lives, which were filled with abundance and good times. Besides, who could worry about those Commies with Herb Philbrick, the wily double agent of *I Lead Three Lives*, on the job? Old Phil always outwitted any who would seek to destroy our way of life.

Baseball was truly America's favorite pastime. As noted earlier, Mickey Mantle, my all-time favorite baseball hero, burst onto the scene in 1951. In 1950, he had played in the Class C league in Joplin, Missouri, where he won the league batting title. Casey Stengel, the crusty old Yankee manager, recognized Mantle's great potential and had him called up. Mantle was the first Yankee player ever to jump from class C to the major leagues. He would eventually replace New York Yankees' center fielder Joe DiMaggio, and go on to a have a storied career. He played on two damaged legs, one the result of a high school football injury, and the other the result of tearing tendons after falling into an outfield drain cover in the 1951 World Series. I just knew he would break Ruth's home run record. Maybe he would've if he'd had two good legs and fewer after-game outings carousing with his buddies Billy Martin and Whitey Ford.

Then the Cubs signed two black players, Gene Baker and a guy who was destined to become an all-time Cub favorite, Ernie Banks, "Mr. Cub." The Cubs paid the Kansas City Monarchs, of the old Negro Baseball League, ten thousand dollars for Ernie's contract—one of the greatest bargains ever. But, of course, the Cubs undid all that by trading away a young super star to be, Lou Brock, for a sore-armed, fat-guy pitcher, Ernie Broglio, and a bunch of other losers.

Television had arrived with about one major league baseball game broadcast each week, usually on Saturday. Dizzy Dean was one of the announcers. His speech and pronunciation were deplorable, but he possessed a unique style. We got our television set in 1951 and Dad got the antenna up and the set working after the evening milking.

The first show we watched in our home was a Charlie Chan mystery, a full-length movie. I recall Chan's chauffeur, a black man who, when frustrated, turned white. We thought it quite humorous at the time, but what an awful image.

Rock-n-Roll was a new sound, and one that started a number of arguments as to who was the first, and who was most influential. Elvis, even then, was the King, but his status as the originator was debatable. Bill Haley and the Comets received a number of votes, as did Jerry Lee Lewis—the man who most likely started the whole craze. Unfortunately for him, marrying his thirteen-year old cousin took a bit of the shine off his star. Back in those days, marrying a close family member typically earned you the reputation of being a scandalous hillbilly—even if you did grow up south of the Mason-Dixon line. In 1953, almost everything in America, at least in my worldview, was just dandy.

For the first two years of high school, I rode the bus. Each morning, it lumbered into our driveway and Don Lapp, the bus driver, along with one or two of the strongest boys, assisted in lifting me in the wheelchair three feet up and through the back emergency door and into the space behind and between the two rows of seats. Now, I was no lightweight, and including my wheelchair, the load must have been a lift of close to two hundred-fifty pounds of dead weight. One young guy, Ray Leathers (or Beeb, as we called him, because he'd lost an eye in a BB gun accident) couldn't have weighed more than one hundred-fifty pounds, but he had amazing strength. In spite of a huge appetite, Beeb didn't have an ounce of fat on his skinny frame. I remember, that because of the blindness in one eye, he had very poor depth perception and had difficulty hitting a pitched ball. However, he did find his athletic calling in football. Guys who played against him were aghast as to how hard he could hit. He was fearless, completely unconcerned for his own physical safety, and could absolutely flatten opponents on the football field. Beeb was one tough guy, and I'm glad he lived in my neighborhood.

Thinking back to riding that bus each day, I can't believe that would be permitted in today's world. I can imagine the hysterical cries, "He's blocking the emergency route!" or, "That skinny, visually challenged kid and the bus driver need to file a work-related injury claim." or, "My son's back is ruined! Get a lawyer—we're gonna sue."

Once we arrived at school, four strong guys carried me up the two flights of stairs to the second floor. I usually remained there for the entire school day. Only for such events as a fire drill, an all school assembly, or early dismissal did the boys take me down to ground level before 3:30 in the afternoon. I used a manual wheelchair, a brand new Everest and Jennings, which was the standard model in the 50's. With hard rubber tires and a heavy frame, it was a rugged and functional piece of equipment. Even with the terrific abuse that my buddies and I inflicted on that chair, it still lasted nearly five years. I had given up using crutches in high school. With close to two hundred teenagers jammed into a relatively small area, I would have been knocked flat the first time I entered the hourly stampede between classes.

Dakota High School was not a large school; it was kind of out-in-the-boondocks and probably was not the first choice for many aspiring educators. While we had some excellent teachers during my four years, there were also a good number of types who probably didn't finish at the top of their college class. In every profession there is someone at the very top of the class, some in the top 10%, top half, bottom half, and someone is last; the 0-1% rank. I think some of them ended up at Dakota. It didn't take the student body long to size up a new instructor. Teaching is not an easy profession, they are underpaid, under appreciated, and often the biggest problem with the teachers was the students. While we had some instructors who were really very bright, that didn't necessarily translate into effective teaching.

One of the smartest guys who taught at Dakota in the sciences had a difficult time relating to the students; we called him Gravy Legs, a play on his name. Another rather eccentric lady liked to demonstrate flamenco dancing in her English class. The performance was usually quite lively until DV, the principal, happened to stop by the class one day.

John Messing, a math teacher and coach, was one of the best teachers I ever encountered at any level. He made math easy and fun. Not only did he excel in the classroom, but each year he also took a ragtag group of fresh-soph boys and molded them into a winning basketball squad. Under his guidance, I recall his teams won four consecutive Fresh-Soph tournaments, with such notable characters as Slip Slamp, Charlie Eichmeier, Dick Mullican, Big John Trimble, Norm Untersee, Gary Beck, Joel Wells, and others. His teams weren't big, not too fast, they couldn't jump (all white guys), but they won.

Eleanor Neuberger was a flamboyant lady who taught English, including the senior level class. I can't say that she didn't like men, but Ron Schradermeier, myself, and Marv Braasch, were the only three guys in her class. We sat far in the back row as Eleanor conducted her class surrounded by bright, pretty young girls upon whom she showered her praise and affection. I never got a grade higher than a B. For one assignment, Ron wrote what I thought was a classic theme on the subject Autumn leaves; however, instead of it being nauseatingly romantic, as Eleanor liked it, his rendering was a great satirical piece, cynical and clever, that had Marv and me in tears. Eleanor was not amused, and she gave him a D- for arguably the most creative theme of the year.

Bill Yates, another science teacher, had been an immigration agent along the U.S.-Mexico border, and we quickly discovered the consequences of goofing off in his class. I did, once, but never again. Mr. Yates, (emphasis on the Mr.), as we called him, was a big man, maybe 6-3, and a solid two hundred-forty pounds. He was also an assertive fellow and was not at all bashful about letting students know when they were out-of-line. One afternoon I was in study hall, in my wheelchair, some twenty to thirty feet from the science room door. Someone had a pack of BB's and a number of us began rolling them down the study hall aisles. The wooden floor was not level, so as the BB rolled along it would jump, making an audible sound. The study hall monitor would rush to the sound and sometimes discover the BB. However, the culprit remained unknown, as by the time the teacher heard the thing rolling, it had traveled a good distance from its starting point. I noted that the science room door on my right had quite an opening at the bottom of the door, maybe ¼ inch with no sill and after a few misses I became quite proficient at rolling them under the door. I had made three or four in a row when abruptly the door opened and out charged Bill Yates! He never hesitated, coming directly to me, his face in a fearsome scowl, holding several BB's in an open palm.

"Well, what do you have to say for yourself?" he demanded.

"Well, I stammered, what do you mean?"

"Now look, Kloepping, I know exactly where those BB's came from; the angle of their trajectory leads straight back to you, remember I teach physics so I know something about angles and straight lines." He made sure he spoke loudly enough for everyone in the now hushed study hall to hear every word. I was shocked and embarrassed and didn't know what to say.

"Well, do you have anything to say?" he asked again.

I managed a rather weak, "No."

"Well, I'm not amused with your foolishness, so let's have no more of these silly antics; is that crystal clear?"

My "yes" was even weaker than my "no."

"What's that, what did you say?" he continued.

"Yes, sir," I managed.

"All right, that's the end of it then."

He wheeled around, stalked back to his classroom, and punctuated his "public dressing down" of me by closing the door with authority. The study hall was absolutely silent; he had not only scared the crap out of me, I'd bet the majority of the students in that study hall made a mental note not to mess with Mr. Yates.

DV Johnson, the principal, was likewise a fellow one had to handle carefully. The majority of time he was an amiable, pleasant guy. He had a rambling sort of style in speaking with lots of "ahems," giving a combination cough, chuckle, ("a cough-ahem"), a good number of "heh, hehs," and "Well, what I'm saying is...." We sort of thought he was kind of a nerd, but in reality he was a good man and really quite a bright individual. But if you got him angry, an amazing transformation occurred. If he did lose his temper, this slow-talking, shuffling guy in a baggy suit, who sometimes seemed in a daze muttering to himself in the hallways, underwent a complete metamorphosis. Suddenly before you was a man who's shoulders squared, a massive bull neck emerged, the wrinkles left his suit, and his speech became fluent and articulate. His movements were swift and graceful, with no hesitation. When he had finished his machine-gun-like outburst, the place was hushed, and each and every directive was carried out in detail. Then he would leave. When he returned to the scene, he seemed to have a twinkle in his eye and his speech patterns had again reverted back to lots of "ahems," and "uhs" with a few "let me see nows" thrown in.

It was Fred Verdun who especially encouraged me to go on to post-secondary education. He had polio (contracted while in the Air Force), and was particularly concerned about my career goals. He liked to argue, so did I, and he suggested law as a career goal.

A final teacher who comes to mind is coach Frank Pfeiffer. I

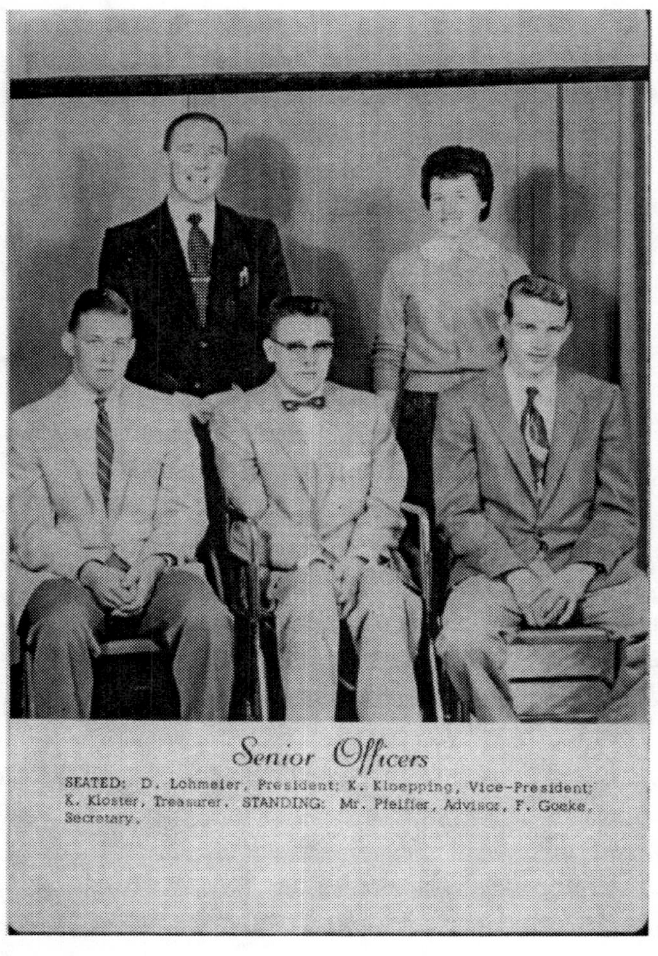
Senior Officers
SEATED: D. Lohmeier, President; K. Kloepping, Vice-President; K. Kloster, Treasurer. STANDING: Mr. Pfeiffer, Advisor, F. Goeke, Secretary.

Senior class officers and coach Frank Pfeiffer (1957)

attended every high school athletic event that I could, which only the boys played back then. As softball and baseball games were usually afternoon affairs I had to get special permission from DV, the principal, to leave school early. Then my senior year, Coach Pfeiffer named me the scorekeeper for those sports, so I had to attend. It was a thoughtful, kind gesture on his part. He took a job at another high school after I graduated. Tragically, several years later, he was shot and killed by another hunter while deer hunting.

I didn't drive, so my transportation to games for the first couple of years was my older sister, Carol. Dad had a new 1951 Mercury, gray, not very fast off the blocks, but it was a heavy car and with Carol at the wheel, we usually had it up close to a hundred MPH racing to the game.

I remember telling Carol, "faster, faster."

"Oh, I can't," she'd reply, but she did. One of her classmates, Karlene, always tried to outrun us in her lighter, sleeker looking little Chevy. But we always caught her and roared by like a runaway freight train. We were careful not to let our parents know about these rural road races, as each year there were horrific accidents at unmarked rural crossroads. We were foolish, but driving fast and racing was what everyone did in rural America in the 50's. Gasoline was a bargain, frequently less than twenty cents a gallon, and cars were built for power and speed. Who can forget those 57 Chevy's, 58 Pontiacs, the last of the Studebakers—the Golden Hawks, a whole range of powerful machines? It seemed like almost every male member of my senior class had a car, and many of them were new.

My last two years of high school, my great friends Gene Shippy, Ron Schradermeier, and Dick Fiene hauled me to school in the mornings, and made sure I got to almost every athletic event of the school. Gene, a lifelong friend, was particularly loyal and was always on time. If he said, "I'll be there at 6:30 for a 7:15 game," he was there with time to spare. My family was always late going anywhere. We kept our clocks set about fifteen minutes fast in an attempt to be on time, but it never worked. But Gene was always prompt, and since he didn't play basketball, he was always available to take me along. Most gymnasiums back in the 50's were not wheelchair accessible, so there were steps to negotiate wherever we went. No matter—we'd get to the town, find the school, they would drag the chair and me upstairs or down or both, and I'd crawl up to the last row of bleachers.

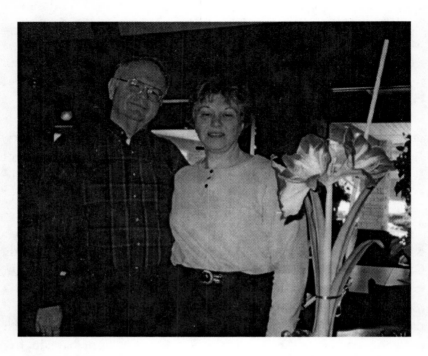

Lifelong friend Gene Shippy with a new "best buddy," his wife, Beth (1999)

Occasionally, I would stay for basketball practice and get a ride from another friend, Dick Rockey, and sometimes stay overnight at his house. Dick became an outstanding athlete during his school days, and while we remained good friends, we each ran with a different crowd for those four years. Basketball games were probably the main source of entertainment from November through February. Our small high school, while playing good competitive basketball, never advanced to the state's final tournament.

During my sophomore year in school, the varsity basketball team did win the conference title and tournament. Almost the entire team had nicknames. The team featured "Goose" Hoover, "Moose" Moore, "Satch" Kincannom, "Rock" Rockey, "Tiger" Miller, and "High

Pockets" Kneubuehl. I don't recall if Jim Yoeman, John Anderson, or Bob Atz had nicknames. The final team member, "Little Ernie Miller," was only 5-1 when he entered High School, but then he began to grow, and continued to stretch upward for the next four years. He didn't stop there, I'm told. I haven't seen him since high school, but my father described him as a "big bugger." For all I know, he's still growing.

Most of the high school athletic events were in the evening and attending the games was only the opening round for the late night activities. A favorite after-game activity was playing cards; bately was a simple three-card game with a trump suit. The game usually had seven or eight players with an ante that was divisible by three, as each player received three cards and declared to be in or out. If you were in, you had to get at least one trick, or you had to equal the pot. Often four or five guys stayed in the hand and sometimes two, three, or even four didn't get a trick. With a fifteen-cent ante, the beginning pot would be only $1.20, (if eight guys were playing); however, if, say, four guys didn't get a trick, the pot leaped to $4.80. Then the next round if two guys didn't get a trick, the pot was suddenly $9.60. The larger the pot, the more greed began to distort reason and the greater amount of bluffing and bravado entered the game. Sometimes the pots reached twenty or thirty dollars or even more. It's a very simple but dangerous game.

One of our favorite hangouts to play cards was at "Gabby" Quick's trailer. Jimmy, his real name, was a quiet kid, who had a little trailer behind a service station and even though some nights he was in bed, we'd wake him up and start a game. He'd cuss, but always let us in and frequently we stayed and played cards all night. He was one year ahead of me in school, from a family that struggled financially. To his credit, he had left home and was supporting himself while still in high school. Gabby was a fry-cook at Joe Fulton's Chuck Wagon Cafe on Route #75 just outside of Rock City, and he usually worked the night shift.

After a basketball game (maybe over at 9:30-10:00), we'd all race back to the Chuck wagon for a $.25 burger, $.25 fries, and $.25 malt. The burgers were huge, with lots of onion and mustard. Gene and I never missed getting back to the Chuck Wagon. Ron Schradermeier and Dick Fiene would come along if they didn't have a date. Also some of the jocks like Dick Rocky, Ernie, and Tiger Miller usually showed up. When the Chuck Wagon closed at 11:00 P.M., we'd drop down about a mile to Gabby's trailer.

Sometimes if a game was forty to fifty miles away, Gabby may have already closed shop for the evening. No matter, usually Dick, or Ernie, both classmates of Gabby, would volunteer to roust him out of bed, drag him back to the Chuck Wagon, open up, and cook burgers for everyone. Gab would really get pissed, read us out, and then would go absolutely silent. When he arrived back at the restaurant, his face was set in a grimace. He wouldn't utter a word the entire time we were there. It's amazing he didn't commit some type of mayhem on someone, at least once anyway.

We most times had beer for the bately games and everyone relieved himself out-of-doors, as Gabby would tolerate us for an hour or so, and then lock himself in his bedroom, where the bathroom was located. I don't readily recall a card game breaking up with him present. We cleaned up the mess, shut off the lights, and left. If we had any beer left, we'd often leave the remaining beer for Jim as a token of thanks for intruding on him. We had bately parties at other places, but the most memorable evenings were spent, jammed into Gabby Quick's fifteen-foot trailer; everyone in the place smoking, drinking beer, telling jokes, passing gas, talking about girls (who will and who won't), and fast cars. Ah, those were the days.

Frequently, my friends and I would engage in post-game activities in the "other room" of my rural farmhouse. The local German community called the room in your home that wasn't the kitchen or the parlor the other room. At about twelve years of age, I began to experiment and invent ways that I could participate in activities with my peers. Perusing the Sears catalog one day, I found a small sized basketball hoop, maybe half the size of a regulation hoop, complete with nets, and basketballs. Mom and Dad were unbelievably patient in accommodating my pursuit of playing basketball. Dad mounted a large plywood sheet on the west wall of the other room. He then attached the basketball hoop about forty-eight inches from the floor. This height was not simply a guesstimate of a proper height; it was based on careful calculations. I was about twenty-eight inches tall from my rear to the top of my head. A regulation basketball hoop is ten feet from the floor. I assumed an average player to be six feet tall (mighty short by today's standards). By figuring out the ratio of the hoop height to the player height, I then applied the same formula using my height to figure out how high off the ground to hang my basketball hoop. I played the game sitting on the floor—not from my wheelchair—because I was more mobile and could simulate more basketball moves (I actually learned to back in with a dribble by scooting on my butt backwards on the highly polished waxed floor).

Once I had my basketball court, I spent hours practicing. I was deadly accurate from anywhere on the court. I could hit from the left side (by the kitchen door), or the right side (up against the bathroom door), or anywhere from out front. The room was about 12x15 feet with the east wall (which I considered mid-court), twelve feet from the hoop. This distance was almost out of my range. Free throws? Well move over Mr. Rick Barry; I could make ten, twenty, even thirty in a row without a miss. I don't recall my all-time record, but it was around seventy I think.

After a high school basketball game, Gene and Ron would stop off at my home and stay to shoot some hoops. They stayed standing, but I moved from my wheelchair to the floor. It was usually after 10:00 or 11:00 P.M. when we'd arrive home, and for the next two hours or more we would bounce basketballs in the other room directly beneath my parents' bedroom. I don't think there's any way they could have slept through the racket with the ceaseless bump, bump, bump of the ball. They never once asked us to stop.

Gene was a devout Irish Catholic kid. There weren't many Catholics in our community and "fish eaters" was a local common slur; there were always priest-nun stories circulating among the majority Protestant community. I recall when John Kennedy ran for president, a standard anti-Kennedy line was," Well do you want the Vatican running America?" Gene was what I'd call a Catholic of conscience; He fully embraced his faith and never in my years of association with him did I observe him eating meat on Friday. That prohibition (no meat on Friday) seemed to rankle Protestants, and for many, established clearly that there was something not quite right maybe even sinister with persons of that faith. It's probably a good thing *The DaVinci Code* wasn't published back then.

As many basketball games were on a Friday night and Gene could not eat meat (and he was a hefty guy, always hungry), along with our shoot-around in the family room, we ate toasted cheese sandwiches. Usually two apiece, with one-quarter to one-half inch slabs of Colby longhorn cheese, cut from the fourteen pound round of cheese in our refrigerator. Gene didn't drink alcohol at the time (he did later) so he washed down the gooey, cholesterol-laden sandwiches with whole milk, several large glasses. He's still alive today. Maybe his wife made him change his diet. Ron and I probably ate the same amount.

A final note on family room basketball involved my friend Dick Rocky. He had become a star basketball player at Dakota High, and many times he'd stop in for a quick game of family room basketball—sometimes even on the morning of a game. He would sit on the floor so we could go one-on-one. He was a very competitive guy, and I think watching me hit shot after shot, he felt compelled to challenge me on my terms. We'd spend several hours playing H-O-R-S-E. One night at the high school game, Dick had a terrible shooting night and couldn't hit anything. Coach Pfeiffer took him aside and talked with him about his shooting, which was usually very fluid, especially a high arching jump shot. That night he looked awkward throwing up line drives. Somewhere in the conversation, family room basketball came up, at which point the coach told him "no more pre-game shooting with Kloepping."

When school let out for the summer, the illicit consumption of alcohol by my friends and I increased dramatically. We rarely went out with the intent to just drink. Rather, drinking was an adjunct to whatever we happened to be doing that evening. Always wanting to be included, I never turned down an invitation to attend a ball game, drive-in movie, local carnival show, town celebration, holiday celebration, Wednesday night movie in Davis, Illinois, or any other excuse to get out for the evening. In addition to beer, a variety of homemade wines, some hard liquor and the famous Kloepping applejack, were also available. My brother Larry made a fifty-gallon barrel of the stuff and while it tasted like plain delicious apple cider, it packed a legendary wallop. It seemed that almost everyone drank, whether they liked it or not. Typically, after only a couple of beers, the guys started to act goofy.

In retrospect, I'd wager that much, if not most, of our worst behavior was not as much a result of alcohol intake as it was trying to live up to the expectations of the group. Most evenings, guys who weren't dating came to the local hangouts. I was usually the only guy in a wheelchair, and typically six or seven of us would end up piling into one car to cruise the local towns. Trunks didn't always accommodate the chair (especially if there was a choice between hauling my chair or beer). Better than half the time, my wheelchair was left in the cafe where we all had converged. The rest of the time it would be locked in Gene's trunk. Not having the chair along would, at times, lead to some interesting consequences for me.

There was a German community called Epplyanna, whose boundaries were roughly defined by people in the area who attended the church of that name. Many of the families were related, the descendants of German immigrants who came to America in the 1800's. They were hardworking, thrifty, church going people who liked to have a good time. The Epplyanna Dutch was one large clan. The unwritten but well-understood code for those of us on the outside was that if you had trouble with any one member of the clan, it meant you were in trouble with the entire group. In light of this, I made a point to develop many friendships within their community. They were genuine relationships, and many remain today. Now, the Epplyanna folks could party. Many grew up on good, homemade wine, with a beer thrown in for special occasions. The Lohmeiers were a highly visible and respected family in the community, and three of their kids were in my class. One wonderfully warm June evening, I was riding around the rural countryside drinking beer with a carload of the Epplyanna boys when someone yelled that he needed a pit stop. A fragrant alfalfa hayfield was selected as the place for the stop and everyone piled out, including me. I crawled a short distance from the car for a little privacy, and the next sound I heard was laughter, doors slamming, and the car taking off with me on the damp ground and my fly open. They eventually came back, but not before a half hour or more. I cussed them heartily, had a brew or two, and all was forgiven.

One night I accepted a ride with two of the wild and crazy guys in our class, Rog and Til, who took me for a joy ride in Til's old coupe. He would accelerate that jalopy to forty or fifty MPH (on a gravel road) pull the emergency brake, and simultaneously crank the steering wheel as far as it would go. The result was a horrific slide and a 180-degree turn, which scared the tar out of me. The ride continued into Schneeberger's Timber. As Til was backing up to turn around, we hit a tree stump with a terrific jolt. He shifted into drive, but the car wouldn't go forward. The impact was so forceful that the rear end of the car had hung up on the stump. They decided to put me behind the wheel and press the gas while they attempted to lift the car off the stump. They couldn't do it. They huddled briefly, snickered, started walking away and said, "See you later, Kloep." Of course my wheelchair was back in town, so I was stranded. Fortunately, they left me some beer as they began the three-mile trek back to Davis for help. I sat there a good hour or more after the last sounds of their hysterical laughter died out. They brought several cars and ten or more guys to get the car off the stump. As I think back on these incidents, it occurs to me just how much they included me as one of the gang. Sooner or later everyone was a target of the group's mischief, and my disability never kept me from being in the crosshairs.

I lived in Stephenson County, Illinois, that bordered the Wisconsin State line and at eighteen years of age you could buy beer in Wisconsin. Many seniors in high school turned that age during their final year in school, and thus the traffic across the line to buy beer got pretty heavy on Friday and Saturday nights.

The first time I crossed the border to buy beer was unbelievably on a bitterly cold January night of my senior year in high school. I had returned home that December after a mind-altering stay in Illinois Research Hospital in Chicago. That partially voluntary banishment to inner city Chicago had resulted in an unforgettable four-month adventure. The next Chapter, VI, recounts some of my observations and experiences in that unique hospital ward inhabited by an equally uncommon collection of souls with whom I lived.

My return home was, I believe, the rationale for my friends Ron, Dick, and I deciding that ice-cold beer sure sounded good. It had to be fifteen degrees below zero, the roads were icy, but no matter, it was off to Brodhead, Wisconsin, some fifteen miles north to buy beer. The tavern we selected had steps both front and back so Ron and Dick had to pull me up into the bar. We went in the rear entrance as we thought we would be less conspicuous. Sure that made sense, three young squirts, two of the three underage, probably none of us shaving, two of them hauling a fat kid in a wheelchair through the back door; we were about as subtle as a drunk at a WTCU (Women's Christian Temperance Union) meeting.

Ten feet inside the back door, a loud voice yelled, "Well, my gosh Kent, how are you doing?" I was so nervous I about jumped out of the wheelchair; it was Glen Earlywine, my mother's first cousin; he was in the bar having a beer and playing euchre, a favorite card game of the locals.

We chatted briefly; he grinned slyly and asked, "Are you here to get yourself a beer?"

"Oh no," I replied nervously, "just getting a case for Dad."

"Oh, I see, beer for your dad." And amid the smirks and winks, we forged ahead. The bartender was also skeptical about our intent. "Got any 'ID' young man?"

"Yes, I do," I stammered.

"How about those two?" the bartender quizzed.

"Oh no they are just helping me in as you have steps, they're not here to get anything."

"OK", he said, I'll sell you the beer but I hope it's not for you and your buddies." With a case of Hamms in tow, we headed for the back door.

"Well, take it easy, Kent, good to see you again," boomed out Glen,

"Yup, yup, see you later" I barely croaked out. What a fiasco, everyone in the whole damn tavern knew what we were doing, and word would get back to my folks.

Ron was driving his 1947 Mercury that had a lousy heater, and barely kept the temperature above fifty degrees, but we had our beer and were off drinking the elixir from the land of sky blue waters. I don't remember how much we drank, maybe all of it, eight beers apiece. Whatever we drank, it was enough to get Dick sick and barf in the back seat of Ron's car. He did have enough sobriety left to heave on the floor, not on the seat. Well, that ended the party. The inside of that old Mercury smelled something terrible after Dick emptied his innards. We rolled down the windows to let fumes escape, but had to crank them back up as a minus thirty degree wind chill in your face for a minute or two and your eyeballs began to frost over. "Jesus Christ, let's go home!" Ron yelled. We crept back to the farm, Dick, prone on the back seat, Ron singing a ribald classic of which he knew many, and me with my bladder about to burst.

We didn't stop to relieve ourselves, as exposing oneself in this kind of weather was hazardous business. The sidewalks at home were covered with ice, snow, and gravel (tracked up from the driveway). Pushing me to the house, Ron slipped and fell, and dumped me out of the wheelchair (no permanent damage). He got up, righted himself, and got me into the house. We had just gotten through the front door, when Ron's wet shoes went out from under him on our worn linoleum floor; he uttered a string of epithets and slowly got up again.

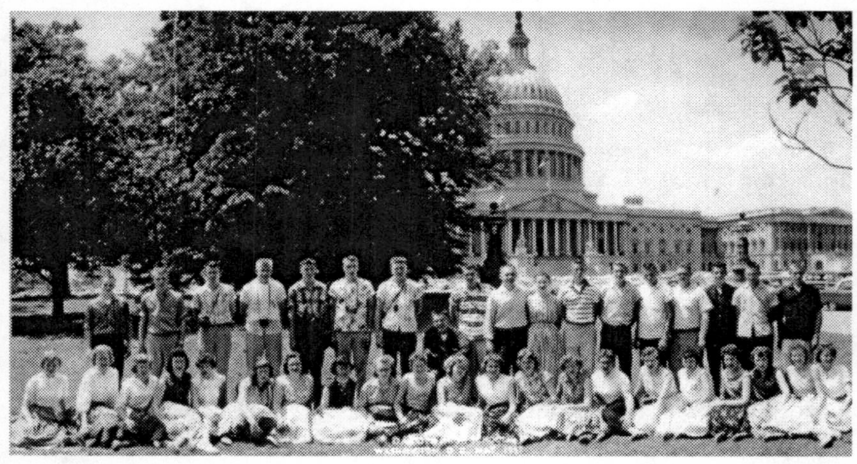

Senior trip to Washington, D.C. (spring, 1957)

He and Dick did get home safely, although Ron had a tough time waking Dick, who had lapsed into a deep sleep (passed out that is) making sure he got into the house. Ron told me several days later, he thought he was going to have to also carry him to the house.

The next morning, at breakfast, Mom inquired about "All the racket last night when you came home."

"Oh, Ron just slipped on the sidewalk, no damage."

"Oh, well, where did all that gravel come from that was on the floor?"

"Hmmm," I mused, "must have come in on my wheels."

"Oh I see," she replied with a faint smile. We had no further discussion on the matter, and I was glad we didn't.

In the spring of 1957, our class took a senior trip to Washington, D.C. and New York. It was to be our final fling together before graduation. The trip included a bus ride to Chicago, a train ride to New York, then another train to D.C. The return trip was a train to Chicago and a bus ride back to Dakota. I had made the decision to stay home because not only were buses and trains not accessible for wheelchair travel, but New York City and Washington D.C. were, likewise, not very accessible for a person using a wheelchair. It was almost a decade before the Civil Rights Act, and the Americans With Disabilities Act would not be enacted for another thirty-five years.

I often thought how strange that with Franklin Roosevelt having had polio in 1921, and essentially being a full-time wheelchair user, that he, or in concert with others, hadn't taken the initiative to at least begin the process of making the city more wheelchair accessible and usable. To the contrary, Roosevelt did little if anything. He took great pains to hide his disability. There are only two known photos of FDR using a wheelchair. With the power of his office, he could have set in motion major changes for people with disabilities, as Eleanor did for people of color. Sadly, he chose to hide or deny his disability. Maybe he felt, or was advised, that if his disability were to become highly visible, his opponents could point to it as a weakness.

Despite my reservations about the trip, my classmates strongly urged me to accompany them. Any time I expressed doubt, or tried to explain the problems that I would face, their reply was always, "Hey, that's no big deal—we'll manage. We'll take turns helping you." So I went with them on the trip, which turned out to be an unforgettable adventure, especially for me. Without the magnificent effort on the part of my classmates, the trip would have been impossible. It seemed nothing was accessible for wheelchair use. I was lifted, all one hundred-eighty pounds of me, along with my sixty pound wheelchair onto the bus, off the bus, onto the train, off of the train, etc. The process was repeated time and again at each stop. There were bus rides in New York and Washington, and transportation to and from daily sightseeing tours; then it was up the stairs and down the stairs and then up again and down. The Lincoln Memorial had one way up—hundreds of stairs. The same was true for the Jefferson Memorial, the Mint, Ford Theater, and the house across the street where Lincoln died, the Capitol building, and the museums. Everywhere we went there were steps. In spite of the hot and muggy weather, which daily seemed to hit record highs, they tirelessly lugged me up and down. Someone always stepped forward and said, "Ok my turn to help."

High School was probably the most carefree four years of my life. My disability, while an inconvenience at times, had not separated me from my peers. It was a period of significant personal and psychological reconstruction as an individual. I don't mean to suggest that I didn't have hang-ups, I did. Relationships with girls, for example, were still a difficult matter, because anytime I thought about a girl as more than just a good buddy, my disability entered the picture. I had many friends who were girls, but I was unable to risk an attempt at a boyfriend-girlfriend relationship. But my classmates provided a supportive, therapeutic environment that nurtured me for four years. They helped me feel like one of the gang, like I was normal, in spite of the obvious challenges in my life. Their collective kindness and help they gave me, the pranks they played on me, and the accountability they required of me were critical in the development of my feelings of self-worth, optimism, and the belief that I could and would succeed in life. To them, I owe a debt that I can never fully repay. I cherish those days, and although in my heart I know what they did for me, many of them probably don't. But it is my hope that one day they will understand how important they were for me.

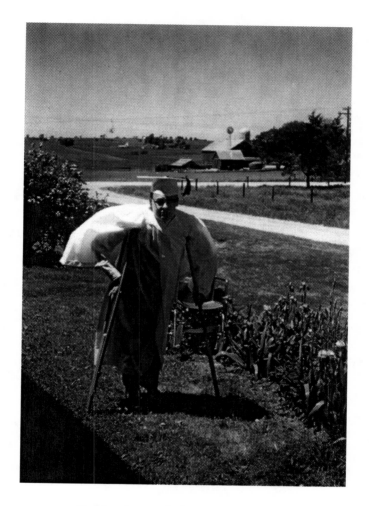

Graduation garb (Dusty Lane, 1957)

VI. Illinois Research: A Summer In Chicago

When I was ready to begin my senior year in high school, I considered myself to be a pretty clever fellow who was quite worldly. Then I moved to Chicago and hung out with a bunch of "brothers", a few "hillbillies," some Puerto Ricans, a couple of murderers, thieves, gays, a psychopathic sexual deviant, and some flotsam of society. There were also a few regular, middle-class types, some Jewish fellows, and one really nice Polish Catholic guy named George Pogvara. After being there a couple of months, I began to realize that I wasn't as smart as I thought I was, especially when it came to people.

In late summer of 1956, I entered the Illinois Research Hospital in Chicago for what the doctors euphemistically labeled corrective surgery. After five months of being sliced and diced by a number of their young physicians-in-residence, I'd label the practice "experimentation."

My parents had the best of intentions for me. Their desire was to prepare me as best they could to meet the physical rigors of my life ahead, and I concurred that the proposed procedures would most likely be beneficial. Before the course of treatment began, the doctors laid out three major goals: 1) straighten my legs, as I had rather pronounced flexion contractions at both knees; 2) perform muscle transplants in my hands in an effort to improve functioning; and 3) rotate my right arm with a surgery they called a Tubby procedure.

The doctors put both legs in casts, and daily for six straight weeks, they added small wooden wedges to slots cut in the casts behind the knees, gradually forcing my legs straight. My legs ached twenty-four hours a day. In my left thumb, a tendon transplant resulted in about 50% improvement in mobility, so they started on my right arm. Step one was a bone graft to fuse the right wrist. Unfortunately, the surgery was botched pretty badly, and only one side of the fusion healed properly. The radius (the outer bone in the lower arm) did not attach at the wrist, as it was intended to, and still floats, unattached, to this day. The next step was to surgically rotate the arm below the elbow (the Tubby procedure) because it had turned over from the polio. That was to be followed by a fusion of the right wrist in a 45-degree upright position. Finally, I would have tendon transplants in all four fingers (moving the tendons from the back of my fingers to the front).

It was August when I arrived at the hospital, across the street from tenement housing where the residents were all black folks. Many of the patients and the staff in our ward were also people of color. The next several months would result in some major changes in me as an individual, and the people and dynamics of that ward were to have a profound impact on me. Talk about culture shock. It was quite a change of scenery for a rural country boy, who was more accustomed to the sounds of cattle lowing contentedly in the far pasture, their bells tinkling melodiously, the neighborhood dogs answering their fellow canine calls from miles away, the sounds of crickets, and the gentle whoosh of wind through the huge maple tree that sheltered our house. I had to carefully think about my comments, as the neighborhood folks and the hospital ward I was in was ethnically mostly black people

"Good morning, boys. Rise and shine. Let's all get ready for breakfast!" It was Mack the male nurse. He was so bright, cheery, and enthusiastic in the morning that he pissed off the entire ward.

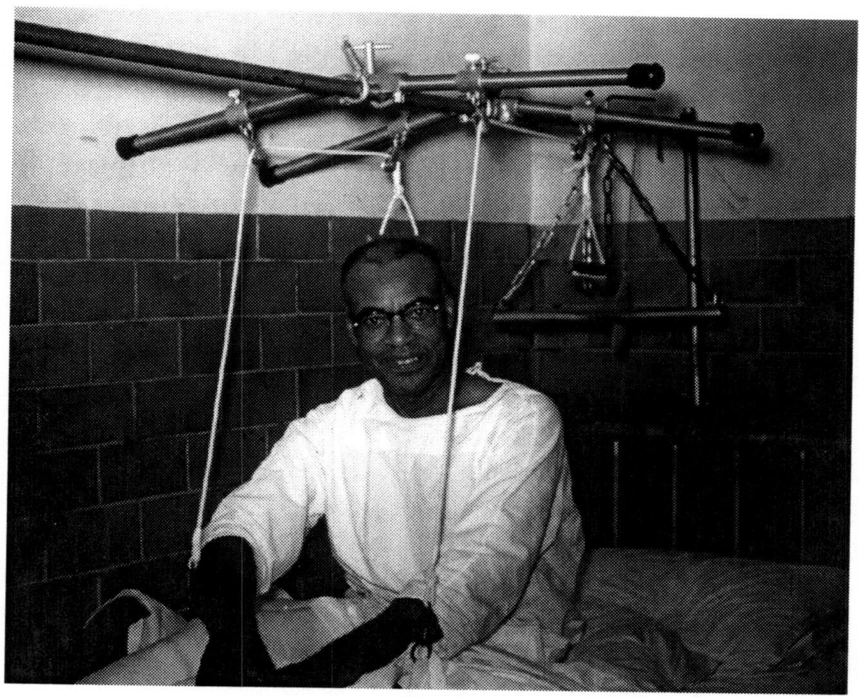

I don't recall this wardmate's name. A really nice fellow. (1956)

Meticulous in appearance and dress, he smelled wonderful, but I don't think many of the guys ever told him that. You see, he liked guys a whole lot better than gals. He was out of the closet at a period in time when many called people of his persuasion queers. He was a highly competent professional, and easily the best nurse we had. The medical staff often asked his views on a particular patient problem during their daily rounds.

It was hilarious to observe the dynamics between Mack and individual patients. Most of the men responded to him as they would to any nurse, but a few bristled, scowling and glaring, when Mack approached. One good ol' boy from Kentucky would growl, "Keep your damn hands away from me you fag!" Mack just smiled and swiveled his hips a little more as he pranced away from the Kentuckian. The way he glided through the ward, I fully expected him to do a little ballet-type leap (and hear bells jingling) ala Red Skelton on his

TV comedy show. Clearly a ribald gesture on Skelton's part, but he got it past the censors. Mack was quite a dandy, and although he wore flamboyant clothing, he always looked like he had just stepped out of a fashion magazine. All the same he was, I'd guess for the majority of the guys on the ward, their first choice for responding to a complicated medical complaint.

I had been in the hospital for over a week and had had several consultations, evaluations, and other seemingly meaningless encounters with a variety of medical personnel before they began to really focus on my case. My personalized course of treatment began with a particularly distressing event. Early one morning, without prior warning, I was put on a gurney, given a Perry strap (designed to cover one's genital area, which it didn't), a hospital gown thrown over me, and was carted off deep into the bowels of the Illinois Research Hospital.

I quizzed a tough but lovable old warhorse of a nurse as to the purpose of the ride, and she somewhat nervously replied, "It's clinic with Dr. Fox, and you need to behave yourself."

"Huh? Who?" I asked.

Shortly, I was wheeled onto a stage under the glare of numerous floodlights. Then I realized I was in an amphitheater, full of people peering down at me from the darkness. Dr. Fox was front and center holding court. My hospital gown was removed, and I was covered with only a two-inch wide strip of cloth while Dr. Fox began an analysis of my anomalies—sort of like grading a poor-quality of beef.

After he completed his highly esoteric performance, he turned to me and with a smirk remarked, "Now, as you all can see, he's grossly obese (pause). Why is that, young man?" The question was terribly humiliating and I didn't know what to say. I remained silent as he continued, relentlessly.

"Well what do you intend to do about your weight? There's no use in us wasting our time if you won't commit to doing your part," he said. I stayed silent, as my only defense seemed to be to not respond or acknowledge his assault.

"Well, what are you going to do?" he continued. I felt my heart racing. I thought, "Hell what have I got to lose?"

Looking directly at him, I replied, "Well now, Doctor, you're the big-time expert. What do you think I ought to do?" My remark surprised him, and I could tell by his incredulous expression he wasn't used to someone biting back. He actually staggered backward a bit, mouth open, but no words came.

There was a hush in the auditorium, and almost instantly the head nurse appeared, along with two orderlies, asking deferentially, "Is that all for this patient, Dr. Fox?" He nodded, glaring at me, and I was unceremoniously whisked off to the sidelines. I didn't get a curtain call.

Nurse "Brunhilda" was visibly shaken, "Jesus Christ, do you know who that was? What are you thinking, speaking to Dr. Fox in that manner?"

She regained her composure a bit on the long ride back to the ward.

"Don't ever do that again," she said forcefully, then added softly, "Will you promise me?"

"Well, I won't, if you don't ever take me back to that meat market," I retorted.

I never again spoke disrespectfully to the esteemed orthopedic surgeon (who also happened to be the chief medical officer on the Chicago Bears staff), but likewise, I was never again hauled on stage to be hung out like a carcass of freshly slaughtered beef for Dr. Fox's amusement and analysis.

As nasty as old Dr. Fox was, there were others who were very supportive, like a young Jewish doctor named Fred Feiler. He was a tall, rather handsome, soft-spoken fellow, who was a terribly nice guy. He was a great listener with whom I could share my most private concerns. When I was really feeling low, he'd listen to my complaints with a mind towards helping. He was a good dude.

Most of us had copious amounts of free and idle time, as the machinery and decisions of a state/public hospital moved slowly. Major daytime activities included watching the Cubs on TV (with Jack Brickhouse, the announcer with the jowls like a bassett, doing the play-by-play), playing penny ante poker, playing checkers, reading, and just sitting around swapping stories—50% of which, I suspect, were lies. Interspersed were surgeries, treatments, occasional death, and the ubiquitous visits from the gray ladies, so named because the uniforms of these upbeat volunteers were a pale gray.

After the evening meal, the ward began to buzz with activity. There was lots of talking, playing checkers and poker, guys going out, and keeping a close watch on the tenements across the street. About the time the sun began to go down, the streets came alive. There was a scramble in the ward to get a front row seat at the large bay windows overlooking the street to the four-story tenement houses. It was drama unequaled by anything on television, and we were rarely disappointed by what happened. There was always music, drinking, drug deals, dancing, and much talking and yelling. Conversations invariably escalated into arguments, and shouting matches often lead to fisticuffs and fighting. Sounds of breaking glass, screams, explosions, the occasional burst of gunfire, and flying trashcans, all shattered the stillness of the cool, damp night air. Soon thereafter, sirens started wailing and the police arrived. They separated the more combative types, broke up confrontations, attempted to restore order, and occasionally hauled people away.

Some of the more entertaining scenes were arguments among people hanging out of windows. There were usually multiple parties involved, with verbal harangues and abusive language flying in all directions. Those screaming matches were always punctuated with sarcastic commentary from the audience milling around on the street below. The best interchanges involved themes involving sexual misconduct. Innuendoes and accusations abounded about who was fooling around with whose girlfriend, boyfriend, wife or husband. The exquisite timing of the taunts and barbs, coupled with the inner city black dialects, often resulted in hilarious commentaries.

I'm not sure when African-American comics began to come to national prominence (via television), but those nightly exchanges would have been fabulous training grounds for them. I never heard anything really new in Richard Pryor's comedy routines, because I'd heard most of it on sultry summer nights at Illinois Research Hospital.

The Cubs were losing, as usual, but a major highlight of the October World Series was New York Yankees pitcher Don Larsen's perfect game against the Brooklyn Dodgers. That's twenty-seven consecutive outs: no runs, no hits, no walks, no errors; in baseball parlance, "nothing across." I still remember him striking out Dale Mitchell for the final out, and Yogi Berra jumping on Larsen.

The poker games were serious business, and although we played with pennies, the games were hotly contested because the games were viewed as contests of cunning, guile and masculinity. One fellow who played regularly, Clarence, was a Sonny Liston look-alike, not only in physical stature and facial appearance, but also in his ominous and sullen demeanor. No one messed with this brother. I recognized early on that keeping silent during the game, especially when Clarence was in the pot, was advisable. One afternoon, Clarence and a wisecracking young man named Rodney were the only two left in a rather good-sized pot. The game was five-card draw with deuces wild.

With the betting completed, Clarence growled, "Flush."

"Oh," his young adversary chirped, "I have two small pair, two fours, and oh yes, two deuces."

Clarence looked up briefly, reached for the pot and said venomously, "Yeah? Well now, a flush beats two pairs, don't it?" He scraped the large pile of pennies into his cloth sack.

"Hey wait a minute." Rodney protested, "I've got four of a kind."

"No," interrupted Clarence, "you called the hand two pairs and it stands. Nothin' more to say. Deal the cards." That was the end of the discussion—no one challenged or argued with Clarence.

There were plenty of light moments in the ward. I spent many hours watching Cubs baseball and playing checkers with an older fellow we called Pops. He was an odd-looking guy. He was skinny, had half his teeth missing (though several prominent lower ones always showed when he talked), and was partially bald with tufts of bristle-like gray hair that stood straight up between the bald spots. He had problems with psoriasis, including patches on his head and nose, which resulted in his face having a splotchy appearance. He always had several days of growth on his face, which, like the hair on his head was spotty, giving him a decidedly unkempt and ragged appearance. He had a deadpan facial expression, and his eyes, wide and staring, made you think he must have just witnessed something terrifying. However, old Pops was crafty. He spent summers in Florida at a V.A. hospital, and winters in Chicago at Illinois Research at the expense of the public coffers.

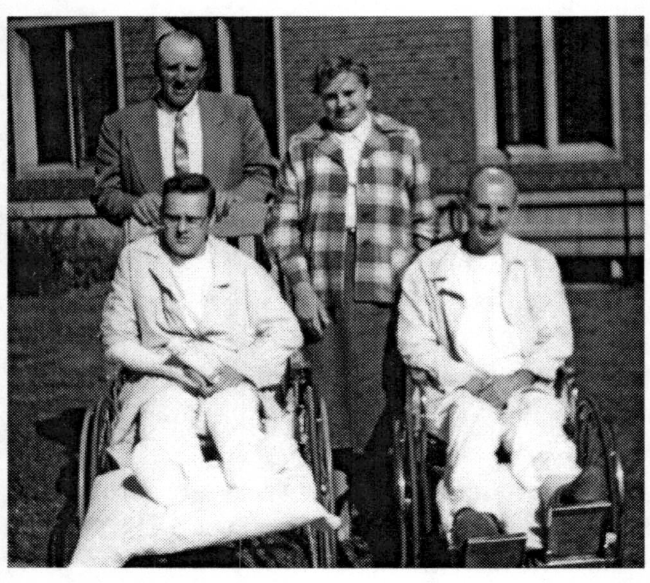

My father and sister, Jolene, and I at Illinois Research Hospital, with "Pops," the self-appointed checkers king (summer, 1956)

He had an unusual bathroom fetish, which I discovered quite by accident. After having a bowel movement, it took him thirty to forty-five minutes to clean himself. It was a daily ritual that began with dry toilet paper, but then progressed into toilet paper that he wetted in the sink. He alternated between dry and wet until, presumably, he was clean. I didn't observe this process first hand, but Pops informed me of the value of proper hygiene after elimination. I did time him on occasion and he would, on some days, approach an hour in the john.

We split about fifty-fifty on our checker games, and between the two of us, we could usually defeat any and all comers on the ward. That was until one morning, when a grizzled old guy casually asked if

I wanted to play a game or two of checkers. "Sure," I cockily replied. Well, the guy proceeded to annihilate me. I didn't come close to winning a single game as he systematically wiped me out. He didn't say much, had a forearm that had been shattered by a lead pipe (I never got the story), but he was an amazing checker player. I asked if he would play Pops and he agreed.

After about three games, Pops said, "That's enough, I don't want to play anymore."

The fellow simply said, "Okay," and walked away.

Out of earshot, Pops barked quietly, "What the hell, was he cheating?" Now, Pops took his checkers playing seriously and did not like losing. I told Pops that I did know one thing about him. He had told me that in his competitive checker- playing career, he had once tied the reigning world checker champion.

"Well, that son-of-a-bitch! I won't give him the satisfaction of beating me again," Pops snorted.

One of the fellows in the bed next to me, Harold, was a person of mixed race, the politically correct term for an individual of mixed heritage who is African American and American Indian. An American Indian friend of mine, who is a writer, once told me that animals are mixed breeds; people are mixed blood. Anyway, Harold and his wife and family were terribly nice, soft-spoken middle class folks. His heritage particularly interested me because I naively thought black people and Indians didn't intermarry. My information on that subject came from two sources. First, the folklore from the community I grew up in, and secondly, from the book *Cimarron* written by Edna Ferber.

The setting in the book was Oklahoma territory in the mid 19th century. In the novel, a young black kid meets an Indian girl while working for the same employer. She gets pregnant and when the child is born, it becomes apparent who is the Father. The young woman, the baby, and the father all pay a terrible price. He is staked out, and rattlesnakes are tethered with rawhide just beyond striking distance. As evening approaches and the night dew falls, the rawhide stretches enough for the snakes to reach him. The girl and child are sewn into the skin of a freshly slaughtered buffalo and as it dries and contracts, they suffocate.

Well, the story and the folklore I had learned were fiction, but Bill and his family were real. I learned from him that, in fact, there was a great deal of intermarriage between the two groups as people moved west. Bill was a rather excitable guy who had a chronic problem with a hip that caused him to walk with a pronounced limp. One morning old Dr. Fox came in to examine him. Bill was jumpy as a cat—Fox intimidated everyone. Things deteriorated rapidly when Fox ordered Bill to walk up and down the ward so he and the interns could observe his limp. Clad only in a short hospital gown and a Perry strap, Bill started off. His rocking side-to-side gait set off a rhythmic swaying of his crown jewels, which, unfortunately, hung down on either side of that damn two-inch wide Perry strap. Each step he took increased the pendulum-like swing. Bill hesitated, stopped, and tried to alter his gait, anything to stop the swaying of his exposed manhood. "Don't stop Bill, keep a steady pace." barked Dr. Fox. Bill endured, persevered, eyes straight ahead, looking like he was in shock (I think he was). The only outward sign of his distress was a slight reddening of his entire body from his rich red-brown natural coloring. Charitably, none of the guys in the ward made any comments, partly out of respect for him, but mostly due to the general consensus that Dr. Fox was not a nice man.

Although I was eighteen years old and had all the normal fantasies concerning girls, I was very inexperienced in anything more than casual relationships with women. I had many girls who were friends, but I carefully avoided any attempts to move friendships beyond the good buddies stage. Though I had read titillating novels, seen pornographic magazines and cartoons, heard thousands of raunchy jokes, and thought I was quite sophisticated, I was soon to learn otherwise. The first clue that I was in someone's cross-hairs was a casual conversation in occupational therapy. My schedule brought me in contact with a forty-year-old black woman named Theresa. Physically, she was a mess. I never knew what the origin of her maladies was, and I didn't ask. She was small, emaciated, in a wheelchair, had a constant wheezing cough (but still smoked), and generally looked close to kicking the bucket. But her mind was clear, and with her rapier-like wit could and would quickly scorch anyone who offended her.

One morning she said rather coyly to me, "Kint (that was her 'Chicagoese' for Kent), ah know sumpin' you don't."

"What's that Theresa?"

"Oh, it's 'bout a lady," she said slyly.

"Yea, what about this lady?"

"Oh, you don't know it, but she got her eye on you."

I was a tad flattered, but also flustered. "Who is it?"

Theresa was pretty cagey, but eventually she let me know. "It's Grace. She on the floor above you, and she going to introduce herself."

Theresa was apparently designated to play the role of icebreaker, letting me know about the lady who had honed in on me. Sure enough, Grace, with curly black hair, a pleasantly chunky physique, black eyes, a big smile and other impressive attributes, introduced herself to me one morning at the entrance to my ward. A number of guys observed her initial move. She scared the hell out of me. She was very pleasant and not at all unattractive, but I couldn't handle it. Grace was a persistent young lady, and I started getting phone calls, written notes, and frequently, she would meet me on my gurney at the door to the ward. Word got around quickly among the guys in the ward. They began to watch me, ask sly questions and make casual references about my lady friend. For such a worldly fellow as I considered myself, my performance, from a male perspective, was abysmal.

One afternoon, Hank, a tall, lanky black man, stopped me at his bedside and with a twinkle in his eye asked, "So Kent, how's it working out with the lady?"

I fumbled, "Huh, oh yeah, well, okay, I guess." Hank always averted his eyes when he began to speak to you, but if you looked away, when you looked back, he would be gazing intently at you. He could read body language like no one I've met since. He sensed my struggle, Grace's aggressiveness, my inability to respond, and my fear that I could become the laughing stock of the ward.

Hank asked, "Hey, man you aren't like Mack, are you?"

"No," I stammered.

"Well, then just relax man. Be cool, go with the flow. It'll work," he advised.

Fate intervened on my behalf. Grace was well enough to go home and was dismissed from the hospital. The docs saved me. However, one evening before she left, she cornered me in an elevator. An orderly had me on a gurney and when the elevator door opened, she came in the elevator wearing not only very tight-fitting pajamas, but also a lecherous smile. Almost, as if on cue, the orderly jumped off the elevator at the next floor, and there we were alone. “Kent, how do you like my jammies?” she purred. I was freaked. I recall keeping up a barrage of chatter and wisecracking until the door opened and another staff joined us. My complete testosterone tailspin, combined with my chagrin, kept me from telling the guys about Grace’s trap.

Speaking of women, almost fifty years have elapsed and although many of the images of people on the ward and hospital staff have faded, I can still clearly picture one woman in my mind. She was one of the head nurses, a tall, slender black woman with large beautiful eyes, very short, tightly curled light brown hair, and lovely white teeth. A “good morning” with a coquettish smile from her turned most of the guys into jelly. She strolled gracefully through the ward, never seeming to be in a hurry, efficient, and despite her quiet demeanor, was clearly in charge. Half of the guys on the ward hit on her, and the other half fantasized about it. She deflected all the boys’ advances with charm and a wonderful laugh. It eventually occurred to me one day that she was undoubtedly one of the most beautiful and sensuous women I had ever seen. She was in the movie star class of gorgeous gals. But women like Marilyn Monroe and Rita Hayworth weren’t on my ward. I had difficulty looking at her when she came to my bedside and asked how I was feeling that day. I must have blushed a crimson red. She had an exotic fragrance about her, and her hands felt like velvet as she held my hands and she spoke to me. After seeing her daily on the ward for those few months, my idea of beauty changed rather dramatically. Strangely, as vividly as I recall her face, I can’t remember her name.

In stark contrast to that lovely nurse was a tough looking patient, a brother who was a quiet fellow with a large, angry scar on his face. The scar started on his forehead at the hairline above his left eyebrow, angled down through the brow, over the eyelid, traversed his nose, and ended on his right lower cheek. I got in the habit of making daily rounds talking to all of the twenty or so men on the ward. I had become fascinated with the diverse background of the guys who came into the ward. Not only was there significant ethnic diversity among the men and staff, but also many of the guys had experiences I’d never dreamed of, and had done things I would have been far too afraid to try. Though the fellow with the scar would communicate mostly with a "ya" or "no" or just a grunt, his monosyllabic dialogue didn't deter me from visiting him daily. One morning I summoned the courage to ask him about the origin of the scar.

He paused for a second (during which I wondered if I'd made him mad), and then looked directly at me and very matter-of-factly drawled, "Well, you see, this dude cut me."

"Geez how'd that happen?" I asked, eyes wide.

"Oh, we had a disagreement, had a fight. He pulled a blade and he got me."

"Gosh, what did you do?" I asked incredulous.

"Well, I killed the motherfucker," he replied, without a hint of emotion.

I gulped and got out a barely audible "Oh, I see."

Needless to say, that ended our brief morning discussion. I retreated quickly, unable to think of anything more to say. I'd guess he noticed that his answer had shocked me into silence—an intended result, as he had had enough of my inquisitive nonsense and my invasion of his privacy. He made his point, and I was very careful in the future to not ask him any more personal questions.

There was a young brute of a guy, whose name I won't use, a drug using, sexually obsessed guy who probably fit the definition of a psychopath quite well. When asked about his injuries, his standard line was, "Oh, I hit a five-hundred pound hog running away from the cops in Arkansas and I shattered my legs. But you ought to see the hog!" He used drugs on the ward, and propositioned every—and I mean every—female who came close enough for him to ask. One evening he disappeared from the ward and the hospital. We learned later that a fifty-year-old gray lady had succumbed to his sexual overtures and had literally wheeled the guy out of the hospital on a gurney in his full chest to toe, body cast. He returned to the ward one morning about a week later, chuckling and grinning lecherously about his escapade, and we never did see that gray lady again.

We also had a "one-armed bandit" on the ward. It wasn't a slot machine, but a guy named Ernie who had lost an arm when he grabbed onto a live high line wire; we called him Orville Hodge, for the Illinois State auditor who had recently been indicted for embezzling state funds. Ernie was extremely lucky at penny-poker; hence his nickname, Orville, for always running off with our money. He really didn't care whether he won or lost, and was liable to stay in any pot regardless of his cards. Occasionally he'd have an outrageously lucky draw and win. He laughed a lot, win or lose, and made the games fun with his unpredictable and unorthodox style of play.

There was a violent-natured young fellow from the hills of Tennessee, a recent arrival in Chicago, who had joined the influx of hillbillies who were migrating to Chicago and other northern big cities. He was an outspoken racist who hated blacks, Mexicans, Jews, and anyone he deemed a foreigner. This included almost anyone who wasn't kin. He had a pleasant, innocent face, and he looked and sounded a lot like the singer Jimmy Dean, but with the fury that burned within him, I'd wager he was bound for self-destruction as well as the destruction of others. On one occasion, I recall him hissing to me, "Where I come from, niggers move off the sidewalk when I'm coming. They know their place in my hometown." The venom in his words was chilling.

Leonard, another fellow on the ward, was a handsome young Italian man who had incurred a terrible brain injury. He was mostly physically intact, but he was no longer the man his wife had married. He had apparently undergone a major personality change after his accident, and had lost a good bit of his ability to exercise self-restraint. Compounding the problem was the fact that his judgment was terribly flawed. He became almost uncontrollable when his wife arrived for a visit, openly pursuing her, fondling her when he cornered her, and trying to coax her to accompany him out of the ward to a private place in the hospital. More than once she left in tears and left Leonard wondering why she'd gone. Sadly, he did not recognize that his behavior was humiliating for his wife, and frankly, embarrassing for the guys on the ward.

There was a guy on the ward, a patient, we called the "Merry Mexican;" no not Lee Trevino, the golfer, and besides he was actually Puerto Rican. His family sneaked booze in for him almost daily, and he taught me my first dirty Spanish words. His wife also brought in wonderful smelling Mexican food and he always wanted me to taste everything. That brief exposure to a whole new way of cooking only whetted my appetite for those spicy dishes.

One day a tall, gentle fellow who was legally blind, came to the ward. His name was Ashley and he spent his days spouting obscene poetry and making up raunchy limericks. He was very creative and used his quick mind to gain attention and make friends. He had no family (though I don't recall the circumstances), was unemployed and seemed adrift. He seemed sort of lost in a world that he didn't understand, and some days wandered aimlessly throughout the hospital. Every day he recited his bawdy stories, sayings, and poems, including the ribald classic, *Piss Pot Pete.* He always wanted me memorize each one, smiling approvingly when I could repeat the lesson of the day. I've forgotten most of them except the saga of Pete. I don't remember when the gentle poet arrived on the ward or when he left. His life seemed to be that way; he kind of materialized out of nowhere and then just faded away.

Day after day, a freckle-faced old gent with fading red hair lay quietly in his bed rarely speaking, only responding when he was addressed. His face looked like he had been battered repeatedly with his nose broken and squashed at an awkward angle. We wondered if he had been a boxer because of the damage to his face. There was a rumor on the ward that he had been an MD. or Ph.D., but no one was sure; what we did know was that alcohol had destroyed his life. He had been found in a Chicago alley, only half-alive, and brought to the hospital by the police. We knew nothing else about him or his life, and I never recall him making a single reference to his past.

I felt extremely sorry for him, as I think the entire ward did, and I wished there was something I could do to help him. At one point, I thought about asking my family to take him back to our farm where he could work for Dad. He'd have three meals a day, a safe place to live, and although we wouldn't ask him about his former life, eventually he would tell us his entire life story. But I didn't approach my parents with the idea. I was afraid to. One day he left the hospital. I bought him two cartons of Lucky Strike cigarettes, and when I gave them to him he whispered a quiet, "Thanks." A tear rolled down his cheek and he turned and walked away. Maybe I should have said something to my folks about him.

John Johnson, who had lost both legs and one arm to cancer, was a man with great courage and a deep personal faith that God had a special plan for him. With his one remaining arm, he would push himself to chapel services every Wednesday evening. He never complained about his situation and was always optimistic that a cure would be found. I spent a lot of time talking with him the last days of his life. Despite being loaded with painkillers, he died in terrible pain, his body ravaged by the cancer. His great faith remained strong until the end, and he left this world with his spirit intact.

I also remember another fellow with cancer who came into the ward. He was a quiet, young, twenty-one or twenty-two year-old chunky kid with a round face and a chalky-white pallor. He walked in with his street clothes on, and changed into his hospital gown to become one of us, a patient. Although he was terribly pale, I didn't think he looked too sick. But when I questioned a nurse, she admonished me to not ask questions, as he was a gravely ill young man. He was, however, quite upbeat and talkative. He excitedly informed us that he was there for a new experimental, but almost surefire treatment. "It's going to work," he said. "I know it will." He had the treatment every day for the first week he was there, and it made him so sick they moved him to a private room. He died early in the second week. I was stunned by his sudden death.

One day it struck me that Christmas was only a few days away. Fall had melted away, and half of my senior year in high school was gone. I was still in the hospital with many more procedures (surgeries) to go before I could leave. With the doctors continuing to fart around, trying to decide when and who got the next whack at me (remember, this is a teaching hospital), I informed my folks and the hospital I was leaving very shortly. If I had elected to stay, my entire senior year would have been gone. Furthermore, in considering the outcomes of the surgeries I had, I began to think that those so-called surgeons might be better suited to cutting up beef and pork at Krogers instead of practicing on me and the other guys in the ward.

I went home in January with a cast on my right arm, which my dad and I removed about a month later using his heavy-duty tin shears. I had an appointment several months later for an evaluation and to have the cast removed. The medical team with whom I met was appalled that I had taken the cast off, and made it sound like I had committed a major felony. But I wasn't a happy camper either, and I told them my experience as an unpaid guinea pig hadn't really been all that much fun. I asked them rather pointedly if the outcome of the wrist fusion was what they had really intended. That question, I think, ended my relationship with them, and brought to a halt any further treatments from the good folks at Illinois Research.

Now, some fifty years later, as I think back to that time, and especially to my fellow ward mates and the staff, I wish I had kept a journal of my days there. I had become so desperate to return home and rejoin my classmates that I had focused completely on leaving and was mostly unaware of the changes that were occurring within me, changes that were set in motion by the people and the environment I had encountered there. The atmosphere in the ward was highly charged, and emotions seemed accentuated and raw. There was terrible grief and despair, unbelievable courage and compassion, fear and deep hatred, wonderful fellows, and others without a shred of morality or values, men who lied, cheated, and stole at every opportunity. I had never before encountered people like that. Neither had I previously lived in a community as ethnically and culturally diverse as that ward in Illinois Research Hospital. I was amazed, at times, by not only the humanness, but also the depravity of the people who were there. Many of my preconceived notions, particularly about folks who were not the same color as me, or who grew up in very different environments, or had no families, didn't ring quite as true to me once I returned home.

I wasn't a huge fan of Martin Luther King, but one thing he said still resonates with me today. In his August 28, 1963, *I Have a Dream Speech*, he said, in effect, We should judge (people) by the content of their character, not the color of their skin. I think I began to understand his earnest entreaty during my brief stay in that hospital ward. I'm not sure I'll ever completely comprehend how those four months at Illinois Research Hospital changed me, but my time there began a metamorphosis that would shape the person I am today.

VII. University Of Illinois: A Brief Visit Across The River Styx

You always pass failure on your way to success. (1)

I arrived on the campus of the University of Illinois in 1957 for the fall semester after what I thought was a rather spectacular four-year career at Dakota High. I was ready to take on the University and all it had to offer. I met people easily, and readily (I believed) impressed them. I had been a class officer in school, finished third or fourth academically in a class of forty-plus kids in spite of rarely studying, had won an athletic letter jacket as scorekeeper for the baseball team, was an accomplished storyteller, played a mean game of cards, was a sports trivia expert—I mean, what else was there? I just knew I was one of the most unique guys to ever hit the Urbana Campus.

I began to think I might make as big a splash as two fellows named Governor Vaughn and Manny Jackson, newly recruited freshman basketball players for Illinois. Their notoriety stemmed from the fact that they were the first two black basketball players at the U of I. Incredible as it may seem, it wasn't until that fall that the University of Illinois was able to identify two individuals of African American descent who were good enough to play for them. Two great high school players from Freeport, Illinois, McKinley "Deacon" Davis and Carl Cain, both black, had become all-Americans at the University of Iowa before 1957. Davis, who led Freeport to the 1951 State High School Basketball Championship, apparently didn't get any interest from downstate Illinois. Cain led Freeport to the "Sweet Sixteen" the next year, but was not recruited (at least very seriously) by Illinois. So there we were, Governor, Manny, and me.

I arrived on campus with high hopes, but in less than three months my world would crumble around me. While Vaughn and Jackson went on to great careers at Illinois, I quickly slipped into oblivion. By Christmas break, I was so personally devastated that I did not return to school. I was confused, depressed, and my ego was crushed. My massive reservoir of confidence and cockiness had completely evaporated.

My father, who was a wise fellow and a good judge of people, picked up the first signal of potential disaster the day he, Mom, and I first visited the campus in midsummer to meet with Tim Nugent, the director of the Disabled Students Program. Tim had been a pioneer in the early days of services for kids with disabilities in colleges and universities. He began his work in 1948, establishing a program on the Galesburg campus of the University of Illinois. Nine years later, the program at Champaign-Urbana had gained national notoriety and received much publicity, particularly for the wheelchair sports programs in football, track, and especially basketball. Tim was a strong personality and was very protective of his unique position of power. He apparently had the authority to determine suitability for admittance to the University. He exercised his authority liberally, and was not bashful about establishing his position of superiority, which was something he did immediately with my parents and me. He was smart, and quickly sized me up as a country boy and his dirt-farmer parents.

The meeting was simply awful. He made us wait long past our appointment time, and we watched from the lobby as he joked with staff, fraternized with every pretty young coed who happened in the office, and ignored us entirely. When we finally met with him, he was condescending and rude, particularly to my parents. After only twenty minutes, he determined, or perhaps divined, that my life would best be spent as an accountant. We all left pretty upset, but none of us had challenged him on any matter.

When she was stressed Mom would sleep, which she did once we began the one hundred-fifty mile trip back home. Dad, who had said almost nothing during the meeting had nevertheless, sized up Tim. With Mom escaping into dreamland, he said quietly, "Kent, you had best steer clear of that guy—he's a horse's ass." In my view, none of Tim's behavior over the following few months would invalidate my father's initial impression.

By September, when the semester began, I had totally forgotten that midsummer meeting, as well as my father's caution. The initial week on campus before the start of classes was a wonderful introduction to the collegiate experience. It was a beautiful warm early autumn; I met many new people, almost all disabled wheelchair users, as I was assigned to the P.G.U. (parade ground units) barracks. These were one-story tarpaper barracks used in World War II that were easy to remodel for wheelchair use. There were four living units on each end with a common bathroom and shower in the middle, and the only modifications to the building for accommodating wheelchairs were wooden ramps on each end of the building. Doorways were already wide, the rooms were spacious, and the bathroom had several partitions removed between stalls to allow access by wheelchairs.

While these rather ramshackle shacks were easy to access, the dining facilities were quite another matter. They were located on the second floor of a large brick dormitory adjacent to the P.G.U. A very steep, switchback ramp attached to the exterior building was the only wheelchair access. Flushed with excitement of being on campus, I didn't take time to consider what a huge problem the ramp would present for me during the semester. I managed to struggle up several times during that first week, but with all the week's activities, I mostly bought burgers and fast foods at the Canteen, a small snack shop across the street from the dormitory that housed the dining facilities.

In addition to class registration, purchasing books, getting a tour of the campus, and general orientation to the University, there were some social activities. The big event was a day at Lake Springfield in Springfield, Illinois, about sixty or seventy miles from Champaign.

I don't remember what organization sponsored the all-day party for the Illinois "Gizz Kids" (disabled students)—maybe the Lions, Elks, or Rotary, or one or more of them. We loaded up on the buses, the interiors mostly stripped for wheelchairs, and were off to the picnic. There was tons of food, music, beer, and boat rides. It was a very pleasant day, warm and sunny, but the trip to the picnic and the return back to campus left me with a disquieting feeling. I was only a freshman and expected to be low on the rung, but the hierarchical separation of students was much more dramatic than I expected. There seemed to be a distinct caste system, with Tim's favorites at the top and several layers down to the also-rans, which I began to fear might be my category.

The wheelchair athletes were big, strong guys with terrific upper body strength. They were mostly paraplegics (spinal cord injured) and were at the top of the heap. Cute coeds, some cheerleaders, others who were very attractive and those who had the collegiate look in dress and style were the showcase students. There were also some extremely bright students, absolutely tops in their classes, who were a part of the elite mix.

They were the super crips, people with disabilities who excelled despite their disabilities, and most importantly, went to unbelievable lengths to be independent in functioning from a wheelchair; they *never, ever* accepted a push on campus (if you did, and Tim learned of the incident, you could expect a reprimand, as it was not the image he wanted to promote—an image of disabled people not needing any help). Even more ludicrous was the idea that the disabled students on campus were no different than the rest of the student body. Sure, that made sense. We obviously had invisible wheelchairs. Today I wonder how many of those students, in particular those who had polio, now suffer from post-polio syndrome as a result of truly insane attitudes about being independent.

These wheelchair jocks were highly visible on campus. Many wore letter jackets, drove sporty cars, and maintained an overall collegiate look. A particularly big attention-getter was wheelchair athletes and University of Illinois varsity football players tossing footballs to one another in the street near the P.G.U. Canteen in the early evenings. Pretty spectacular, thought the crowds who gathered to watch the boys show off. Wheelchair jocks rifled long passes to the likes of Bill Brown, a star on the varsity football team who later became an all-pro fullback for the Minnesota Vikings of the National Football League. Ronnie Stein, a guy in a wheelchair, had been an all-state athlete in several sports in high school. After a tryout with the Chicago White Sox and a swim in Lake Michigan, he contracted polio and lost partial use of his legs. His upper extremities and trunk were unaffected by the disease, and Ron could reputedly throw a perfect spiral sixty yards from his wheelchair.

I couldn't even grip a football, let alone throw it. It began to dawn on me that image was highly valued. I was a fat kid with a crew cut and an old-fashioned wheelchair with hard rubber tires (I was the slowest guy on wheels). I wore floral sport shirts over plain slacks and had nerd glasses. Nonetheless, I began the first week of classes determined to succeed and shake the feelings of foreboding that had begun to shadow me. Just nerves, I tried to assure myself, and once classes are underway, I'll feel better. It never happened. My discomfort increased with almost every passing day. In my mind (and backed by a good bit of evidence), Tim had separated the sheep from the goats, and where I came from, you didn't want the goat label. I began to get paranoid and even dreamed one night that my wheelchair had a large orange "G" stenciled on the back of it.

There are always cliques, but what made these circumstances so difficult was that it seemed to me that Tim and his staff not only participated in, but also actively fostered the emergence of a caste system. In the initial month of school, struggling terribly and feeling miserable, I made several half-hearted attempts to approach Tim for help. I never did make an appointment; he was always busy with program matters to which he had to attend. It appeared, however, that he had time for the elite students in his program—students who could, and would, continue to foster the "Super-Crip" image.

I recall that the Russians had launched Sputnik that fall, and one starry night I went out after dark to watch the tiny blip of light sail by. It was very chilly and I begin to shiver almost uncontrollably. It wasn't all the cold. I felt awful as I sat there alone in the darkness. I began to look for help, comfort and friendship—anything to bolster my sagging ego.

The guys I lived with, my shack mates in the barracks, were a rather unique collection of fellows. We had few winners in our midst, with one exception. Chuck W., a young black kid from Chicago, was one of Tim's stars. His physique featured a waspish thin waist that spread into a tremendously powerful set of arms and shoulders. He was an impeccable dresser who wore a shirt and tie most days and had a very natty collection of hats. He was simply a dandy. He loved the ladies and they, in turn, adored him. Charlie had a habit of exiting his wheelchair to sit on the ground under a large shade tree, propped against the trunk, blissfully reading his lessons with several winsome young lasses seated close by. We referred to them as Charlie's Harem (hmm, maybe that's where Charlie's Angels came from?). Charlie was assertive, self-assured, and not shy in sharing his views on issues. He was a tough Chicago kid, and polio at a young age demanded that he become a fighter to survive, which he did quite well.

Dan H. lived next door to Chuck in the barracks and was also from Chicago. He was short, had dark hair that he slicked back, and though he was chunky was surprisingly fast in his wheelchair. He liked to tell us stories about his sexual exploits (most of them back in Chicago), and he had a tendency to target practice with his revolver in his room. He'd set a mattress against the wall and blaze away. Amazingly, he never got caught.

Jim P. was an extremely bright fellow who wore a corset that pushed his stomach and chest upwards, and I think, contributed to his breathing problems. He was post-polio, and due to respiratory difficulties, frog-breathed (gulped air). He was a wonderful writer who never got anything but A's on his English themes. He was cynical, caustic, and hilarious in his commentary on political issues. During the time I knew him, he reinvented his personality, beliefs, and values more than once. He was ultraconservative, almost a racist, when I first met him, but five years later at Southern Illinois University, he had transformed himself into a wild-eyed anti-McCarthy liberal.

Two of the nicest people in our shack were Kenny W., a Gimp, and Harry H., an AB. On campus, the standard nomenclature was "AB" for able bodied and "Gimp" for disabled folks. Harry, a skinny black guy from Tennessee, was a cross-country runner who was quite differential to white people (he told me only bits and pieces of the harshness of his life as a result of his color) and spent a great deal of time very carefully sizing up each social situation and responding accordingly. He was a country boy like me, and I found in Harry a kind, genuine, thoughtful, young man who, because of his ancestry, had learned to behave in ways expected by people around him. I often wondered how Chuck W's environment differed from Harry's. How did Chuck emerge so assertive, so much an in your face guy, while Harry was so cautious and wary? Personality was partially a factor, but personality alone didn't account for all of the difference. Maybe it was a simple matter of geography, north vs. south.

Kenny W., a gimp, was a long, lanky, handsome fellow from "Cent" tralia, Illinois. Folks from northern Illinois pronounced the town's name as Centralia, a single word. Kenny, by contrast, a Southern Illinois lad emphasized "Cent"- and the "tralia" (with an extra "t") tailed off. He was a Navy veteran who, only days after his discharge, had a one-car accident, which broke his back at the T-4 vertebrae, and resulted in total paralysis below the waist. He spoke quietly and slowly and always had a story if you had the patience to listen. He smoked Sea Stores cigarettes that were sold to Navy personnel. They did smell and taste a bit musty, but at the price of five cents a pack, I also began smoking Sea Stores.

One evening over several beers, Kenny related one of his stories about leaving his home in Illinois and joining the Navy.

He had never before been out of the state of Illinois and he remarked, "Shit fire, I didn't know anything. I was just a country boy from Cent-tralia." He was shipped by train to California and had to catch a bus to La Jolla.

Kenny said, "You know, I waited for that bus to La Jolla for two hours after the scheduled departure time. Finally I went to the ticket counter and inquired about the delay."

"When is the bus to La Jolla going to arrive?"

"We have no town by that name on our route," replied the agent.

Because he couldn't make the agent understand the name of the city, he finally wrote it down— L-A-J-O-L-L-A.

The agent looked up at him incredulously, then smiled and asked, "You're not from around here, are you son?"

"No."

"Well, I'm sorry, but the bus for 'La Hoya' left two hours ago."

Kenny spoke English, sort of, but Spanish was indeed a foreign language to him. He always had a story, told with his unaffected drawl and a great sense of timing—not to mention a humorous twist. He loved old movies and could recall the most obscure bit-players from years ago. One of his favorite no-name players was Paul Fix, an older guy who usually had two or three lines in old Westerns. Once Kenny identified him for me, I often spotted him in many old cowboy movies.

Tom T., a quadriplegic, lived at the other end of the barracks. I had never seen squalor like the room where he lived. Clothes, books, partially eaten food, cigarette butts, spare wheelchair parts, trash, pop cans, toiletry articles, tin cans, magazines, and newspapers were strewn throughout the room. He bathed and showered about once a week, whether he needed it or not. He was a senior majoring in architecture, and spent most of his time trying to survive. He was a classic example of a guy who really needed help with daily living activities like dressing, showering, and getting to and from class. I don't ever recall him going to the dining hall because either he didn't have a meal ticket or could not get up the ramp. His diet was mostly coffee, cans of soup heated on a hot plate, burgers now and then, and whatever freebies the guys would bring back from the dining hall. He endured a hell of an existence, but he couldn't or wouldn't get help, because at that time it was considered bad form.

There were others whose faces remain, but whose names I don't recall, who frequented our place. They were to become my University family. As I retreated from the larger institutional environment, I looked to them for solace. I learned from them how to survive with minimal effort, how to avoid Tim, and how to essentially fade into the background and not draw attention to myself. Indeed, I had embarked on a self-destructive journey.

The University of Illinois campus was huge, spread out over many city blocks, with the distance from the P.G.U. to the main campus some eight blocks. Getting from one class to another (invariably each class in a different building) also meant a push of sometimes three-four blocks. The Disabled Students Program had a fleet of buses equipped with mechanical lifts that had regularly scheduled routes to and from, as well as within, the campus. Without them, most students would not have had the endurance to traverse the campus on a daily basis. I was greatly impressed with the technology and the efficiency of the system in delivering dozens of wheelchairs to campus. But unbelievably, the bus rides turned into a humiliating experience almost from the start.

Unfortunately, my weekly class schedule coincided with the schedules of two of Tim's favorite wheelchair jocks. They were big, sharp dressing upperclassmen with extremely large egos. They singled me out the first day I rode the bus with a barrage of questions. Each day the questions became more personal, with references to my weight, the clothes I wore, what my parents did, what I was going to do as a career, my experience with women, and worse. In a few days, the questioning stopped and the unsolicited self-improvement suggestions began to be offered. They were fairly malicious, and I found myself too embarrassed to respond. I finally refused to acknowledge them, and silently endured their snickers and smirks. I couldn't imagine that the situation could get much worse, but it did.

Two of my classes were easily accessed by a long, gently sloped ramp. But getting to the other classes was a nightmare. Although billed as a wheelchair accessible campus, the ramps which led to my two other classes had a heavy door halfway up with no level landing to stop, open the door, and continue going up. The proper technique was to push up to the door, hold yourself and chair with one hand, reach for the door handle, roll back far enough for your chair to clear the door, and simultaneously keep the door open while proceeding up the ramp. It was almost impossible for me. The very strong guys and many of the girls who had full use of their arms and hands were adept at the procedure. I had neither the strength to negotiate the ramp nor the hand dexterity to grab and grip the door handle to get through the door. As the weather turned cold and it rained or snowed, ice began to form on the ramps. My hands became numb and I lost all dexterity. Some days I was unable to get up the dining room or classroom ramps, and with no one to ask for assistance, I felt quite alone. With an increasing sense of despair and my growing anger at Tim and the entire program, I turned my energies to other pursuits.

THE IMAGES ON THIS AND

THE FOLLOWING PAGE

REPRESENT THE SUM

TOTAL OF FOND MEMORIES

FROM MY DAYS AT THE

UNIVERSITY OF ILLINOIS.

By late October, six weeks into the semester, I began to realize that my first incursion into higher education was already in the toilet. I also had discovered that my feelings and circumstances were shared by a fairly large number of other students, some of whom lived in my shack. Initially, as the probability increased that failure was imminent, we began to focus on finding activities to occupy our time. Our attendance in classes had dropped off dramatically, and some weeks I did not attend a single class.

Poker games were a favorite diversion. Since many of the guys who played had money from accident insurance claims, or were veterans on disability pensions, penny ante was a thing of the past. The games we played were often in the five to ten dollar betting range. Sometimes the pot for a winning hand was a hundred dollars or more. A typical big winner could make four to five hundreds dollars and occasionally there would be a guy who left with a thousand or more. Likewise, there were individuals who lost similar amounts. I was extremely cautious, and played only in games in the fifty to one hundred dollar range. I was a good poker player and most times did not lose, winning from five to fifty dollars per game, which was almost every night. Thus, I had solved the problem of not being able to get to the dining room. I existed on burgers, fries, malts, and other junk food. Alcohol was not allowed in the barracks, but our resident counselor Stan, whom we affectionately referred to as the Commandant for our Stalag, and the residents had agreed on a pact of "don't ask, don't tell." If booze was discovered in our barracks, we would accept full responsibility and leave Stan out of it. The arrangement worked for us and after that alcohol was always available.

One evening in the midst of some heavy drinking, Jim P., who had a very creative mind, came up with the idea of opening a pornographic movie house in our barracks. He had sources who ordered 8 mm black and white, silent movies. A bunch of guys chipped in and we ordered a projector, screen, and a half dozen ten minute flicks with exotic sounding titles like "Brigitte Bares It All" and "Humping Hannah." Well, we got the movies and were sorely disappointed. They were beautiful girls all right, but not nude. They were attired in skimpy two-piece bathing suits and spent the entire ten minutes gently swaying and gyrating about as lewdly as a bunch of Baptists at a senior prom in Dallas. What a disappointment. No bumping or grinding, no skin, and nothing really lascivious or disgusting. The films were actually quite boring. Well, no matter, we got the word around that for a dollar we'd give you a half-hour porno (three movies) show that would awaken your testosterone. We had a fairly good business initially, but word spread rapidly that our advertising was misleading and you could see more skin walking across campus. Jim continued to buy new films, (the new ones guaranteed to titillate even the boys at Penthouse Magazine) with the same result. With the poor quality and nothing lurid to show, our paying customers evaporated. We hadn't challenged Larry Flynt's position as a porno king, so it was time to return to the drawing board for new ideas.

We had created enough problems already and had begun to hear reports that Tim and his staff were unhappy and were looking to ferret out troublemakers. That feedback only served to fuel a now-growing agenda to undermine Tim's authority, as well as the sycophants who served him. We began a calculated program of disinformation for his stooges to feed Tim and the staff.

Like the night eight or so of us loser types were drinking at Phrens, a favorite campus beer joint, and began making frequent and regular trips to the alley outside of the bar to drain off the large amounts of liquid we were ingesting. As the evening wore on, we became much less inhibited about our activity. In groups of three or four, we began taking aim at a nicely trimmed hedge on the yard of a residence bordering the alley. The next trip we would encircle a stately Maple tree and simultaneously douse it from east, west, north, and south. Somewhat later, a young waiter came to our table and whispered to us, "If you wheelchair boys don't stop using the lady's yard next door as a bathroom, she's going to call the police." We did have a legitimate problem as the restrooms were up stairs with no access. However, we could have been more discrete in the matter. Once we received the warning, our behavior became even more obnoxious. We loudly announced that we were from Tim Nugent's program and repeated the Center's phone number for her to call in the morning. We continued the foolishness and while the police never did show up, we hoped that our obnoxious behavior had cast a cloud on the program.

We began a systematic boycott of activities sponsored by the

Center, especially wheelchair basketball games and other organized gimps only affairs, like the fraternity for disabled students, DSO (Delta Sigma Omicron), an organization which we all joined and then promptly ditched.

The Center had two six-man wheelchair football teams, blue and white, which served the basis for further humiliation in my brief career at Illinois. They literally had a draft of incoming and returning males who could participate in wheelchair football. Can you guess who was the very last draft pick? My ego was so damaged that I didn't feel like I was last. I felt like I was left over

Increasingly, we began to get attention from the Center, mostly negative, but, hey, that was better than being ignored. One night Dan H., Jim P. and two gals were caught drinking in a local cemetery by the police. Tim was furious. Our shenanigans seemed to be infectious, and a barracks several blocks away hired two young ladies of ill fame from Cincinnati and set them up in one of their suites. They did a thriving business for about a week. Word of the "red-light stalag" spread like wildfire. The gals caught a train out of Champaign back to Cincinnati before the police arrived.

Since many of us were missing multiple classes, we began to get notices from the Dean's office concerning our absences. Jim P. was a master at concocting what appeared to be medically valid excuses for not being in class. Someone had stolen a prescription pad from the Student Health Center, and with each visit to the Dean's Office, we carried a hand-written official medical document excusing us from class. We had master forgers, and simply presenting the note to the Dean's secretary ended the visit.

Strangely, although I had hoodwinked the Dean's office with my medical excuses, I recall a feeling of having been cheated, and once again, summarily dismissed. Was our deception so sophisticated that further investigation was unwarranted, or were we not worth the trouble? I never saw a Dean, and was never asked to account face-to-face with a person of authority for my absences. I truly felt adrift in a sea of misery, vacillating between hostility and self-pity. Primary responsibility for the entire debacle rested on my shoulders, as I needed to take the initiative to find alternatives out of the morass. But I was a naive nineteen year old who had enjoyed academic success without much effort, was accustomed to the spotlight, and was in possession of an over-inflated ego. I wanted help desperately, but saw no alternative. Tim and his cronies had become the enemy.

One day in November, as a group sat chatting, someone casually mentioned a town named Calumet City, located in the Chicago Metropolitan area. The place had a notorious reputation, as it was a Mecca for all those seeking debauchery and sin. The main street was lined with bars and strip joints, all reputedly controlled by the Mafia. As the discussion continued, and tales of past excursions by members of the group unfolded, I listened with growing interest. In retrospect, I think the boys had decided it was time to wring the remaining "country boy" out of me and had orchestrated the discussions for my benefit. Serious planning began for an early evening departure to Chicago. There were six guys in wheelchairs in three vehicles, each car carrying two people and two wheelchairs. I rode with Tom T., the senior architecture student. Jim P., Marv C., and a slick dude we called "JR," and Bill F. were the other five on the trip. We rented one hotel room for the six of us and hit the bars sometime around midnight.

Tom, the guy I rode with, had terrible spasms in his legs and lower torso, which is not an uncommon phenomenon for people with spinal cord injuries. A typical spasm involved one leg spontaneously beginning to "dance" on the wheelchair footrest. Hitting a bump in the road, being startled, a sudden blow to the leg, anxiety, a variety of things could set off the spasm. Arms and hands could also become involved. Usually, grabbing the limb that was beginning to spasm and holding on to it would relax the spasm. Tom was well known in the gimp community for the severity and duration of his spasms. He was the spasm king on campus. First, one leg would begin to shake, and if he didn't get it under control, the other leg would take off. Failing to stop the increasingly severe jerking, Tom would lean over, wrap both arms around his legs, and hang on. Unfortunately, on occasion, his lower torso would also begin to spasm. We knew he was in trouble when he yelled a drawn out "Ooooh Shiit!" Most times he just hung on and eventually got them under control, but not always.

One Saturday night, Tom had a date with a cute little gal who lived in a real brick dormitory (not a shack) across the campus. Tom spent hours getting ready. He took a long, hot shower, washing away a weeks worth of dust, grime and body grunge. He had gotten a haircut, and with a precise shave and mustache trim, he actually looked fairly presentable. He had a new colorful sport shirt, worn with the top button undone to prominently display his impressive chest full of honey brown hair. Shoes were shined and he smelled wonderful. He was terribly nervous. This was his first date with this gorgeous gal. Several of us "propositioned" him before he left, trying to help him get over some of his increasing anxiety. Tom left with flowers in hand. This was going to be a night to remember. Well it was, in fact, quite an auspicious occasion.

Every gimp on campus heard the story of what transpired. Tom arrived in plenty of time to pick up his date, almost beside himself as he headed in the front door of the dorm. As his chair hit the threshold of the heavy glass door, one leg shot straight ahead in a violent spasm. Tom dropped his flowers and desperately grasped for the leg, which only served to set off the other one. As he struggled to get his legs under control, his torso decided to jump into the act. Shaking violently, a number of coeds had gathered, asking and offering assistance, which only further exacerbated Tom's growing sense of impending disaster. We heard later that the entire first floor heard the familiar, "Ooooh Shiit" as the spasms became so severe that they pitched him head first out of his chair and onto the floor of the lobby. Several guys also picking up dates rescued him by getting him back into his chair. He followed through with the date, but he was so distraught at the threshold disaster that he fumbled his way through the entire evening. We were playing poker when he arrived home, and after more than a few beers, Tom related the story.

Now this is the guy who's driving me to Chicago. He drove with hand controls, of course, but I had visions of his legs taking off while we're doing seventy on the highway. I knew I was doomed. I was going to die on a trip to a Mafia-run strip club on the south side of Chicago. Trying to appear cool, I casually asked Tom what he did if he had spasms while he was driving. "You know it's the funniest damn thing, once I get in the car and plant my feet on the floor boards, I never have a spasm," he marveled. It was true; He didn't even have a tiny quiver for the two hundred plus mile trip north.

We hung out in the motel room for several hours after we arrived, drank a few beers, had a burger, and then headed for State Street in Calumet City. The place was as billed: a collection of sleazy bars, with equally sleazy girls, bartenders, bouncers and barmaids. Beer was a buck a bottle for Fox Head. It was terrible stuff, but we all drank it because that was the only kind the mob sold. You couldn't go into a bar without buying drinks. You could stare, drool or gawk at the naked ladies promenading on stages behind bars, on elevated runways through the seating areas or, in some clubs, on a stage about head-high for a close-up leer, but only if you were imbibing.

There were two kinds of girls working in the bars—the dancers, and the bar girls, or b-girls as they were called. B-girls approached everyone who entered, wanting to spend a little time with the customer in return for a drink, usually two or three dollars for watered-down whiskey. They were girls whose job was to hustle drinks, and they would go to extremes to get the men to ante up. Their hands immediately began to grope the customers, and they weren't at all bashful about their behavior. My mentors for the trip had given me a lengthy lecture on the many techniques these unscrupulous types would employ to fleece a naive country bumpkin like me. They had me so spooked I hid most of my money inside my socks, half on the left, half on the right. And when a b-girl approached me, I immediately bought her a drink. In particular, I was cautioned about not trying to purchase any "flesh." They'll just take your money, and besides, you'd be a fool to end up in the sack with one of those gals because you'd probably get more than you paid for.

Notwithstanding their advice to me, two of the porno pros, Jim and Dan, who had made numerous trips to Calumet City, did succumb to lust and hired two young ladies for a "party." They paid their money and were directed through a door at the back of the club that entered a dark, dimly lit hallway. The door at the end led them to their ladies in waiting. A bouncer accompanied them to help with the door. As he opened it, he quickly pushed Jim and then Dan through the door and out into the alley. That ended the transaction. They got out of the alley, came around to the front, and reentered the front door of the club to protest. They were quickly asked to leave, as quite amazingly no one in the club had seen them before. The bartenders, girls and bouncers were incredulous at their story, saying, "Don't push it boys. Your story is bullshit and you'd best leave." They did, because none of the folks who ran those bars had a very good sense of humor. Their sole interest was to separate you from your money. There were no complaints, refunds, or discussions about the quality of customer service.

Given the sordid nature of the place, it would seem improbable that humor would have played any part in the evening. But in the early hours of the morning, all six of us wound up at the same club sitting around a large circular table. Marv, a handsome, virile-looking fellow was regaling a b-girl with stories of his sexual prowess and escapades. He was suave, and I think, had sparked a bit of interest and admiration in the young lady who was at that point sitting on his lap (both in his wheelchair). He would whisper in her ear, and she would giggle and repeatedly say, "Oh, really?" in mock surprise. Marv eventually got around to explaining to her his powers of concentration and his ability to control himself sexually. He explained to her in great detail that as a student of Eastern Philosophy, through meditation and study, he had learned complete control of his body. For example, if he chose, he could not be sexually aroused. The young woman, although not too bright, was also skilled in her craft and advised Marv that her techniques were so well developed that no male could resist responding to her caresses. He asked her if she was a student of the Kama Sutra, which she thought was some kind of karate school.

"I'm a betting man," Marv challenged. "What's it worth for you to learn just how highly developed my powers of self-control are?" By this time, the girl had informed the bartender of his boasts, and after a quiet discussion, the bartender announced they would entertain a wager. If Marv failed to get aroused, drinks were on the house. Well, the little b-girl proceeded to empty her arsenal of tantalizing titillations upon Marv and his body. Nothing happened. Marv remained calm and collected, continuing to smirk and sip his Jack Daniels. After exhausting her arsenal on Marv, she gave up, truly astounded at his self-control. We left the bar together, and I'd bet she told more than one customer the story. We laughed heartily at Marv's little charade. Marv had a spinal cord injury, which had resulted in total loss of sensation below his waist. Nothing worked from about mid-chest down. It would have been a miracle if Marv had developed an erection, and the young woman in question didn't appear to be the type who had studied neurology. She didn't know that what she was attempting was physiologically impossible. Years later, when our paths again crossed at Southern Illinois University, Marv was still fond of retelling the incident.

Sometime later that morning, probably close to dawn, I became separated from the group and headed down to a section of bars and clubs that seemed much less busy. Few people were in the area and the lighting was poor. As I crossed the alley to the sidewalk, a huge black (6-8 or more) fellow stepped from the shadow of the doorway.

"Where you going?" he asked.

"Oh, down to these clubs. I haven't seen them." I replied.

"Look man," he warned, "you don't want to go down there. Those people are bad."

"What? I'm not worried." I said with bravado.

"Now listen to me. If you go down there alone, the best you can hope for is a knock on the head and waking up in an alley with everything you have gone. If you're not lucky, you might not come back at all. Those people deal and use drugs. The girls live there, they sleep on the tables, and they don't have homes. Now I'm putting you back on the sidewalk across the alley. Don't come back, because next time I won't stop you. You've had your warning." He lifted the wheelchair and me, (probably two hundred and fifty pounds) up onto the curb like I was balsa wood. I thought of arguing with him, but even with a couple of six-packs of Fox Head swirling through my system, an alarm went off. I suddenly felt very chilled. I slowly made my way back up the sidewalk into the mob of people milling in and out of the clubs, many in advanced states of inebriation. Suddenly I had become very sober. I found Jim and Dan and stayed close to them for the rest of the time.

They had latched onto a very attractive blonde gal with a terrific body. They were both drunk and were buying her multiple drinks. Jim had her phone number and was discussing helping her find a pony for her little boy back home. I observed her systematically fleecing the boys, now only wanting my adventure in sin city to end.

I thought I was having a wonderful time and had already begun to think about the next trip, but the encounter with the bouncer was like being doused with ice water. The more I thought about how close I might have come to disaster, the worse I felt.

We returned to the motel room shortly after daybreak, slept for several hours, and headed back to Champaign. I never returned to Calumet City, although several groups made additional trips before Christmas. They urged me to go along, but I used being short of money as an excuse. Over forty-five years later, I still have flashbacks to that giant of a man stepping from the shadows. Whoever he was (and I think I know who his employers were), there remained in him a vein of compassion that may have saved me from a disastrous outcome.

The semester seemed to drag on, and I made a last desperate attempt to salvage my classes by cramming for mid-semester examinations. Jack Coleman, a kid who lived across the road from our farm back home also attended the U of I. He was a sophomore or junior, a good student and a bright guy. I called him and asked him if he would tutor me for my math class. He spent three or four hours with me one evening, but I had fallen too far behind, missed basic concepts, and was probably going to bomb the test, which I did. I was barely hanging on with a C or D in english, failing economics completely, but unbelievably, my accounting class was still potentially a C or possibly even a B.

One of the few individuals who was supportive during the semester was my accounting instructor. He called me in to his office and talked with me at length about my performance in class and the semester in general. He was a pleasant, soft-spoken man who, as I recall, looked like Dean Rusk, the former Secretary of State under Eisenhower. He strongly suggested that I attend class on a regular basis, saying encouragingly, "What work you do turn in is good. Much of what you complete is B or A work, and you obviously have the ability to readily grasp the concepts. Are things not going well for you in school?" I came close to breaking down, wanting desperately to spill out all of the humiliation, despair, and anger that I felt. But I had become so mistrustful of the program and had lost so much confidence in myself that I retreated into my own protective shell and was unable to respond to his invitation to unload my troubles.

In 1957, the University of Illinois and other schools with strong academic reputations had little compassion when weeding out the students who were marginal scholars. I remember statistical data, disseminated with a bit of pride, which stated that 20% of the freshman class would be eliminated. That philosophy, coupled with the elitist philosophy of the Disabled Students Program, made me expendable, and my behavior sealed my fate.

It's hard to fool mothers. Two hundred miles north of my tarpaper barracks, Mom began to fuss about me. She had a feeling that all was not going well. I hadn't written home much, and though I did call sometimes, I was careful to avoid telling them that the semester was destined to end in disaster. My older sister, Carol, a nurse, had a day off, so they drove down to see how I was doing. I was sick with the flu and running a fever. The barracks had no heat, as the oil burner at our end of the barracks had gone out. Most of the guys couldn't or wouldn't light it when it did go out, which it did with regularity.

Mom and Sis were appalled at not only my condition, but also the situation in the barracks. It was not very orderly, and there was absolutely no food or drink readily available. Jim P. had an electric fry pan, which Mom used to fix me something to eat. She went to the drugstore for cold and flu remedies. They spent the day trying to fix me up, and although the visit was welcome, it served to remind me that soon the semester would end and I would have a great deal of explaining to do for the complete debacle of this educational opportunity. For the entire semester, the only support I can recall was the kind words of the accounting professor. Oh, I had the camaraderie of the guys I hung with, but those were mainly diversionary pastimes that helped us all avoid the reality of our worlds coming apart.

The last weeks of the semester were a blur of partying, playing cards, drinking, and general carousing. We drank openly in the barracks, began to have marathon poker games—sometimes twenty-four hours straight—and kept ourselves busy with a variety of antics, while rarely attending class. In spite of our fun, the semester would end in tragedy.

With the Christmas break upon us, there seemed to be an urgency to end the semester in style. There had to be a final fling, because we were certain that a number of us were not going to survive academically. Stan, our barracks counselor, was a graduate student and his classes either ended several days before most of us undergraduates, or he had completed his work-related responsibilities and wanted to leave early for the break. He gathered us together to exact a promise from us that if he did leave early, we would agree not to blow the whistle on him, and further, that we would stay out of trouble. There was unanimous consensus that Stan had been a good sport, had looked the other way for most of our transgressions, and that we should make excuses for his absence should anyone ask. Stan skipped town early, thanking us for our support, and issuing a final warning to stay out of trouble. The latter advice didn't work.

The day he left, the partying began in earnest. Card games and drinking that lasted all night and late into the next day became the norm. But unfortunately, one day the events escalated to a tragic and climactic end. Late one afternoon, two brothers dropped by our barracks to join in a game of poker. One fellow was post-polio and the other was an AB who had been drinking heavily at a barracks next door, and had decided to come and take our money. They were good card players, but they played as a team and were cheating. We couldn't catch them or prove that they were using signals for when to bet, raise, or drop out, but their consistency in winning and the unorthodox style of play made it quite apparent that their winning was more than chance. We finally tired of their antics and told them to get lost. They weren't pleased, but both had more alcohol in their systems than needed, so they staggered off in a huff, calling us a bunch of sore losers.

As the evening grew late, the rowdiness increased. A very strong fellow, a paraplegic with a massive upper torso, decided that having to open the door to enter the bathroom was an inconvenience. In his state of inebriation, he probably did have difficulty getting the door open and passing through. His solution was to break a new passageway to the bathroom through the plasterboard wall partition. Using only his hands and fists, he knocked a hole in the bathroom wall through which he could easily drive his wheelchair. We thought it was hilarious.

The craziness accelerated as Dan and his friend JR, both of whom had small-caliber pistols, decided to set up a firing range in Dan's bedroom. We all took turns shooting the pistols into two mattresses that had been stacked against one wall. Not to be outdone, one of the fellows next door who had a .22 caliber automatic rifle demonstrated, several times, just how rapidly he could empty a large number of shells out of the magazine. He was careful, only aiming the rifle straight up and riddling the ceiling with a barrage of bullets. It was impressive, and I'd guess there were many dozen holes in the roof before morning.

The two brothers who we had expelled from our card game earlier ended up next-door and continued to drink and play cards. The fellow with polio, I think his name was Jim, had extensive loss of functioning in his hands and arms. He also had rather significant respiratory involvement from the effects of polio, and his normal style of breathing was somewhat labored. Sometime during the early morning, he had reached the point of complete intoxication. He was unable to continue playing cards, as he couldn't keep track of the game or hold the cards. The fellows told him he would have to quit because he was too drunk. They told him to go to bed and sleep it off. Jim protested, saying he hadn't had nearly enough to drink, and producing a bottle of hard liquor, proceeded to drink the entire contents. Shortly, he passed out and the guys playing cards managed to get him into a bed and close the door behind them. They returned to the game and continued to play late into the morning.

From what we later learned, Jim had so much alcohol in his system that his body could not get rid of it fast enough through respiration. He suffered swelling of the brain, and in his agony, he rolled out of bed, thrashed about wildly, bruised his body and head terribly, and finally succumbed to alcohol toxicity. His brother had gone home sometime after Jim was put to bed, and when he did not return to his home, his brother had come to the barracks looking for him. Tragically, he discovered the body. Initially, he believed that foul play had been involved in his brother's death because of all the bruising.

Harry H., the cross-country runner, woke up my barracks mates and me; he opened my door, shook me awake and, pleading in his Tennessee drawl now with a deadly hush, he whispered, "Kent, get up! The 'po-lice' are all over the place. Someone died last night in the barracks next door. Tim is over there and he's like a wild man." I bolted from my bed, dressed, and completely straightened my room in about ten minutes.

When Harry first sounded the warning, the barracks was a shambles. There were empty beer and liquor bottles, litter, food, chunks of shattered wallboard, papers, and all kinds of trash and garbage strewn about. We all pitched in, and Harry filled two huge laundry bags full of bottles and trash. He slipped out the south end of the building at about the time Tim barged into the north entrance of our barracks. He was so angry he was white, his lips quivering and his entire body shaking as he confronted each of us, vehemently demanding to hear what we knew about last nights events and what each of us had done the past ten-twelve hours. Tim was extremely distraught, and must have felt that much of what he had worked for was in jeopardy. When he was satisfied that I had not been in the barracks where Jim died, he stopped the questions and began lecturing me for having chosen the wrong people as friends. He also made it clear that I would not be returning next semester to cause him further grief. With not only the barracks in a shambles, but my life as well, I viciously vented my frustration towards Tim and his program, particularly his elitism and lack of support for many of us. Already in shock from the tragedy of the day, and surprised by the vehemence of my outburst, he did not respond and stormed out of my room. That was the last time I spoke with Tim, and although I would eventually head a major program for disabled students, we never met, spoke, or communicated professionally.

I left school at the Christmas break and did not return for final examinations. I think my parents had figured out that I would be staying home, and they didn't press me for details. The final degradation of the semester came with a visit to the Offices of the State Vocational Rehabilitation Agency that had fully financed my semester at the University. Room and board, tuition and fees, books and supplies, and other incidental expenses were paid by the agency. My brother took me to the meeting in Rockford, twenty-five miles from home. It was a cold, dreary, overcast January day, and the ensuing meeting was equally dismal. My brother was in the room with me when the counselor reviewed the lowlights of the semester.

"What happened?" my counselor inquired. "I would have bet my last two bucks on you making it, and further, why did Tim Nugent recommend—now listen to this—'that this student *never* be considered for readmission to the University of Illinois under any circumstances'?"

I had no comment for the counselor or my brother who later asked me, "What the hell did you do?"

I could only muster a weak, "Mostly made bad choices, I guess."

I deserved to get the boot from the University, as did a good number of my cohorts, but I think Tim was a bit vindictive. But in his position, he had the power to ensure that I never returned. I brought little to enhance his program's image.

When the fall Semester of 1957 had begun, I could only envision good things ahead for me. But with all the promise for the future, it didn't work. To paraphrase Charles Dickens, "It seemed to be the best of times, but it became the worst of times; it was to be an age of wisdom, but it became a time of foolishness. It was the spring of hope that sank into the winter of despair." I had fallen from grace and retreated back to the safety and serenity of my country home to lick my wounds. There were some dark, long days ahead as I contemplated the lost opportunity and what was ahead for me. My parents were not harsh with me, nor did they reprimand me for failing. My mother and I had one lengthy discussion about what had transpired during the four months at Champaign-Urbana. She concluded the talk with a bit of simple, yet powerful wisdom, remarking, "Well Kent, we will have to see what happens now, but maybe it was a blessing in disguise."

And it wasn't all bad. In the months ahead I learned a new vocation. I wasn't able to become a farm hand and work out of doors, but inside the home there were opportunities. I learned the basics of cooking, I could vacuum floors, I did a great mop and wax job, I cleaned sinks and toilets, I learned to dust and polish furniture, and I became the primary dishwasher in the family. I began to slowly regain some of my self-confidence and sense of self-worth as the downstairs maid.

VIII. Southern Illinois University: Redemption In Little Egypt

This fellow, Jerry, was really a good driver even though he was blind. All we had to do was have Charlie Brown (not the cartoon character) ride in the front passenger seat and tell him where to go.

In the Bible, the gospel of John, Nathaniel asks Philip, "Can there be any good thing come out of Nazareth?" The question reflects the low-esteem that Jews held for the city, but for Christians, it was the home of the Savior, Jesus.

In the fall of 1958, after my quick exit a year earlier, I returned to the Illinois campus for a one-day visit. As in the biblical question, I wondered if anything good could come from this place, particularly for me. For believers, salvation did come out of Nazareth, and strangely, out of the tarpaper jungle at Illinois emerged a man who would also open doors for me; not for salvation, for this fellow was far from sainthood, but as the key for my return to higher education. Bill Fife had been accepted as a graduate student in Rehabilitation Counseling at Southern Illinois University in Carbondale.

Bill had been at Illinois when I was there, and he had been an active participant in many of the follies that fall semester of 1957.

He was, however, more mature than many of us, and while he had a wild streak, he also made sure he attended to his academic responsibilities. Thus, Bill became the conduit by which a number of us U of I rejects would be resurrected and re-enter college. The first step for me to return to a college was a letter of contrition. Along with the application to Southern Illinois University, I was advised by Bill to include a letter to the Dean acknowledging my reckless, self-destructive behavior while at the University of Illinois. The letter had to demonstrate the complete overhaul of my personality and how sanctimonious I had become. Furthermore, if I were not accepted into college, I was headed for either a monastery or the priesthood. Two problems, of course, were a) I was Protestant, and b) monasteries were probably not wheelchair accessible.

I'm not sure if the repentant tone of the letter helped, but I was admitted. I don't recall if Southern accepted me based on my application and letter, or if final admittance was contingent on a visit to the campus and a meeting with a pugnacious Dean named Zaleski. Whatever the case, Southern Illinois University was in a major push to increase enrollment, which likely played a part in my acceptance. In any event, Mom, Dad, Mom's sister Aunt Esther, and I made the trip to Carbondale, Illinois, in late summer of 1959 to meet with University people and complete the admission process.

Esther and Uncle Hub were especially supportive, and inserted themselves in my life at critical times. Esther, who I thought (and still do) was probably one of the smartest people I ever met, seemed to recognize intuitively when she could be helpful to me. I know that she prompted Hub to take me fishing when she saw I needed a break in my routine. After I was summarily expelled from the University of Illinois, she gave me a job at their Chevrolet dealership as a bookkeeper and taught me the fundamentals of the General Motors Accounting System (GMAC). That job and related experience was a crucial step for me in regaining a semblance of self-confidence. She also went with me to get my first driver's license. I'd also guess she was a thoughtful, supportive ally for both of my parents as they struggled with decisions concerning what kinds of rehabilitation programs and other services might be helpful for me.

When we arrived at Carbondale, we stayed overnight in rustic cabins at Crab Orchard Lake and returned home the second day with my admission signed and sealed. As he had done two years earlier (after our visit to the University of Illinois), my father gave me some simple but sage advice. All he said was, "Well Kent, you now have a second chance. You know what you need to do, so do it."

In 1959, Southern Illinois was a school of some eight thousand students nestled in rural southern Illinois, in an area known as Little Egypt because Cairo, Illinois, was located at the confluence of the Illinois and Mississippi rivers some sixty miles south of Carbondale. The University had a new president, Delyte Morris, who would become a legend in higher education circles. He was a hard-charging, charismatic fellow, under whose leadership the Institution would blossom, doubling in enrollment during my six years in attendance. Southern Illinois University had a totally different attitude regarding students with disabilities. They saw and treated us simply as students. There was an office on campus that handled disabled student issues and where Bill Fife worked to coordinate services. But unlike Illinois where Nugent's program orchestrated every aspect of a student's life that they could, Southern was a hands-off community. They saw us as adults and would only intervene if needed. Most importantly, as students, we were expected to utilize existing University resources just like all the other students. The difference in philosophy was immediately apparent, and I felt again as I had in high school—a whole person whose disability was not what defined me. I would not be used to serve the agenda of others. Many, if not most, of the students who had been at Illinois and then transferred to Southern, expressed the feeling that going to the University of Illinois had mostly served to make them feel different from the rest of the student body.

The first several days on campus, there was an all-University orientation and many get-acquainted activities, highlighted by a watermelon feed at the President's home. I met and spoke with Delyte and his wife, as well as hundreds of others. What a contrast to the Illinois gimp ghetto mentality. I was assigned room 110 Brown Hall at the Thompson Point Housing complex, one of six new three-story dorms on Thompson Point Lake. It was a beautiful setting, with trees lining the shores of the lake and a footpath encircling the entire forty-acre body of water. The tri-level dorms had some twenty rooms on each floor, all on the same side of the structure, with a lounge area on the opposite side running the entire length of the building. The lounge area had floor-to-ceiling windows overlooking a lush grassy area behind the dorm, bordering the lake.

Thompson Point had a central cafeteria where everyone ate. Unlike the cafeteria at Illinois, this entrance was ground level and the small snack bar below was accessed by a gently sloped ramp. There were four residence halls for men and two for women. In 1959, there was no mixing and matching of boys and girls in the same dorm. The University took the matter of personal morality very seriously, particularly for their young coeds. Delyte and the rest of the administration would not tolerate a Clintonesque carnival of corruption at Southern. To demonstrate their commitment to these high standards, the women of Thompson Point were locked in their residence halls, Steagall and Bowyer, at 10:30 P.M. sharp. The enforcer at Steagall Hall was a sharp-tongued little lady, Mrs. Mullikin, who stood by the front door, key in hand, ready to drop the hammer at exactly 10:30. If a woman was late, even one second, it was a study hall sentence for an entire week, 7:00-9:00 P.M. More serious infractions resulted in more severe penalties, including one reported instance of locking a girl in the broom closet for several hours. Mrs. Mullikin was well known on campus for her obsession for the rules. A member of the men's swim team would sexually maul his girlfriend in front of Mrs. Mullikin, simply to agitate the old gal; he'd moan, groan, make outrageous sucking sounds while nibbling on his girl's neck and ears, all the time groping her entire body. Mrs. Mullikin glared silently at the scene (with either murder or lust in her heart), and as the bell rang for 10:30 P.M. curfew, she stalked to the door, putting an end to the indecency.

During my first year at Southern Illinois, I became fully invested in the college experience. My first priority was getting passing grades in all my classes and although I wasn't a very serious student, I had the ability to cram for final exams. Though I was doing C and B work for the term, I was often able to raise my final grade a full letter C to B, B to A sometimes even two steps, C to A, by cramming. I had learned how and what to study, I really had lots of free time, and in retrospect, probably did not use it very prudently. I did a lot of partying, played poker (I earned most of my spending money at nickel, dime, and quarter poker games), played bridge, pinochle, and hearts, and shot pool. I won the Thompson Point chess tournament one year, swam nights in Thompson Lake, went to all kinds of University athletic events, and had a hilarious time. While I met hundreds, maybe thousands of students, and knew many girls, I still didn't date.

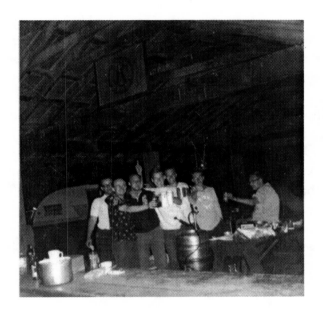

A beer blast at the Carbondale city reservoir; I'm on the table (1960 or 1961)

Unlike the U of I where no one gave you a push in your wheelchair, I developed a surefire method of getting a lift—and usually from a girl. Pushing up some of the hills on campus was really not easy. To get a push from someone, there obviously had to be students in the vicinity, which there usually were. Before beginning the ascent of the hill, I'd slow down and wait for a good concentration of females going in my direction. Timing was critical. I'd have to start up the hill before they passed me or they could miss seeing me struggle. It worked 99.9% of the time. I never felt guilty about my ploy, as everyone won in the process. I got a push, I met some great students, and invariably they felt good about helping me out. Maybe it was the first time they had interacted with a person who had a disability. Gosh, there I was, helping to break down attitudinal barriers and didn't realize it. Nice rationale huh?

There were far fewer students with disabilities at Southern, particularly the first couple of years. Out of six hundred students at Thompson Point, there were probably only a dozen who had disabilities, and I recall only six or seven other students who used wheelchairs. I knew all of these students, but we didn't cluster based on disability. Rather, each of us had a distinct group of friends, almost all of whom were non-disabled. Many more students would come to Southern in the following years, not only based on outreach by the school, but also from the gimp grapevine which was amazingly effective, not only regionally, but nationally as well. There were not that many schools in America in 1960 that had facilities, programs, and an open door policy like Southern, and the word got around quickly that Southern Illinois University was a great alternative to places like the University of Illinois.

Over the next several years, the number of disabled students increased steadily. A number of my former buddies from Champaign-Urbana who left or were kicked out of school landed at Southern. Jim P arrived at Southern, a flaming left-wing liberal decrying "McCarthyism," and one evening he and his entourage of long-haired hippie types crashed a meeting of the House Un-American Activities Committee at the Thompson Point cafeteria, shouting down the panelists, accidentally (they claimed) unplugging the 16 mm film being shown, and totally disrupting the proceeding. My God! Here we had a mini-insurrection led by a guy in a wheelchair. The campus police arrived and escorted Jim and his motley crew out the door, with Jim bellowing about fascist police tactics, rights of free speech, and other ad nauseum. That would never have happened at the U of I. The attitudes toward disabled students at Southern was strongly reinforced that evening. Even gimps could act like assholes at this Institution. He was colorful.

Another Illinois expatriate who arrived soon after Jim was Marv C., a handsome, smart-talking guy who could coax young coeds into most anything This was, of course, the same Marv of Calumet City fame. He was bright, articulate, and a terribly cynical fellow, a great storyteller, and always a must-guest at parties.

Although I had met and became quite good friends with many girls, I was still very cautious (okay, afraid) of trying to establish a significant relationship with a female. My dorm buddies, constantly on the lookout for me, suggested this girl or that girl. "Hey, I'll ask her for you. Come on—we can double date," they'd say. In the fall of 1960, my second year, there were several new girls in wheelchairs at Thompson Point. Shirley, a very attractive black girl, was way too wise for me; another attractive girl in a wheelchair was a complete snob and dumb as a box of rocks.

Another little gal, Janie, had severe cerebral palsy with a good bit of spasticity. She was a nice girl, but someone I didn't consider dating. It was not because of her disability; she simply wasn't at all my type. She used a motorized wheelchair, a relatively new machine on campuses in 1960, and it had a tendency to catch on fire. The wiring was very poor on the early power chairs, and regularly we'd hear someone yell, "Get a fire extinguisher, Jane's on fire again!" Everyone kept close track of her and made sure that if she got into trouble, someone could quickly come to her rescue. She really liked the guys, but she would develop severe spasms when a guy talked to her, or worse, teased or touched her. One evening during dinner in the cafeteria, Janie was eating with us—probably six to seven other people at a large round table. Dessert was apricots. Janie had a large, juicy half of an apricot resting in her spoon on the way to her mouth (she had to move slowly to control her spasticity) when a handsome jock walked up behind her, placed a hand on her shoulder, and crooned, "Well, hello, Janie." Have you ever seen the lightning release of a medieval catapult when the lever was tripped? When the guy touched her, Janie literally jumped up in her chair, her wrist flexed violently and the apricot flew (on a line) a good fifteen feet directly into the face of an unsuspecting fellow a couple of tables away. It was hilarious. I'm not sure anyone told Janie where her slippery fruit landed, or if the guy it hit ever knew where it came from.

There were girls, a number who were not disabled, that if I'd asked likely would have accepted an invitation to go out with me. But there were very real logistical problems that confronted me in the social-dating arena. I didn't have a car, and walking (pushing) downtown was a long haul to take a date to the movies. Furthermore, many theaters had steps at the entrance, and worse, once inside, there was no place to park a wheelchair. There were just too many hassles. Under extreme duress from one of my roommates, I did agree to a triple-date with a lady from Toronto named Roberta—whose nickname was "Bunny." She was an attractive Jewish gal who the guys claimed came from money. While her financial status remained unknown to me, her bounteous bosoms were quite apparent. Well, the one date was really kind of a bust (no pun intended), and Bunny eventually found her man—a nice fellow with an outrageous name, Dave (that's okay) Trebilcock (that's not). Some of the guys in our dorm started calling him "tremblecock," but eventually we settled on "crumplecock." The name really didn't fit him, as he was quite an energetic, animated guy, but we thought it was clever. I enjoyed women, but I just didn't have the courage to pursue any romantic adventures. Thus, I confined my social activities to mostly all-male adventures, or when girls were involved, group dates.

I lived in Brown Hall, which housed approximately one hundred twenty men. My roommate that first fall semester was a dandy named Harvey Grandstaff (and he said he had one), a guy who knew every angle ever devised to get through school without breaking a sweat. He loved to play golf, but in his own words he was a lousy golfer. However, for every game he played he was dressed like an English country squire in full golfing regalia, as if he were off to St. Andrews itself. He told me, "My opponents don't know how bad I am, but when they see me dressed like this their golf game has a tendency to fall apart."

I don't recall much about most of the fellows on the floor that first year. However I do remember my suitemate, a Chinese fellow named Ching Ma, because he had almost become an outcast in the dorm. He was from mainland China. Some of the guys resented Ching and liked to antagonize him. He was a strange fellow who did not speak English very well and had a difficult time in the dorm. He had taken a more American sounding first name, but his choice, Ferdinand, only served to make him a target for more abuse. I felt sorry for him and often intervened on his behalf to end harassment. He began to visit me late in the evenings, usually after 10:30 P.M., and we drank something he called "medicine tea." It was awful-tasting stuff, but he was in need of friendship, so I drank it—usually several cups. He told me about his family and life in Communist China, always speaking in almost hushed tones. One time, after he left the dorm, he had me over for dinner in his tiny squalid apartment. Dinner was meager, but he made me feel like an honored guest. I lost track of him when I started graduate school four years later.

Brown Hall was one of the four male residence halls on Thompson Point, with Bailey, Felts, and Pearce the other three. From the very beginning of my first semester there, it appeared there was an unspoken competition between the men's dorms for who had the rowdiest hall. I recall stories circulating about the pranks that individuals, floors, and entire residence halls had orchestrated. Bailey Hall, hands down, was the winner during the 1959-60 school year. Dorm water fights, panty raids, nights of parties at Crab Orchard Lake, in-dorm drinking (which was prohibited), mooning people from dorm windows, and violating all manner of campus rules and regulations were the kinds of essentially attention-getting behaviors we all wanted. These antics were not only reported in the student newspaper, *The Egyptian,* but also in the local papers, on radio/TV (if you were fortunate), but best of all, was the campus grapevine. One evening, the Bailey boys stepped beyond the usual collegiate misbehavior standard by starting a brawl in a local bar. Several of them were arrested and jailed overnight. A football player, Dave M., a really nice guy until he began to drink alcohol, may have started the fracas. He used to entertain bar customers by breaking beer bottles on his head (don't try this at home). Initially, it would be all fun and games, but the situation could just as readily turn into a bar room brawl.

Bailey Hall had a gimper named Jim Greenwood, a guy who would later rise to a very high corporate position with IBM, who served as one of the leaders in all their shenanigans. Jim had some sort of neuromuscular disorder and had very limited use of his hands. He had a deep, gravely voice, and reputedly could drink most of the other guys in the dorm under the table. He dressed mostly in shorts, sleeveless sweatshirts or other ragged tank tops. All over campus, he was known as a "cool" gimp. He even joined a fraternity.

The school year ended on a positive note for me. I had successfully passed all my courses, made many new friends, and although I knew the summer would be a good time carousing with my buddies, I was already looking forward to the fall quarter.

I returned to Brown Hall for the 1960-61 school year, and early on there was excitement on campus; visits from presidential hopefuls Richard Nixon and John Kennedy. Nixon's visit (October 28) was kind of a dud. After his presentation, I was able to wheel up to him, shake hands, and speak to him for a few moments. But, earlier, when JFK had come, (October 3) a football stadium full of frenzied students and supporters greeted him. Sitting in my wheelchair in a sea of screaming admirers, all I could see was butts, boobs, arms, legs, and torsos. Then, unbelievably, the Secret Service man leading Kennedy to the podium (walking backwards through the crowd) turned Kennedy just as he reached my wheelchair. The future thirty-fifth President of the United States sprawled over my wheelchair and me. His penetrating eyes looked directly at me, he smiled, and said, "Oh, I'm sorry son." I was speechless. As he backed away all that came out was a mumbled, "Oh that's okay Senator."

A number of the guys who lived in the Hall the previous year returned, and there were also some rambunctious new fellows who immediately decided they wanted to make Brown Hall the most outrageous dorm on campus. Major players were guys like Ron Cecchini, Tom Gohlson, Ted Farmer, "Drew" Chagnon, Sam Martin, Lloyd Dinkelman, Don Hequembourg, John Davis, Ken Desotell, Dick Motley, Bob Profilet, Larry Devantier, Ken Pedersen, "Swede" Fredrickson, and the most unlikely character of all, the University President's nephew, Charlie Brown. There were many others from the dorm who were not instigators, but were willing participants in helping Brown Hall earn the title of most notorious dorm on campus.

The key person who would ensure we reached our goal was Mel F. our resident fellow. Although he was a Ph.D. candidate in college personnel administration and a very bright fellow, he knew nothing about relating to forty highly energetic guys. Unfortunately for him, fate had also given him charge of a group of unusually high-spirited fellows who were constantly looking for new challenges. He began his reign with a laundry list of petty policies—no cussing, being fully clothed when in the (all-male) lounge, no feet on the furniture, etc., etc., etc. We had weekly floor meetings, which were essentially

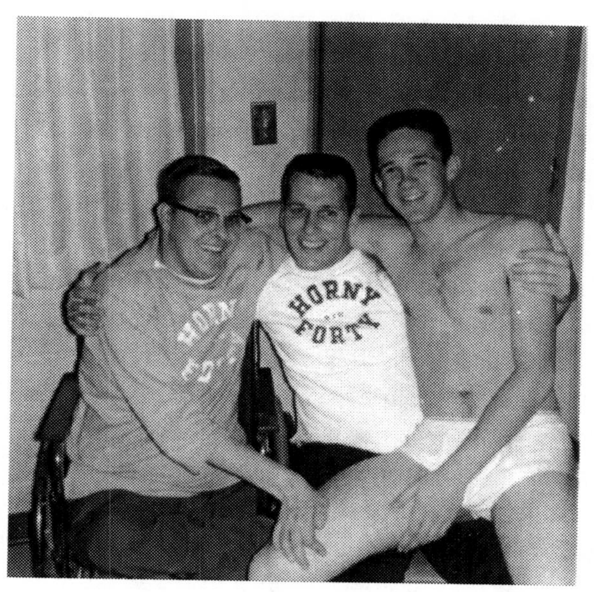

Brown Hall pranksters: Ted, Art, and me (1962)

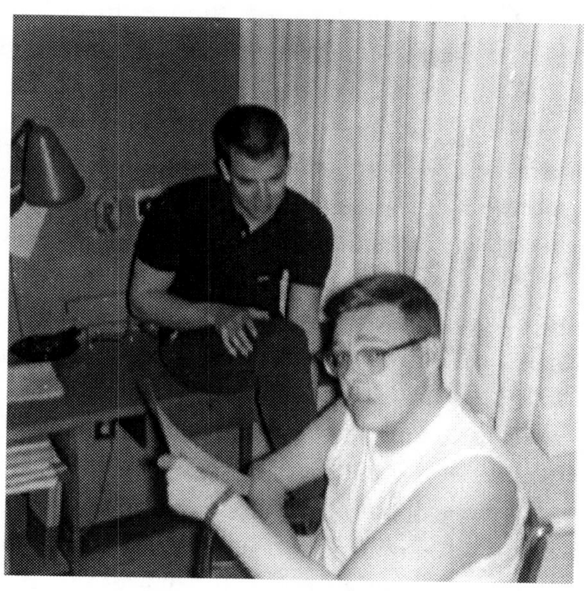

Don Hequembourg and me at Brown Hall (1962)

a platform for Mel to read us the riot act and come up with some more rules. He successfully alienated the entire floor of guys by the end of the first month. His zero-tolerance policies only served to fuel the growing animosity and unleash our creative energies in schemes to oust him.

The first major catastrophe was an all-dorm water fight. It began one Saturday evening while Mel was off premises. By the time he arrived on the scene, there was water running from the third floor to the second floor, and the first floor was two to three inches deep in water. Mel freaked, called the cops, rousted us all out for an emergency meeting, and laid out a dozen new rules. Despite all his bluster, not a single resident was punished.

Not long after, on a Saturday night, we "buried" him in Thompson Point woods. We made a cardboard headstone, complete with an epitaph, and placed his grave in a prominent place. The student newspaper picked up the story, but it didn't faze old Mel.

One of the most effective nerve-jangling tactics we employed to harass Mel was a lighted bundle of cherry bombs dropped from the third floor, into the incinerator chute. The guys had the timing down so precisely they would explode across the hall from Mel's door on their way to the basement. One concussion was so strong it knocked the glass cover off the hall clock outside his apartment. That incident shook Mel up pretty good. The incinerator chute was metal, and when the firecrackers went off, the entire building vibrated. In spite of our ever-increasing creative methods to rile him, Mel refused to talk, negotiate, or come halfway towards resolving the mounting tensions.

The incidents continued throughout the year. The final stroke of genius, the coup de gras, was filling his room with crumpled up newspaper. With the help of our lady friends from Steagall Hall (who saved their newspapers for weeks), we spent the entire weekend filling his apartment, probably ten thousand cubic feet of space, floor to ceiling with newspaper, while he was off campus at a conference. Mel turned a chalky-white color and almost collapsed when he forced open his door. He left quietly that spring quarter without fanfare or farewells. I never felt too guilty about the troubles we caused Mel, because while he wasn't a bad guy, he was sneaky, elitist, antisocial,

Can't Swim

Resident Fellow 'Mourned'

Have you ever had the feeling that you weren't wanted? One resident fellow at Thompson Point recently got the idea.

His residents, who termed him "too strict," erected a tomb in his honor Tuesday night near the agriculture building.

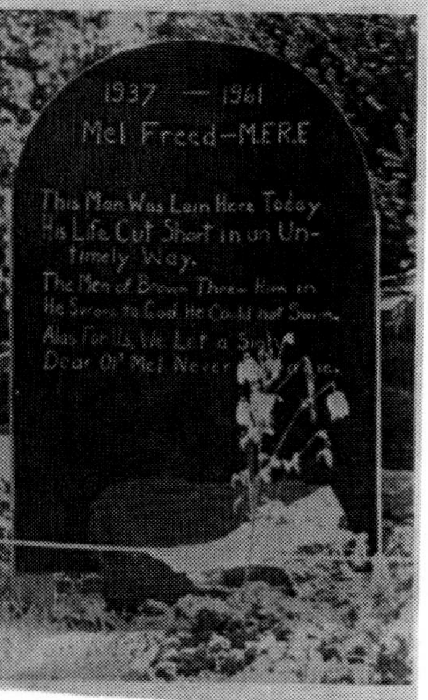

The tomb consisted of a cardboard backing containing his epitaph and an appropriate stone and flowers. Residents on this unfortunate fellow's floor said, "He's really strict about University policy."

One of the students declared that the resident fellow is not very popular.

"We filled his room with paper to the ceiling one time when he was gone; it took him almost three hours to clean it out," said one student.

The epitaph on his tomb reads:

"This man was lain here today, His life cut short in untimely way. The men of Brown threw him in, He swore to God he could not swim. Alas for us, we let a sigh, Dear ol' Mel never told a lie."

"Dear ol' Mel can't swim," said one disgruntled resident. "We've threatened to throw him in the water, but he said he would take action against anyone who did."

The students hope that the "deceased" will reevaluate his methods in the future. By reevaluating his ways, the students feel he will become a latter-day Lazarus.

and terribly egotistical. I hope he learned something about human nature from that experience, and that he became a nicer guy and had a brilliant career. He undoubtedly had the brains, and hopefully his time at Brown Hall taught him a little about matters of the heart.

In each of our lives, there are incidents or events that in retrospect we might label as life changing. It's like driving down the smoothest new freeway of life, in cruise control when, without warning, you hit a giant unseen pothole. The impact not only jars springs and shocks, but sometimes the wheels come completely off your limousine. The spring of 1961 was such a time for me, and it began innocently in Sociology 101 in the Old Main building. After almost two years of academic success as a Saluki, a riotous social life, and complete reconstruction of my self-confidence and ego, I signed up for a five-unit class in Introductory Sociology that met M-F at 2:00 P.M. It was a relatively easy class, not too stimulating, and by Friday it was tough to sit through another fifty-minute lecture. But the prospect of an easy grade was a draw. The very first class, a blonde gal in a wheelchair sashayed (and that's hard to do in a wheelchair) into the room with a tall, willowy blonde walking at her side. I quickly began to move over to give them space to sit, as students in wheelchairs were parked in the corners of the classrooms at the front or rear of the room. Well, they both kind of smirked and wheeled/strolled right on by me to the opposite front corner of the room. Oh, I thought, a couple of wise guys.

The class was also filled with jocks, which usually indicated a course that would translate into an easy C. The instructor, an athletic young fellow, had been a track star, but unlike the two mystery broads, was very approachable. I had become a hard-core athletic groupie and knew many of the campus athletes across all sports. It didn't take long for me to get to know a number of guys in the class, and within a matter of weeks, I was tutoring several of them, including a lanky wide receiver who went by the name "Bonnie." He was a prototype split end, 6-3, with great speed, large hands, and long, slender arms and fingers; he had the makings of an All-American. Unfortunately, while he caught everything in practice, in game situations, wide-open, he would frequently drop a critical pass. It was as if his hands had been sprayed with silicone lubricant—the ball slid right through. It was a psychological thing with him, a lack of confidence and concentration. In our tutoring sessions, I got to know him quite well, and it became clear that the dynamics of his life and experiences as an African American were inextricably interwoven with his performance as an athlete. He was a powerfully built handsome fellow, but he had a fragile and bruised soul.

The class was easy for me, and I had made a deal with the instructor to do pro-bono tutoring in exchange for him allowing me to skip Friday classes to attend University track meets. While I missed the majority of the Friday afternoon classes, I rarely missed the other four class periods. I have to admit I found myself looking forward to the class and seeing the two still-unidentified blondes. They must have guessed my interest, and no matter what technique I employed to learn their names, they foiled all my initiates. They smiled, said "Hi," and sometimes even, "How are you?" but never stopped to chat. The more I schemed to get their names, the more elusive and evasive they became. I tried to fake them out by offering to read their test scores that were posted by initials after the first exam. I managed to get the initials M.S. and S.H. out of them, but no names. I finally gave up trying to learn their names, and sometime after they made a point of introducing themselves, Marlys Sternberg and Sue Hackley.

We began a sometimes ragged, unorthodox relationship, which eventually became a friendship and ultimately led to the abandonment of my bachelorhood.

They vacillated between being sweet, charming and oh-so-friendly to being aloof, exasperating, and beyond smart aleck—approaching the smart-ass level. Every time we had a quiz or exam, they feigned despair that they had probably flunked. But when the grades came out they would giggle, roll their eyes, and exclaim almost breathlessly, "Oh, my, I didn't expect another A!" They were masters at agitation, and by the end of the quarter, I had had enough of them jerking me around. I had a B average going into the final and they both had A's.

I became obsessed with besting them. I had to at least match them with an A for the course. I spent hours studying for the final; I memorized the textbook we used for the class, my notes, and notes I'd borrowed from others as well. Never before, in my entire college career, was I so well prepared for an examination. And then fortune smiled on me. Marlys and Sue, while studying at the library, picked up, or were picked up by some guys, and they went drinking. It was the night before the final exam, and they got home late, their minds blurry. They must have been foggy for the 8:00 A.M. exam, and I expect they bombed the test, because they both dropped to B's. I'm not sure that I missed a single question, and gloriously, I got an A. It was sweet revenge.

Even to this day, Marlys and her buddy Sue accuse me of some kind of collusion with the instructor. They insist that I had forehand knowledge of questions, or even a copy of the exam. They theorize that either the instructor or a somewhat disreputable friend of mine who was a clerk typist in the sociology department had filched the exam for me. But none of those accusations were true. I simply smoked them, fair and square.

I went home for the summer to rejoin old high school buddies for drinking, softball games, fishing, and all the usual pursuits. While the summer was a carefree respite from school, I frequently found myself thinking of those two gals, one tall, one short, the latter with smiling blue eyes and an intriguing and sometimes sinful-sounding laugh. I began to count the days until fall semester 1961 and wondered if they would be there.

Well, the two blondes, Sue Hackley and Marlys Sternberg, were both on campus when I arrived, and were even haughtier than last year. So, too, had many of the old Brown Hall gang returned, with some new faces peppering the crowd. With two good years under my belt, I was pretty cocky and ready for a good time. I arrived on the campus, my usual rotund self. For some strange reason, it suddenly occurred to me that I needed to lose some weight. I can't imagine why. I told no one of my plan, but committed to becoming slim and svelte. I gave up sweets, second helpings, and a variety of fattening foods,

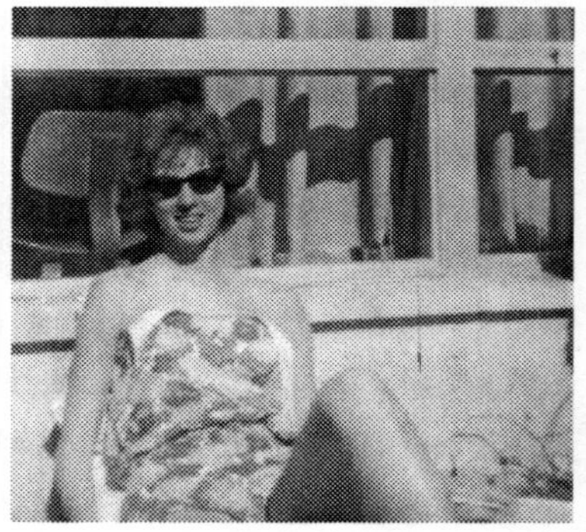

Sue (Hackley) Poppaw catching some sun at Steagall Hall. A college buddy and my manuscript typist. (1962)

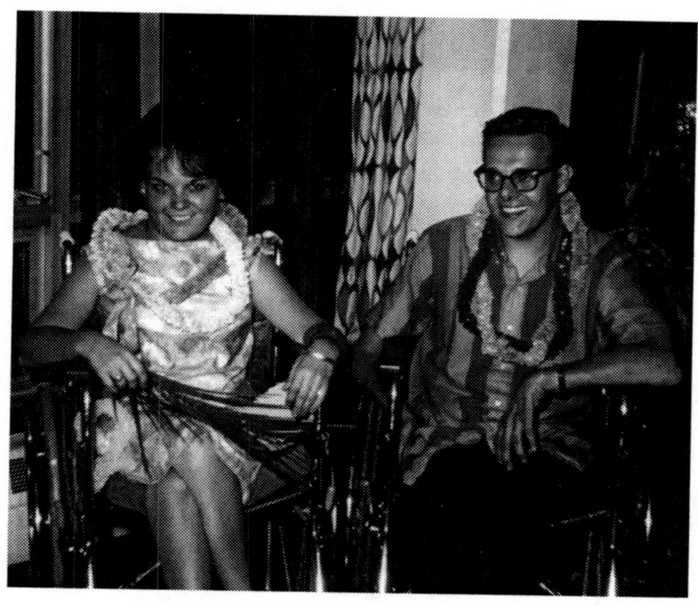

A "foxy" gal (Marlys) and me at a Brown Hall luau (1962)

but NOT beer or alcohol. No reason to go overboard on the matter. By the next spring, I had lost probably fifty pounds

The school year 1961-62 was a fun-filled year. I tried very hard to not be obvious about my interest in what Marlys and Sue were doing. Two of my best buddies were Lloyd Dinkelman and Don Hequembourg. We were known as "Heq, Dink, and Klop." We ate, went to movies, sporting events, and played cards together. During the same period, a rather large loosely connected group of guys and gals began to hang around and party together, and Lloyd, Heq, and I became a part of the mix. There were smaller sub-sets of the larger group, and each sub-group usually included the same people. Whenever there were both men and women involved, invariably I was there, as, more often than not, were Sue and Marlys. There was a mix of people with disabilities and non-disabled individuals. Unlike at Illinois, however, where we were so conscious of being either an AB or a gimp in the group, disability was never a focus.

A truly unforgettable Hawaiian fellow named Al Naukanna was

the leader of one of the sub-sets. His torso had been nearly cut in two in a dock accident, but miraculously he had survived. A longshoreman, he had traveled the world, and his phone rang regularly with calls from India, England, Japan, and remote Pacific Islands. Al loved the ladies and in turn, they rapidly succumbed to his charm and swarthy good looks. His parties always included a good number of gimpers—me, Marlys, her friend Peggy, Marv, Jim P. and others. Usually four or five non-disabled folks were also in attendance. Al was a personal friend of Dave Brubeck of "Take Five" fame, and one night he let me chat with Dave on the phone.

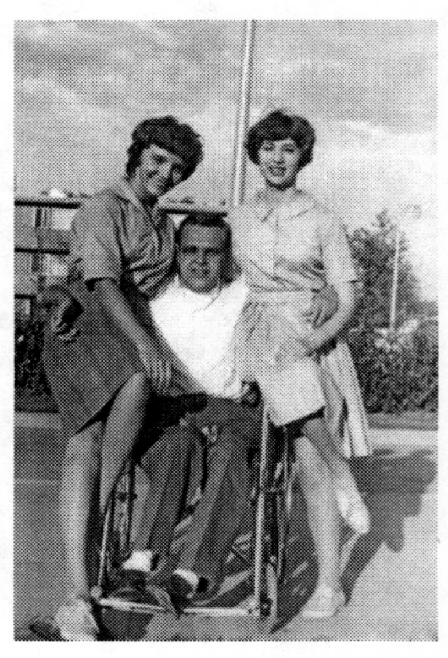

Wow, a lot of woman! Sally Metzlaars, Lucy Klaus, and lucky me (1962)

Yoshimichi Ueno, a tall tan charming fellow from Japan, is another memorable fellow that I still correspond with, at least yearly. He was a graduate student in International Relations and I'd guess, was an extremely bright guy. He crossed cultures easier than anyone I ever met. We became great friends and drinking buddies, and spent hours discussing politics, religion, cultures, families, history, honor and integrity—every topic one could imagine. I explained every idiom, slang

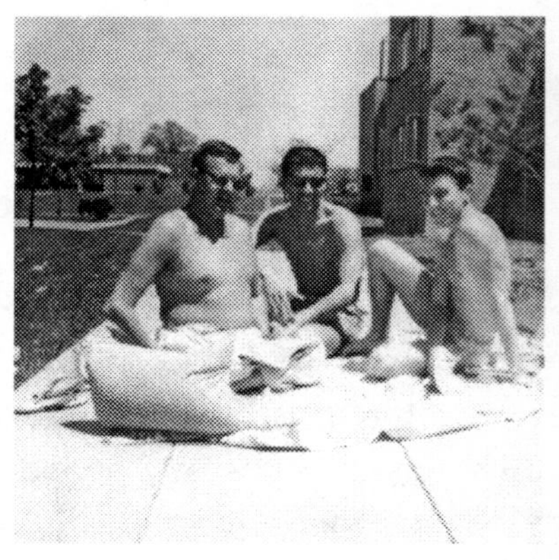

The backyard of our resort-like community; tough times in college. Yoshimichi Ueno, Lloyd Dinkelman, and me (1962)

word, and colloquialism he brought to me. Our best work was done drinking beer or sake, and when Yoshi finally understood a word I'd been trying to explain, we raised our glasses in a grand salute and exclaimed, Kampi! "Beating around the bush" was a tough one for Yoshi, but he was a quick learner. He visited my home on numerous occasions, and was much admired by both my family and the community where I lived.

A favorite local college bar in Carbondale was the Rumpus Room. It really began to jump late Friday afternoons. Carbondale had a strong Southern Baptist influence and thus, dancing was not allowed in public places. But by 7:00 or 8:00 P.M. on Friday night, the entire place was rocking. One typical Friday, Charlie Brown and I were enjoying the festivities and happened upon two fellow collegians, Dave and Jerry. They lived at Thompson Point and both happened to be blind—Dave from birth, and Jerry as the result of an accident with firecrackers when he was about fifteen years old. They were first-rate partiers and they could really sop up the suds. Well, this particular evening Charlie, Jerry, Dave, and I were to become fast friends. The action slowed at the bar so we left, but we were not ready to go home. We considered our options and came up with Carterville, a town due east, and a dive called Skinheads.

Jerry mentioned off-hand, "Well, let's go."

"Hey man," asked Charlie, "where do we get wheels?"

Jerry replied, "No problem I have one parked about two blocks from here." It seemed odd that a blind guy would have a car, but in his small rural Iowa hometown, he drove regularly with his younger brother as his pilot (eyes).

"I'll drive," chirped Jerry. And he did, about ten miles on the main highway east of town with Charlie as co-pilot, describing the roadway to him. He was amazingly adept at interpreting Charlie's directions into a smooth ride to Skinheads. He did pull one stunt that panicked everyone in the car. At the last stoplight going out of Carbondale, one of Carbondale's city police cars pulled along side to our left. Charlie warned Jerry to be careful and not arouse suspicion.

Jerry asked, "What are they doing, Charlie?"

"Jesus Christ, Jerry, they're looking at you."

"Really?" he smiled, and turned his face to the two policemen in the car, smiled and waved.

"For God's sake..." Charlie sucked in his breath. The cops grinned, waved back, and made a left turn as the light changed.

Amazing as his skills were, we didn't let Jerry drive the return trip home. He was too drunk. One might say he was blind drunk. Charlie drove home safely and helped dump me in bed. It was a warm evening, and lying in bed my head began to swim and my stomach began to churn. I got up, threw a pair of slacks on, and headed out for some fresh air in Thompson Point woods. The result was the following headline and article that appeared in the next morning's student newspaper.

Student Injured

Wheel Chair Crashes

A Southern Illinois University student was knocked unconscious when his wheel chair overturned early Saturday in Thompson Point woods.

Admitted to Doctors Hospital, Carbondale, for observation was Kent Kloepping, a freshman from Juda, Wis.

SIU Security Officer Tom Leffler said Kloepping's wheel chair ran off of a small bridge at the bottom of a hill in the woods about 1:35 a.m.

The wheel chair students often allow the chairs to coast down the hills.

Fireman Elmer Rodgers who took Kloepping to the hospital in the emergency truck said he apparently landed head first. Kloepping was found by another student, Bill Sulheimer. Leffler said he apparently had not been there very long.

Doctors Hospital officials said Kloepping was in good condition. He was to have been released Saturday.

Kloepping reported he had decided to get some exercise and took off through the Thompson Point Woods in his wheel chair.

Blacktop walks are providel for students through the woods. Kloepping lives at Browne Hall, Thompson Point, southwest of the woods.

It was kind of embarrassing, really. I learned at a later time that my future in-laws, on their first visit to Southern, heard the story of the student crashing his wheelchair. Future son-in-law? It was probably good that we didn't meet until a later date.

The spring semester, 1962, ended more rapidly than I wanted, but shortly before the term ended I learned Sue and Marlys were going to summer school. Well, I soon discovered I could use the additional credits, so I signed up to room with Don Hequembourg in Southern's tarpaper jungle, Chautauqua. Unbelievably, at the end of the spring semester, my father arrived in Carbondale to take Yoshi and me home in a brand-new, 62 Chevy two-door hardtop, with hand controls.

"What is this?" I stammered.

"It's yours." The stars had aligned, and my fate and future was sealed.

The summer school session was five weeks long, and ended around mid-July. I signed up for two classes, with the last class session on Thursday morning of each week. This meant I had almost four days before my next class the following Monday. How fortuitous. I had arrived back on campus for the start of summer school in my brand new 1962 white Chevrolet Impala coupe with a robin egg blue interior. Listening to the "oohs" and "ahhs" from the boys and more importantly the ladies at the other end of the barracks, I began to feel quite studly. Yes, I thought, this sleek, shiny little machine might turn out to be more than just transportation. My timidity barometer in approaching women immediately began to sink quite rapidly.

My roommates for the summer were Heq, another guy in a wheelchair (I can't recall his name) and his attendant, a young dude named Bill B. We lived on the north end apartment of a Chautauqua barracks with a single girl in the middle unit and Sue, Marlys, and two other gals in the apartment on the south end. The young woman in the middle, Nancy, was a very friendly, attractive girl in a wheelchair. She was rarely home and when she left—day or night—she was always dressed very nicely and painted up like she was heading for a party. We guys decided she was a handicapped hooker, but none of us had the courage to investigate further. She didn't go to classes, and her lifestyle and activities remained mostly unknown.

Chautauqua was a large collection of these barracks/shacks, and during the regular semesters, many married students lived there. I didn't know where the word Chautauqua came from, but I looked it up, and I learned from *Webster's' Third New International Dictionary*, that the definition was, "a traveling or stationary institution that flourished in the late 19th and early 20th centuries, providing popular education usually combined with entertainment in the form of lectures, concerts, or dramatic performances often presented outdoors or in a tent." Someone named Lancaster Rollard said, "It is no more, its place taken by the radio everywhere."

Reflecting back on that summer, a whole bunch of us (including us four guys and the four girls in our barracks) were usually in attendance at whatever Chautauqua event was happening. Yes, our summer of activities definitely fit the criteria for a Chautauqua; we were sometimes stationary, often traveled, education was in the form of classes attended (minimal), no concerts as I recall, and lectures mostly extemporaneous rambling pontification induced by too much alcohol. These presenters had no credentials to speak on their selected topics, but it didn't matter since the listeners never took notes and could remember very little of what was said by the next morning. Many events were out-of-doors, at the lake, and around a campfire with no tents. Often, there was lots of singing toward the end of the festivities. I have to admit our Chautauqua events were light on education and heavy on entertainment. My Chevy, of course, was the key to the entire summer. I went all over southern Illinois visiting college friends who were not in summer school, and hauling loads of revelers to party locations.

During that Chautauqua Summer of 1962, we sometimes engaged in some foolhardy and reckless behavior. A late fall excursion to Cairo, Illinois was likely one of the most stupid things Marlys, Peggy, and I ever did. Recall old Jim P., reformed racist, former free speech advocate? Well, he had again reinvented himself and had become a fanatical civil rights proponent. He was literally hiding out in the black community of Cairo, Illinois, a town with an abysmal record of civil rights abuses, where black folks lived in one part of town and white folks in the other. Tensions were extremely high in the town, and aroused segregationists fought any and every initiative towards integration. In 1962, there were many folks in the city who could remember a time when a black man was lynched and his body left hanging at the gates of the city for several days.

Unthinking, we had decided to look Jim up in Cairo; we had to drive around barricades into the black section of town, three honkies in a bright new white car. In rather short order we were confronted by a group of grim-faced "brothers" who not-too-politely asked our business. We finally convinced them we were friends of Jim's and sure enough, four big strong guys hauled him out of a house in his wheelchair. "You idiot, Kloepping," Jim sputtered, "You're damn lucky you didn't get shot coming in here, and further you'll be lucky if someone doesn't 'plink you' on the way out." We had a rather abbreviated visit as he was known as a white rabble-rouser in the Cairo community, and didn't like being out in public. We finally realized how stupid we were to nonchalantly drive into the heart of potential disaster, and as I recall, we left town a whole lot faster than we arrived.

Marlys and I began to date, mostly because (I told her) I thought she liked my wheels. We'd often double date, sometimes with two other gimpers. Now, with four wheelchair users in one car, all the wheelchairs stayed home which meant we went to the drive-in movies, a drive-in restaurant, and a drive-in liquor store if we needed alcohol. If we had car trouble and happened to be at the lake smooching, we had to wait for someone to drive up and find us. We often had Marv and Peggy along on our dates. If we did end up at the lake under a

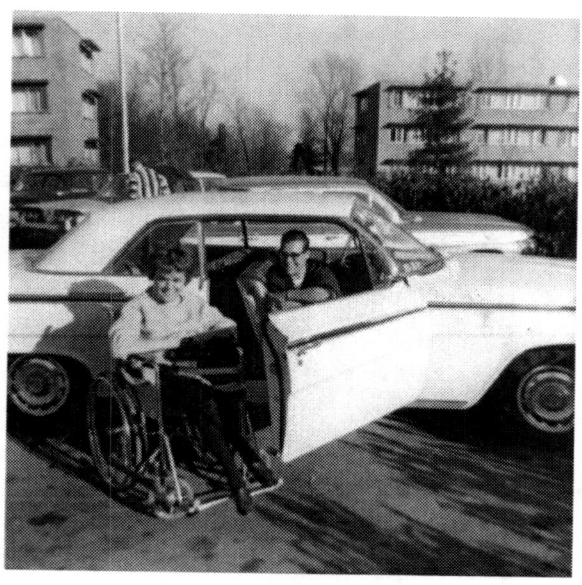

Our wonderful '62 Chevy (1962)

full moon, all Marlys and I got was sore sides from laughing at all the thrashing in the back seat. Marv reputedly had the fastest hands in the West, but Peggy was faster. One night after thirty to forty-five minutes of hand sparring in the back seat, Marv laughed aloud and exclaimed in frustration, "Christ Peggy, I swear you have hands growing on your ass!" Marlys and I were hysterical with laughter.

I'm not sure how much one should recount about the details of courtship, but it wasn't too long before I figured out I had met my life partner in Marlys. What really clinched the deal was probably my first introduction to her family—in particular, her father and mother, Walter and Lydia Sternberg, and her grandmother, Caroline Niemeier—from the great state of Minn-e-so-tah (emphasis on the so).

Walter, my father-in-law, was a bright old purebred German and proud of his heritage, like his entire Gopher State family. Now, I've not seen any of them goose-step to work, and they don't claim lineage to old Kaiser Willy, but they are genuine Kraut, with a few Danes mixed in for flavor. I'm convinced that if every family in America had the work ethic, family values, intelligence, and generosity of these folks and my Illinois family, our country would be basically problem-free. Make no mistake—I haven't found any saints among the group, but as adults, they all get over the hell raising, settle down, marry and become solid citizens.

Walter wrote and spoke fluent German (high) and was also an extremely capable fellow. He was very organized, methodical, and independent in his thought processes and approach to life. He took his time, pondered issues carefully, and once he had reached a conclusion regarding a matter, I doubt one could change his mind. He was a conservative problem-solver; he knew how to fix his machinery, knew when a car or tractor had worn out and immediately sold it. He was cautious, but was able to accumulate a large amount of land by recognizing the right time and price to buy. He established consistently effective routines and had the ability to not vary his approach to daily activities. He was a true German original. Two dominant characteristics that he exhibited, a high level of intelligence and purposeful self-direction, are clearly evident in his following generations.

My mother-in-law Lydia, one of Grandma Niemeier's four daughters, also had four daughters. Marlys, the youngest, is my wife. Lydia was a wonderful cook, and anything she made tasted special. She wasn't fancy about her cooking and didn't try gourmet dishes, but her rice pudding was legendary. All her daughters also make it, and while it's good, it's never as good as Lydia's. She was a quiet, thoughtful, soft-spoken woman who was quite intelligent and always well informed on current events, though I never heard her argue an issue. She was a keen observer of behavior, and never missed or misinterpreted family dynamics.

Grandmother Caroline Niemeier was the stereotypical German Grossmutter. The first time we met she told me, "I came to Minnesota as a sickly child, but here I became a strong, healthy woman. We had come from Germany to Illinois when I was ten, and I was not well. Then we went west to the prairies of Minnesota, homesteaded, and I was always healthy after that." At that first meeting, she quizzed me about my heritage, and liked the fact that I was mostly German. When she realized I couldn't speak duetsch, she began to interject German words and phrases into our conversations. My puzzled looks brought chuckles from the rest of the German speaking family. Her eyes twinkled, her pleasant face wrinkled as she smiled gently, always communicating a bit of approval. Each time we parted, she would gently squeeze my hand, pat my arm, and say in a near-whisper, "Auf wiedersehen," and then ask, "Can you say that?" She was a dear, grand little lady, and our Tucson German buddy, Carol Helnholz told us the Germans use a special term of endearment, Oma, for such a grandmother.

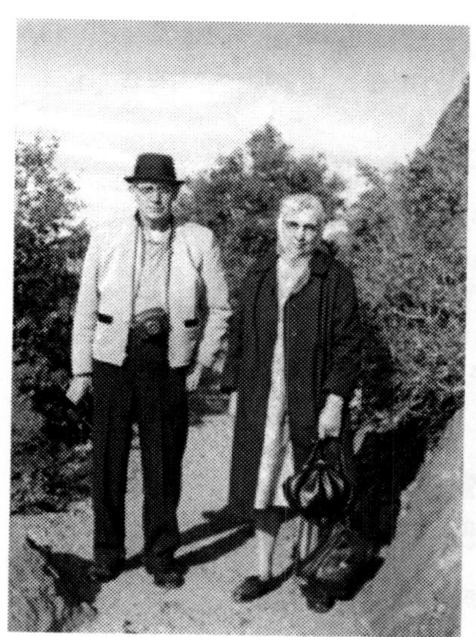

Marlys's parents, Walter and Lydia Sternberg, visiting us in California (1967)

By the end of summer, I knew that I wanted to marry this lass from Minnesota. I thought she was really cute, bright, and never gave me an inch. I had met my match. It was hard to leave summer school, but upon returning for the fall semester 1962, we became inseparable, eventually becoming engaged in February of 1963.

In the spring of 1963, I was accepted into the Masters' program in Rehabilitation Counseling for the fall of 1963. We set a wedding date of September 7, 1963. Our wedding was to be in Minnesota in the Missouri Synod Church; hence, I took instruction in Carbondale to become a card-carrying Lutheran. Previously I had infrequently attended the United Methodist Church, a church that, among some hard-core Lutherans, was viewed as a sort of Christian fringe group. Sue Hackley, our buddy in all the past years shenanigans, was to be in our wedding that fall. She had taken a job at Flaming Gorge Resort in Utah, for the summer, and there had met a handsome fellow named Bob Poppaw. She suddenly developed other priorities and didn't make our wedding. In retrospect, it's lucky she concentrated on the guy at hand. Forty years later, we have renewed our friendship with Bob and Sue.

Reverend Arthur Drevelow, who married us, was an ultra-conservative pastor of the small rural congregation of St. John's Lutheran Church in South Branch, Minnesota. Arthur had a Ph.D. in theology

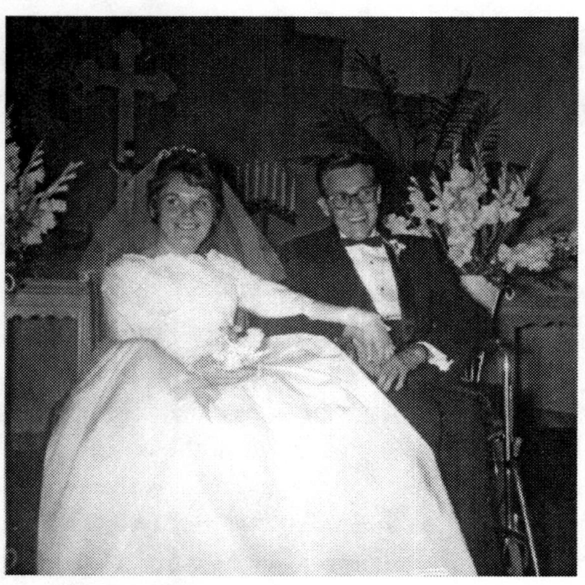

Wedding day, St. John's Lutheran Church, South Branch, Minnesota (September 7, 1963)

and was an extremely bright man. We took an abbreviated weeklong wedding trip to northern Minnesota, cut short when Marlys caught a terrible cold, which she always did when she was stressed. A highlight of the trip for me was sitting on the ground, straddling the source of the Mississippi River in Itasca State Park, and admittedly contributing to the fouled river's pollution problems by taking a whiz in the pristine little stream.

We moved into student housing at Southern Hills, next to also newlyweds Bob and Judy Adams, and I began my two-year graduate studies program in Rehabilitation Counseling. We were officially poverty stricken, with a total income of $180.00 a month. Dad paid our car insurance, but rent (I think $95.00) and all other expenses came out of the $180.00. We were too dumb to understand how poor we were. It's possible that marriage and the exuberance of youth clouded our perceptions of all the calamities that could befall us. We really had many good times being impoverished, and always had enough money for the necessities, plus a little entertainment now and then.

Bob, our next-door neighbor, had broken his neck at a fraternity swim party at Colorado State University his sophomore year. He married his high school sweetheart and was fanatical about not having anyone lift a finger to help him. He would sometimes struggle twenty minutes or more getting his heavy manual wheelchair into his car. Several years earlier, he and I were caught in a driving rainstorm on campus and two young coeds raced to our assistance. Bob literally screamed at the astonished girl, cussing her for daring to touch his wheelchair. We left him struggling in the rain while his would-be Samaritan sobbed over a Coke as my helper and I tried to console her. Old Bob was hard core, no exceptions. He never accepted help.

The graduate program in Rehabilitation Counseling was unlike anything I could have imagined. First of all, my classmates were a strange lot. Dan, an older guy who was legally blind with travel vision, was a Freudian who wanted to do an analysis on every comment made. A single good morning could get him going. Mike, a rotund young fellow, adopted every cliché ever written in psychological jargon. "I can't handle that data," was his favorite line. Allen, totally blind, was a bright guy, but I think his primary goal was to use his training to refine his technique for seducing women. Dorothy, also blind, was lost most of the time. If you surprised her when you said hello, she got disoriented. She was the worst blind traveler I ever met. Bill and Norma English, who were to become lifelong friends, were probably two of the most normal of the group. However, in deference to our friendship, I won't detail any of Bill's idiosyncrasies. Norma was solid as a rock. Then there was me. While I think I did inherit some schizophrenic tendencies, in my defense, I had to struggle with the Missouri Synod Lutherans on one hand and the philosophy of Carl Rogers on the other.

Guy Renzaglia, the program director, was a brilliant therapist. He was actually scary in his ability to discern your most private thoughts and expose the most closely guarded black secrets in one's soul. Weekly, he psychologically annihilated one or more of the pretenders in our group-counseling practicum. Faculty member Robert E. Lee, of Chinese and Irish descent, was a great guy. He allegedly had fifty sport coats. Ernie Doleys was a statistical wizard whose Ph.D. dissertation was only nine pages long. My advisor, Phil Caracena, was the most non-transparent person I ever met. I never had a clue as to his thought processes or thinking.

The program was not easy or comfortable. We were expected to undertake and engage in a process of critical self-examination and be candid in our critiques of our fellow budding counselors, pointing out value-laden thinking that could be counter-productive to the clients whom we were attempting to help to understand their own feelings and thoughts. The counseling practicums got intense and sometimes quite upsetting. But just when our stress levels were highest, there were moments of comic relief. Dorothy would get lost in a broom closet, or Dan would go off on a Freudian analysis of a newscast, or Allen would detail one of his hitchhiking stories. Although totally blind, he'd get dropped off on a highway and hitchhike. One time a cabbie ran over his foot. Allen used his foot to feel how far he was off the pavement, and when the cabbie stopped and backed up, Allen proceeded to whale away on the guy's car with his cane.

Playing bridge with Bill and Norma English also helped keep us sane. We'd buy a gallon of cheap Stag beer, in a tin can that was painted to look like a wooden barrel, and play all night. We'd often break up at 6:00 A.M., eat breakfast, and head for class.

It was a challenging time for me, a newlywed being confronted with radical new professional ideas and membership in a new church. But we had many good times, and despite the lack of money, always had what we really needed.

We never missed a Saluki basketball game. Impressively, coach Jack Hartman took mostly local talent and molded winning teams. A notable exception to local talent was Walt "Clyde" Frazier who led the Salukis to a 29-1 record one year, and later became an all-pro with the New York Knicks.

I did a three-month internship at Anna State Psychiatric hospital and learned to love the patients. There were many whose grasp on reality was far better than that of the staff. The majority of souls were legitimately several standard deviations from reality, living in strange and complex zones only they understood.

The two-year graduate program flew by, and suddenly my course work was completed. I found myself struggling with a final research paper—my masters' thesis. Unfortunately, I did not complete the thesis by the end of spring term 1965, nor during the ensuing summer session. As a result, we lost our nice apartment in Southern Hills married student housing, and ended up in another tarpaper barracks. It was similar to the Chautauqua shacks, except this was much worse. It had no heat, an uncovered broken window in the kitchen, one single bed, a rickety kitchen table, and a leftover Goodwill discard for a living room couch. Marlys typed my thesis, which, in those days, consisted of an original and four or five carbons. And remember, this was long before the advent of the personal computer. One mistake and you had to start over—no erasures or white outs were permitted on the thesis. It was a tough, depressing several weeks, with no money and no heat. Once again living in a dump, we both felt abandoned and disconnected from everything.

Marlys struggled daily, terrified to make a mistake, and I fretted, afraid I'd fail the defense of the thesis. All the while, a damn bird flew in and out of the broken windowpane. Then unexpectedly, one gloomy, windy, night we got a brief reprieve from our pity party.

There was a loud rapping on the door that scared both of us silly. Who would come to our rather secluded barracks late in evening?

"Who is it?" I asked tentatively.

"Hey, Open up. It's Parks."

"Parks, Holy cow!" It was Billy Parks, a graduate student in Special Education who had also done his internship at Anna State Hospital while I was there. What a relief and welcome sight. Bill, who was African American, had become a good friend of mine during our three-month internship at Anna State Hospital. He was a good-looking, cocky young fellow with a great heart. He was very candid about his views on politics, religion and, particularly, on the growing Civil Rights Movement, the relationships between whites and blacks, and their respective group and individual responsibilities.

Bill had grown up in a large city in a big family. He had been poor, but didn't lack any gray matter. He was a bright, astute observer of human behavior who had little time for pretense, but could be very diplomatic when the occasion demanded. He had married a black debutante from Memphis. Before I met Bill, I was not aware of the world of wealthy black society. His wife was a polished and sophisticated lady with impeccable manners; she dressed beautifully and exuded class with a capital C! I didn't much like her, and I wouldn't have been surprised to learn that her take on me was that I was somewhere close to white trash. What a contrast they were. I never did quite figure out how they ended up together. Bill had a heart of gold and a keen sensitivity to others.

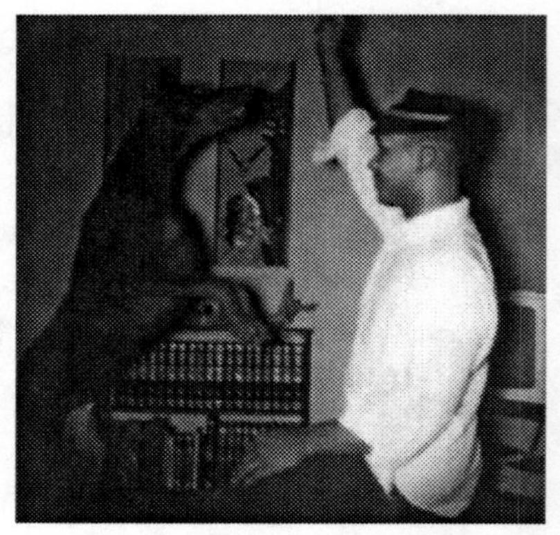

Billy Parks and his beautiful red Doberman at our apartment in Southern Hills, at Southern Illinois University (1963)

He knew Marlys and I were stuck alone in the barracks, struggling to get the thesis typed, living on our last pennies, and suffering in a really miserable situation. He had just dropped by with a bottle of wine to chat and relax. We all got a little tipsy from the wine, and at some point in the evening, we began sharing nursery rhymes—some old, some new, and some ribald variations of old classics. Bill left late, hugging us both good-bye. I haven't seen or heard from or about him in the past forty years. In recalling that late evening visit, I often feel that his visit that evening may have saved both of what remained of Marlys's and my diminishing reservoirs of mental health.

Sometime during my last year in the program, we made the decision to leave the ice and snow of the Midwest winters. Three incidents prompted us to think about the consequences of staying in the Midwest:

1) One snowy, miserably cold night, we left Carbondale to attend a Christmas party for the Rehabilitation Department at a lodge in a State Park some twenty miles south of town. The roads were icy, so we followed Bill and Norma English in their little Volkswagen. Sure as hell, we slipped in the ditch, our 62 Chevy spinning crazily out of control on the slippery, snow-covered road. When Bill and Norma noticed we were no longer following them, they came back looking for us. "Now what the hell do we do," I asked? " We have four people, two wheelchairs, and one small VW."

Bill said, "Don't sweat it. We'll get you in."

I skeptically answered, "No way."

But he insisted. "Come on, let me handle this."

I still don't understand how the four of us, plus the two wheelchairs, fit in that bug. We had a great time at the party and picked up the car the next day, but it made us begin to think seriously about the implications of the two of us living and driving in a climate that regularly had ice and snow.

2) We were to get two more doses of reality during that winter holiday school break. We went to Minnesota and Illinois for Christmas. The trip up through Iowa was beautiful, sunny, and dry. However, during the four hundred mile return trip from Minnesota to Illinois, we had twenty-five miles of bright sunshine, followed by a howling blizzard that accompanied us for the next three hundred seventy-five miles. We made it home about sixteen hours later, aver-

aging about twenty-five miles per hour. We were exhausted and more than a bit shaken.

3) Then on the final leg of the trip from northern Illinois, another four hundred miles south to Carbondale, we were again about thirty miles down the road when the snow began to fall. It became a blizzard, with huge amounts of snow, wind, and bitter cold. About one hundred-fifty miles south, near Bloomington, Illinois, we pulled off the highway to eat a sandwich and drink hot coffee from the thermos we had along.

Unthinking, I drove about a mile down the secondary road—and out of sight of highway #51. When we finished our snack, I turned the key in the ignition and nothing happened. The battery was completely gone. The snow depth outside was a foot or more, and it was still snowing heavily with visibility less than fifty feet, and there was no one on the road but us. We both realized we were in serious trouble. I know the thought crossed my mind that in a few days' local headlines might report that two disabled people were found frozen in their car. Suddenly, through the swirling snow, a slow-moving black shape emerged from the grayness. It was the front of a pick-up. As the well-used, worn old truck crept into full view, I opened my door and jumped/fell out into the snow, waving my arms frantically. The driver, a grizzled old farmer, stopped, got out, and looked at me with a mixture of disbelief and confusion. It was difficult to communicate with the wind howling and his hearing loss, but I conveyed to him the desperation of our situation. "I'll send back the wrecker from the garage in town." he said. Some thirty minutes later, the tow truck arrived and hauled us to the garage. It was Sunday, and not until late in the afternoon did they locate a new battery. We limped home, arriving in Carbondale late that evening. We made the decision in the next few days to follow Horace Greeley's time-honored advice, to go west. We did just that in October of 1965, moving to California, where the sun mostly shines and the snow mostly stays in the mountains.

Postscript

Six magnificent, fun- filled, meaningful years at Southern Illinois University will ensure that I will forever be a Saluki.

First of all, I relearned that I didn't have to pretend I wasn't disabled and never needed assistance. Disabled folks at this school were merely other students, not super crips; we were not isolated or segregated, and our peers treated us like we were normal individuals who happened to have some limitations. I probably had more fun in those years than I've had since or will ever have again. I touched only briefly on some of the antics that my dorm mates and I engaged in while we lived in Brown Hall. For two of those years, our behavior (particularly the first floor guys) was at times pretty outrageous. We weren't quite as outlandish as the boys in the movie *Animal House,* but given another year together and we might have made it.

By the time I left Southern, I had reacquired many things I thought I'd lost. My self-worth and self-confidence had been restored, I had learned about leadership, I had successfully challenged authority when things needed to change, and I had made many lifelong friendships. But among my most prized new riches, were my WIFE, my DEGREES, my MEMORIES, and my new CAR.

I think that's the right order.

IX. The Road West: To Find A Job.

Opportunity is missed by most people because it comes dressed in overalls and looks like work. (1)

"Well, Kloepping, are you getting dangerously close to finding work?" Frank Silva, my brother-in-law had just arrived home from the day shift at Corning Ware Glass Company and had settled into his favorite chair. From behind the San Jose Mercury newspaper, which he held in front of himself (to hide his facial expression I think), he had asked me the pointed question concerning my sometimes-lackadaisical job search.

Marlys and I had been staying with my sister, Carol, her husband, Frank (Ignacio) Silva, and one-year-old Richard since we arrived in the Golden Gate State in early November, 1965. Four or five weeks later, we were still houseguests and my search for that elusive first job had not yet been fruitful. Frank had a well-developed, wry sense of humor with a great sense of timing. I'm not sure that he said hello when he walked in the door that afternoon, but the intent of the question was clear, pointed, and hit my job-seeking starter button with about two hundred volts. Later that evening, I laughed when I told Marlys about the query, but it did get me serious about finding employment. Carol, nine days short of being one year older than me, had gone to California in 1961 looking for work as well as, I always figured, a husband. She was an R.N. and easily obtained a good job—as well as a husband named Frank.

Marlys and I left Minnesota at the end of October of 1965. I was newly armed with a masters' degree in Rehabilitation Counseling and Marlys with a B.A. in Speech Pathology. We both were filled with excitement and unspoken trepidations about truly being on our own. We loaded all our worldly possessions into the trunk of our 1962 Chevrolet, and with both wheelchairs in the back seat of the sporty two-door hardtop, headed west for California. Neither of us had jobs, not even a prospect, but our destination was 425 Cypress Avenue, San Jose, California—the home of Carol and Frank Silva. That was to be our base of operations for a brief period while we got settled and found jobs and a home.

The trip to California took five days, and for two individuals in wheelchairs, it was sometimes quite an adventure. There were few motels that didn't have steps to the front entrance, and once inside the room, a common space-saving aspect of motel design was to cut corners on the bathrooms. Some of them were as small as a phone booth. Invariably we'd have to transfer from the wheelchair to a straight back chair (frequently we had to request one from the office), and literally scoot the damn thing across the doorsill of the bathroom to the stool and sink. Mounted mirrors were always too high (from the seated position), so we carried a small, freestanding circular one.

There were no legislative or statutory regulations requiring accessibility to buildings and facilities for the wheelchair user in 1965, so finding a usable or even accessible room was, at best, a fifty-fifty probability. After driving five hundred miles (a ten to twelve hour grind), I dreaded the routine of getting out of the car to check on accessibility of the motel we had selected. Getting in and out of the vehicle was not a simple matter of opening the driver's side or passenger's door and exiting. We both had to exit through the passenger door. The laborious process was 1) Marlys opened the door; 2) I got on my knees and leaned over the back seat and lifted her manual wheelchair out of the rear seat floor, starting it out over the door frame; 3) Marlys grabbed the chair and eased it to the ground, unfolded the chair, and transferred from the car seat to the wheelchair; (one down, one to go) 4) I got back up on my knees, reached over the seats and pulled my wheelchair off the back seat onto the floor; 5) now seated, I pulled the passenger seat forward, and while hanging between the opening, I backed my chair up and out of the floor, over the frame, and onto the ground; 6) I then folded the passenger seat back and transferred to my wheelchair. (God, it makes me tired just writing about the days of dragging those not-so-light weight manual wheelchairs in and out and out and in, again and again). We'd also developed a system that allowed Marlys to stay in the car while I got out. Rather than both of us going through the arduous process of dragging two chairs and us out of the car (and then back in again), Marlys simply slid under me to the driver's side and I was then able to get out. As we were essentially newlyweds—two years down the matrimonial path—Marlys invariably took advantage of my awkward position while sliding over her by grabbing whatever was hanging loose or getting in a payback goose.

I wish I had kept a journal of the trip. I can't recall anything of our first three days on the road. I know that we probably drove through Nebraska on our way south, and in fact I think we stayed in Salina, Kansas the first night. Then we continued south to highway # 40 to avoid the possibility of snow. Because we took that route, we missed the opportunity to meet some family that we would not get to know until eighteen years later.

I knew that we had relatives, Kloeppings, who lived in Nebraska around the Cozad-Lexington area. My grandparents (Dan and Della Kloepping) used to go out west to visit, but by the time I was old enough to remember, most of the visits had stopped. Then I met Mary, a young Kloepping woman, at my parents' fiftieth wedding celebration in 1982. Her husband was a physician in northern Wisconsin. Mary, the only girl among six siblings, was the daughter of Warren and Anna Jewel Kloepping (Dad's second cousin) from Cozad, Nebraska. That meeting, subsequently, led to regular visits at the home of Warren and Aunt Jewel as Marlys and I were making our annual trek to the Midwest to visit our respective families in Illinois and Minnesota.

A great disappointment in my life is that I didn't get to know Warren and Anna Jewel much earlier. We met the entire family for the first time around 1983, on our way back to Tucson from a summer visit to Minnesota. We parked our motor home in the driveway of their farmstead between Cozad and Lexington, Nebraska, and stayed a couple of nights. We liked them immediately, and since that first meeting, they have become two of my favorite people. They are another couple that Tom Brokaw missed in his book *The Greatest Generation*. They worked hard, raised a great family, and Warren served in World War II. They are bright people with great wisdom and loyalty to family, with an almost intuitive sense of what is really important in life. On one of our first visits, they took us out for pizza at Johnson Lake.

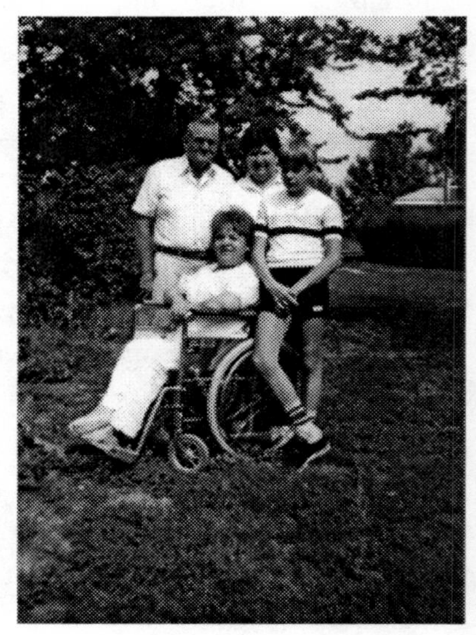

Warren and Anna Jewell Kloepping, Marlys, and Matthew. Cozad, Nebraska (1984)

I wasn't sure about what to drink (gosh, a beer sounded good) and I stammered, "Well, Warren, shall we have a beer?"

He recognized my hesitancy and with his infectious smile and twinkling eyes replied, "Why sure, and maybe more than one!" I know my wife feels as much affection for them as I do. I've often thought to myself, if my parents weren't my parents, I'd want those two, Anna Jewel and "Red."

Once we got to #40, which was originally much of the fabled old Route # 66, we continued west until Kingman, Arizona, where we headed north for a quick detour to Sin City—Las Vegas. With no written record of the trip, most of the events of the five days are forgotten—with the exception of several incidents. I remember that on the third night of the trip we stayed in Gallup, New Mexico. I recall visualizing much of the countryside, especially in New Mexico, as foreboding, desolate, and bleak. I suppose my perceptions of the landscape were influenced by the fact that Marlys and I were traveling alone, two gimps heading west to an unknown future.

In retrospect, I wonder what our parents thought about Marlys and me leaving the Midwest, although neither set of parents discussed with us any concerns they may have had about us traveling alone. We had been married for two years, and prior to getting married, we had both been quite independent. A major difference at this juncture was that we were leaving the Midwest, venturing far beyond the region that had been essentially home territory, a sort of safety zone, where family could reach us in a relatively short time if we needed help. I have to believe that all four parents must have worried about all manner of calamities that could befall us, but to their credit, they did not try to dissuade us from leaving. Nor did they communicate misgivings that could have weakened our resolve to relocate to the West. In fact, to the contrary, their unfailing support and confidence in our ability to meet the challenges we faced were critically important for us. So too, did the exuberance of youth embolden us to take risks that each of us must.

Our trusty 62 Chevy was our lifeline to the world. I thought more than once about the possibility of having car trouble. What would we do if we had a major breakdown in the middle of nowhere? Those were the days before cell phones, and although many truck drivers had CB's, we didn't even have AAA emergency road service. We probably had one major credit card and a gasoline credit card. That we were both disabled and more vulnerable than the average twosome continually crept into my thinking. Of all the possible catastrophes that could have befallen us, none did. Our Chevy Impala purred like a kitten. It was a great little machine with a strong heart. It would never have failed us, and we were in its care.

Today, in my sixties, I'm not sure I could muster the courage to leave the security of the life I've built and embark on a major life change. I have become like an old dog, preferring to stay at home on familiar turf. I've become accustomed to regular meals, and my favorite tree on which to take a whiz is just a short stroll from the shade of the porch. I keep one eye partly open to keep track of all who enter my domain, and I'm a bit suspicious of those I don't recognize or who are strangers in the neighborhood. Life has a quiet rhythm. I think about and contemplate, but don't pursue, new adventures, as the thrill of the chase has past. Ultimate contentment is regularity and a warm bed. Yes I'm a lot like that old dog. But forty years ago, we were riding high on an elixir of anxiety, anticipation, and adrenaline as young dogs racing to find what was on the other side of the hill.

We left Gallup shortly after 6:00 A.M. the next morning. I think we both wanted to leave the bleak landscape of New Mexico behind us as quickly as possible. But on the way out of town, we stopped for breakfast. As I recall, it was especially tasty, the waitress was friendly, and as it was early, there were few customers. At some point in the meal, I began to experience a somewhat unsettling feeling that someone was watching me; how silly, I thought as I glanced around the cafe. Then I spotted a pair of dark eyes peering over the top of the two-way swinging door behind the counter that led into the kitchen. As I continued to stare back at the black eyes, they suddenly disappeared.

We were getting ready to leave, and again I could feel the eyes boring into my chest. I quickly glanced up and there they were, two quizzical eyes beneath a brown forehead and a black crew cut. What the hell is the problem, I wondered.

On the way to the car, I mentioned the guy to Marlys and she brushed it off with, "Don't get paranoid." We began loading into the car, me in first, fold the chair, lift it into the back floor, then on my knees and lift the chair up onto the back seat. Marlys transferred on to the seat and began to chuckle "Don't look now, but I think I see your friend from the kitchen." We were parked behind the cafe which had a hallway across the back lined with windows. As I glanced over to the cafe, there he stood—the cook. He was an Asian guy, maybe Chinese, who stared with a look of astonishment.

I said, "What the devil is he doing?"

Marlys snickered saying, "Relax, he's probably completely dumbfounded with the two of us having dropped into the cafe first thing in the morning."

He was. He didn't move from the window or attempt to hide the fact that he was taking in every aspect of us getting into the car. He was transfixed in place by the scene unfolding in front of him.

We completed our entry, and now having such an attendant spectator, we deliberately slowed down the process to ensure he caught the entire show. I started the engine, backed up slowly and as we turned to leave, we waved to our befuddled friend. He raised one arm rather limply as if all of the strength in his body was focused on his laser-like stare.

Marlys was laughing so hard she was in tears and couldn't speak. As we began to drive away, our friend stood motionless with one hand upright in a catatonic-like salute. As we pulled out of the parking lot, we looked back just as our mesmerized spectator exited out a back door and stood on a cement slab with his hands on his hips. As we headed down the road he turned away shaking his head, gesturing animatedly with both hands as if to say "I saw it, but don't believe it, and now I have to figure this out." He may not have seen many people in wheelchairs, out and about, and especially two traveling alone. In retrospect, once I knew he was watching us, I wish I had performed more for him—like rearing up the front of the wheelchair and wheeling to the car on the two back wheels (I could do that in those days). I often wondered what he concluded after seeing us. Whatever he thought, I'd wager we jarred some myths that he held about people with disabilities.

That day was to be memorable for another encounter, but this one was not at all humorous: It was sinister and unnerving. We were west of Flagstaff, Arizona, and had finally stopped laughing about our early morning cafe-encounter. We were rolling along highway #40, making good time. Again, as earlier that morning, I suddenly had an unsettling visceral feeling that literally caused me to shiver. I checked the gauges on the car, which all showed normal readings, listened attentively to the hum of the engine, which sounded fine, steered into the left lane and then back to the right lane, everything seemed normal. Then I glanced into my rearview mirror. There was a black car following a fair distance away, and I could see two individuals inside, the driver and a passenger.

Just fellow travelers I thought, but instinctively, I decided to accelerate and pull away from the following car. We had been driving probably sixty-five MPH and as our speed increased past seventy-five, it became apparent that the car was not dropping farther behind. I said nothing to Marlys and slowly accelerated past eighty MPH. The car did not fade; in fact, it appeared to close the distance between us. My heart began to beat a little faster as adrenaline began to flood into my system.

I slowed down rather rapidly and Marlys asked, "What are you doing, why did you slow down?"

"Well there's a car behind us that seems to be keeping pace with us." It frightened Marlys (me also), so we decided to get away as rapidly as possible. We were on a desolate, completely unpopulated stretch of highway with only Kingman, Arizona, on the map many miles ahead. We accelerated to ninety and finally close to one hundred MPH, near the top speed limit of the six cylinder Chevy. The ominous black car kept pace. It was an older model car, Buick or Oldsmobile as I recall, and was obviously a more powerful vehicle. We drove at this high rate of speed for probably ten to fifteen minutes and the black car kept pace. Both of us were now beginning to experience something near panic, wondering who these people were and what their intentions might be.

"Oh, maybe they're just goofing off and giving us a hard time," I said rather unconvincingly.

"Yea, and maybe they're not," whispered, Marlys.

A sign indicated a roadside rest area, and we both sighed a bit of relief at the prospect of joining other motorists and hopefully derailing our now apparent pursuers. Unfortunately there wasn't a car in the rest area. It had no facilities and only a half-mile strip of concrete with trash cans at the entrance and exit. We pulled in and stopped at the last trash can located where the strip reentered the highway. We kept the motor running with the car in drive and we waited, hoping that the now ominous black vehicle would go on past the rest area. It didn't. It pulled off onto the paved strip and stopped in the vicinity of the first trash barrel about fifty yards behind us. My heart was pounding and my mouth parched as Marlys began to cry.

"What are we going to do?" she pleaded.

"Just wait," I said, "Let's see what they do now."

The car remained motionless for a time; then, very slowly, began to creep menacingly towards us. Who was in the car, and what were their intentions? We waited and waited until the figures of two men came clearly into focus. I was sick with fear, but tried to maintain some semblance of bravado. They stopped and stared at us, the car twenty feet behind us. We waited, and could see them talking to one another, as if deciding on their next move. Then their passenger side door opened and a sleazy-looking dude wearing a sinister sneer began to slowly slither out, never taking his eyes off us.

"Jesus Christ!" I yelled, "Hang on, we're getting out of here."

I jammed the accelerator to the floor and actually threw some gravel and debris back at the car. Our valiant little Chevy seemed to sprint away as never before, and the ominous black car did not move. Whether they had a change of heart or their car's engine had stopped running, we didn't know. But we flew away out of harm's way and quickly lost sight of them. I kept the accelerator pedal pushed to the floor, and our white steed almost reached the century mark, and we never saw the black car again.

What a wonderful little car we had. We felt as if it had saved us. Dad bought it for me from John Pela's Chevrolet in Rock City, Illinois. John, who ran the Chevy dealership into his nineties, sold new cars but his specialty was a wide variety of "fix-'em-up, move-'em –out" specials (used cars, that is). He would do a minor tune-up, dab a little paint here and there, paint the tires a shiny black (even if they were bald), polish the hubcaps, perfume the interior, put on a cheap set of seat covers, and with his favorite saying, "It runs like a sewing machine," put another satisfied patron on the road, feeling they had made a really good deal.

He was a memorable old rascal who for years sponsored local fast-pitch softball teams that provided many summers of great competition under the lights in rural Rock City, Illinois. He was generous in giving to the community, but always came out ahead in his car deals. He was a talented musician who played the violin into his ninth decade. Although he remained married to the same woman, everyone suspected that he did some extracurricular "fiddling around" in addition to his scheduled musical interludes. The lady who was the object of his affection, a woman who he called his bookkeeper, lived in a city some fifteen miles distant. The relationship spanned quite a number of years and eventually, after his wife passed away, he married his paramour. He was an energetic fellow. Listening to him make that violin sing even in his advanced years, the community consensus was that old John still had a mighty lively bow.

Notwithstanding his business and personal lifestyle, he did have the best interests of the locals in his heart. The car he sold Dad was a special machine. It was the key to finding my wife and dazzling her; it endured our sometimes-tempestuous courtship; it alerted us to potential danger one dark night when a lone stalker was approaching us; and that day in Arizona alone on that desolate road it had surely delivered us from the clutches of evil.

I hope that I told Dad and Mom how much that car meant to me. Maybe they knew, for the folks buying me a car and essentially saying, "Here, this is yours—no strings attached," signaled to me their acknowledgement of my adulthood.

Growing up with a disability, there had been many things that I simply could not do. In rural farm families in the fifties, the family lived and worked as a unit. There was much to do and every member of the family had responsibilities that contributed to the economic health of the farm. I was keenly aware of my limitations, particularly as I approached and began adolescence and watched my male friends assume major work responsibilities on their farms. My parents did include me; I raked hay in the truck, drove the small C Farmall tractor for light duty fieldwork, and drove the truck around the farm, hauling materials, helping Dad build fence. So the gift of the car conveyed a powerful unspoken message for me; I, like my brother and sisters who were all recipients of their generosity, had earned their trust and a gentle blessing that I would find my way. That car, indeed, represented a milestone in my life.

But back to that day in 1965 on US #40, when those two thugs were following us. They had spooked us terribly and cast a pall over the rest of the day—a day that had begun with laughter and mirth thanks to the "Gallup Gawker." That astonished fellow had seen us with innocent and unabashed curiosity; by contrast, the two who pursued us for many miles may have sensed an opportunity to fulfill their malevolent intentions. Who could know what was in their hearts. Marlys and I learned a lesson that day. While we are all vulnerable, she and I were, in some ways, more vulnerable than most other people.

We stayed in Las Vegas that evening and engaged in some small-stakes gambling. I lost, but Marlys won a bucket full of nickels and we retired early, as we hoped to reach San Jose, California the next day. It was a drive of over six hundred miles. We left Las Vegas very early in the morning, probably around 5:30 A.M. and as we rolled down the strip and out of town, we noted a tall, powerfully built fellow in gray sweats, jogging slowly on the right side of the street. As we passed, he turned to look at us. It was the Champ, Muhammad Ali. He flashed a big smile and gave us a wave. We were both so surprised we didn't stop, which I surely would have had I had not been so taken aback. He was there for a fight with ex-champion Floyd Patterson. Ali not only won that fight, he gave Patterson a severe beating. Ali didn't knock him out, which I'd guess he intended, as he was very angry with Patterson. Patterson always referred to Ali by his given name, Cassius Clay. To the media, he would not call him Ali. All during the brutal ten round pounding, Ali taunted Patterson, repeatedly asking, "What's my name?"

We arrived in San Jose late in the afternoon. We pulled into the driveway, and wanting to surprise Carol, I slipped to the ground from the driver's side and crawled up the sidewalk, up two stairs, and rang the doorbell. When she opened the door she initially looked straight ahead and didn't see me seated on the stoop. But a bright-eyed little fellow who did see me was staring at me, eyeball to eyeball. Two prominent characteristics I noted immediately were large brown eyes and the strangest growth of hair I had ever seen—bald in front, with a circle of hair at the back and top of his head, like a permanently attached yarmulke with fringe that danced in the air as he bounced about. That was little Richard Silva, "the bouncing Brown Bandito," who is today a United Airlines pilot.

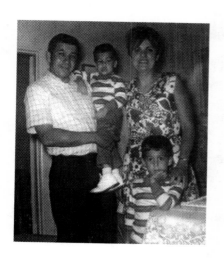

Frank, Carol, Tim, and (in front) Richard Silva. San Jose, California (1969)

My job search eventually led me to Goodwill Industries of Santa Clara County at 46 Race Street in San Jose, California. I had gotten a job offer from the State Disability Determination Office in Oakland, California, some fifty miles north of San Jose on the East Bay. I didn't relish the drive to Oakland, nor did I want to move out of the immediate area. I liked the idea of Carol, Frank, and little Richard being close. After numerous interviews I was offered a job as a vocational counselor at Goodwill, and took the position at six hundred dollars a month.

With a new job, it was time to begin searching for a place to live and allow Frank, my patient brother-in-law, to reclaim his home. Once again, we found our choices limited by the issue of wheelchair accessibility. Invariably, apartments on ground level had steps at the front door. We finally found a four-plex at 240 Richfield Dr. just off Stevens Creek Blvd. The landlord was very accommodating and built two ramps for access. One was about twelve feet long to bridge steps from the parking lot and another six-footer accessed the six-inch step at the front door. Move in was a breeze as all we had was our clothes, some toiletries, a few books, a coffee pot and some cooking utensils. We didn't stay there long, maybe a year, moving next to a duplex at 1310 White Drive in Santa Clara. Again, the new landlord had offered to build ramps, the rent was less and we were closer to Carol, Frank, and Richard.

I have two very distinct recollections of the time we lived at that 4-plex. My first memory concerns a dog named Sassy, an African Basenji, a so-called barkless dog, in whose veins flowed the courage and brashness of her ancestors who hunted lions. She was, without a doubt, one of the most intelligent dogs I had ever encountered, as well as one of the most exasperating animals I ever owned.

I also clearly remember the young couple who lived above us. They had a curly-haired little boy, and on the surface they appeared to be the perfect, all-American family. She was a stay-at-home mom and he was a policeman. She was a pretty gal, sweet and soft-spoken. Her husband was a handsome, powerfully built fellow whose mere presence in the room was intimidating. I thought he was a scary dude the first time I met him, and it didn't take long to get glimpses of the hostility and anger that seeped from a boiling cauldron in his soul.

He loved being a cop, loved his weapon, and loved his badge that gave him power over others. He began to stop in for a beer after work and invariably he would give me the rundown on his day of keeping law and order. He particularly liked to tell me about non-compliant people that he stopped. As he described the encounter, he became increasingly animated; he was a bright guy and was probably very good at escalating the level of antagonism in the situation. As he recounted the incident, his face would flush, his breathing became more rapid, and I'd swear he'd begin to salivate as he described the increasingly confrontational nature of the situation and the likelihood that he might have to draw his weapon, and even better, use it. He told me that he did have to draw the gun on several occasions, and he related the feeling of exhilaration he experienced watching the person wilt with a semi-enraged policeman towering above, brandishing a .44 MAGNUM! I believed it was only a matter of time until he used the weapon with deadly results. It actually gave me goose bumps listening to his stories. Maybe that's why we moved so quickly. Neither of us felt very comfortable with a trigger-happy gendarme living above us.

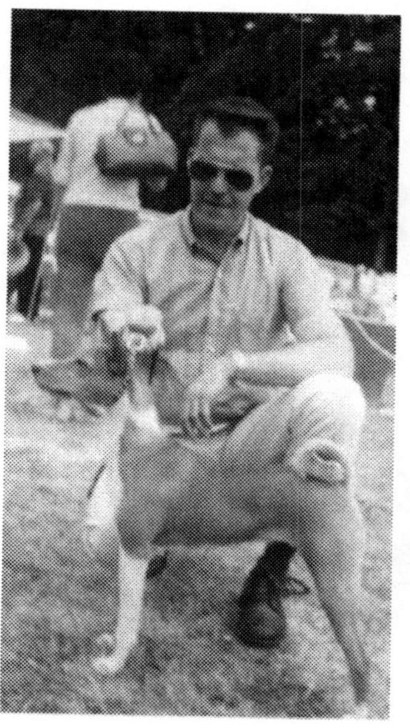

The "freeway pugilist," Ron, with our African Barkless dog, Sassy (1966)

Sassy, the Basenji, not only led us to a couple named Ron and Betty, but also the California dog show circuit. Ron was a bright guy who worked in Silicone Valley's emerging technology industry, and changed jobs anytime he didn't like something at work. He was exceptionally good at what he did, but he was also extremely rigid in his thinking. He controlled his wife, kids, and dogs like a drill sergeant and had absolute rules for running his household and affairs. He was clever and unpredictable and was prone to pulling crazy stunts, like he did one morning on our way to a dog show in Daly City, California, in the middle of six lanes of jam-packed freeway traffic. We were following Ron and Betty, and were several cars back and a few lanes over, and had stopped at a traffic light. When it turned green, several lanes did not move and horns began to blare and people started yelling. That's when we noticed a guy in the middle of traffic dancing, weaving, bobbing, jabbing at the air, and throwing punches at a non-existent adversary. "Oh my God," exclaimed Marlys, "It's Ron." We learned later that Ron got pissed because a guy was following too closely behind him. When Ron had to stop for the red light, he got out of his car and confronted the guy. After a verbal exchange of freeway courtesies, Ron jumped out of the car and challenged the now-freaked-out guy to a fistfight on the spot. Ron was in great shape, had very muscular arms, and from a distance reminded me of a great old middleweight fighter, Carl (Bobo) Olson. In fact, I think Olson and Ron each had tattoos, not common in those days. Well, the other guy never did get out of his car, so we didn't get to see any fisticuffs.

We went to many dog shows in the Bay area, and also traveled to Sacramento more than once. That was always a fun trip as good friends from our Southern Illinois University days, Bob and Karen Profilet lived in Rancho Cordova, next door to Sacramento. Bob was stationed at Mather Air Force base and was a rising star in the Service. After a dog show, we'd often stay over the weekend with them. One fourth of July we had a mini-reunion of Southern graduates with several other Saluki alums in attendance. Bob tried to grill a turkey breast, but we were all drinking heavily, and failed to notice that a stiff breeze was blowing directly into the grill, dissipating all the heat. Six hours later the damn bird was still raw. No one cared at that point.

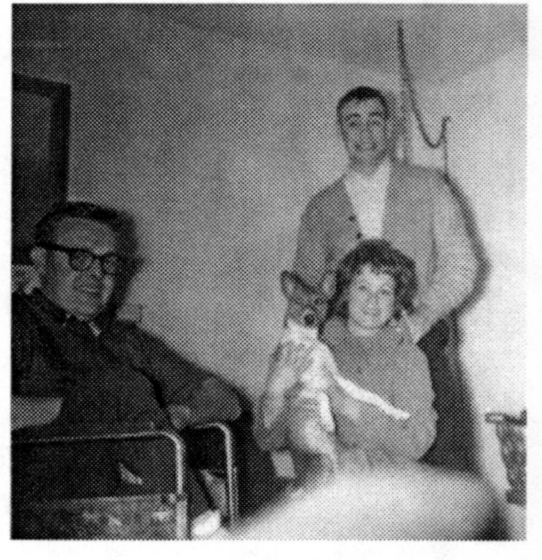

Happy times with Bob and Karen Profilet (and Sassy) at Mather Air Force Base in Rancho Cordova, California (1966)

Ken and Shirley Blaker were also close by, as Ken, a recent PH.D. from Southern had taken a job at Santa Clara University. We had lived only doors apart at Southern Hills married student housing in Carbondale. We had some good times with them, including a memorable Bay Area reunion for Southern Illinois graduates at DiMaggio's in San Francisco. The highlight of the evening was Marlys and I being carried up flights of stairs to the restaurant in a torrential rainstorm. Even with the sizzling entertainment later that evening in the underbelly of San Francisco, North Beach, I never did dry out until the next day.

The main Goodwill office on Race Street was next door to a meat packing operation and many mornings as I arrived at work, several large trucks were parked in front, unloading all kinds of meat carcasses, cows, pigs, calves, and sheep. What a sight—and what a smell! Goodwill Industries had other buildings that housed operations for receiving, sorting, cataloging, pricing and repair of appliances and other items. There were also maybe a dozen outlet stores spread throughout the Santa Clara Valley. The folks who worked as staff for Goodwill and the clients we served were, at times, almost indistinguishable. Goodwill was not quite as exciting as some of Ron's antics, but both the clients and the staff contributed their share of bizarre moments. There were as many unbalanced staff people working for the organization as there were people who we served as clients, people classified as individuals with psychiatric disorders and/or mental health problems. The agency also served other individuals with physical disabilities, developmental disabilities, people with histories of alcohol/drug dependency, sociopaths, and ex-offenders—every classification on the books.

My first secretary, a dear lady with a heart of gold and lousy secretarial skills, looked, dressed, and behaved as if the year was 1942 rather than 1965. Her attire and hairdo were classic Andrew Sisters' style from the World War II period. She drove a two-tone brown 1944 Plymouth sedan, and wore hats, coats, and shoes circa the early 1940's. I never had the courage to press her for answers, but on one occasion, with tears in her eyes, she referred to that period in her life as a time that was long ago, and further, that much had happened in her life. Notwithstanding her mostly absent clerical skills, she was the most loyal secretary I ever had. Her primary responsibilities were typing reports and correspondence for me. Invariably, it took three or four, sometimes five or six drafts to finally end up with a presentable product. She always insisted on taking my letters via dictation, "like in the old days." She didn't want me to write a draft, and if I did, I had to read it to her. I can still visualize her perched on a high stool (probably a donation from a bar), color enhanced dark brown hair, bangs across her forehead, god-awful red lipstick, little circles of rouge on each cheek, a loose fitting button up the front blouse with exaggerated shoulder pads, several pieces of gaudy costume jewelry, a plaid skirt that hung about six inches above her ankles, wearing bobby socks and saddle shoes. It took her what seemed minutes to get herself positioned just right. When she finally stopped wiggling, shifting, and arranging her skirt, blouse and whatever, she would pick up her dictation pad, #2 pencil (easier to erase mistakes), give me a big wide smile and announce, "Ready, sir." She was a sweet, melancholy woman who belonged to another time. She, like many others there, had many hidden scars. She was fragile and vulnerable, and at the same time a wonderful lady.

My boss, a social worker, really had two main interests, arranging for Wednesday morning chapel services and keeping the cook happy. I usually ended up at chapel, because when few people would attend, Lew would come recruiting. The problem with the services was a succession of rather strange volunteer preachers who I'd guess had a lot of time on their hands and needed the practice preaching. Occasionally we got a good one, but generally it was difficult to tell if some of them were filled with the "spirit" or overloaded on Thorazine.

Our cook, I think her name was Hilde, was a solid, stern, but kind German lady. She spoke German fluently and was a marvel in the kitchen. She worked in an appallingly small space with helpers who had little, if any, training in cooking, and who were frequently no-shows for work. The turnover rate in the kitchen was astronomical, partly on account of Hilde's demands on her kitchen workers. When she learned that my heritage was German, she invariably greeted me in the tongue of our mutual ancestors. Then, smiling at me, she would ask," Now, do you know what I said to you?" Of course I didn't, and she delighted in interpreting for me in English. Now my father-in-law, Walter Sternberg, spoke and wrote fluent German. He was a bright old fellow, also prone to rattling off phrases and sayings in German. After working for a period at Goodwill, and returning to San Jose from a visit to my wife's parents' home in Minnesota, I decided to surprise Hilde with a little German phraseology that I had learned from Walt.

One midmorning about coffee break time, I approached the kitchen counter and before she could address me, I blurted out in my best German accent, *"Guten Morgan, Hilde, wie geht es, scheiss?"* By the look on her face, I know I had made a terrible mistake.

"Oh, Kent. I don't think you mean that, do you?"

"Heh, heh," I stammered, "I guess that wasn't quite right was it?"

"No, it wasn't" was all she said as she turned back to her kitchen. That was my one and only attempt at addressing Hilde in German. Some months later, I recounted to Walt what I had said to Hilde. After an uncontrolled fit of laughter, he finally told me what I had asked. Look it up in a German dictionary if you're curious.

I worked for Goodwill less than two years and had many more memorable moments, with not only the staff and clients of the agency, but also in the neighborhood where the main Goodwill office was located. One sunny morning I was on my way to do a follow-up visit with a client who had been placed as a helper in one of the outlet stores. As I was about to enter my car, the scene unfolded. Now, Goodwill Industries, 46 Race Street in San Jose, was located in a tough neighborhood, and all manner of the flotsam and jetsam of humanity inhabited the streets in the area. I sensed I was in trouble the moment I spotted the two unkempt, dirty derelicts staggering up the sidewalk towards me while I was loading my wheelchair in the back seat of my 62 Chevy. I'd done it probably five thousand times in this car, and had it down pat. Open the door, jump in the passenger seat, tilt the bucket seat forward, elevate the front end and wheels, and presto, using the doorframe as a point of leverage, pull the chair into the back in one relatively easy motion.

But when these two chaps spotted me and realized what I was doing they literally lunged forward and yelled in slurred voices, "Hold on buddy, we'll help you." Oh, no, I thought.

Oh, that's okay fellas. I can manage."

"No, no, no, we'll help."

They arrived simultaneously at my open car door, stumbled into the tilted forward passenger bucket seat, nearly knocking me off the seat to the floor, and began wrestling with the chair. Arms flailing, they pushed and pulled, (I heard upholstery rip), staggered and shoved one another, making little progress.

"Here, let me show you how to tilt the front of the chair up so it will clear the hump in the floor," I offered. I frantically grabbed for the chair at the same instant my two helpers decided that one coordinated shove would get the thing in place. It did, ripping a triangular patch in the fabric of my new bucket seat covers, jamming my thumb severely, gouging a couple of nickel sized chips of paint off the door frame, and sent them both halfway into the back seat.

"There you are, bud," they gleefully proclaimed as they got themselves upright.

"Gosh, thanks guys." I remarked, "Here's a buck for your help."

They looked shocked for a second, and then they both chorused in unison,

"Oh, no!" They shoved the dollar back to me and feverishly rummaged through their pockets producing a handful of grimy, sticky coins (I counted seventy-three cents later).

"You take this, bud, it might come in handy."

I was so startled that before I could respond they abruptly turned away, arms over each others shoulders, and lurched away chattering like a couple of magpies. What a disaster—a torn seat, chipped paint, and a thumb that would be tender for weeks.

It was a toss-up as to whether the alcohol on their breaths or their rancid body odor was more potent, but no matter. They left in high spirits, sure in their hearts that they had rescued a disabled fellow on that bright sunny morning. After the encounter with those two Samaritans, I never failed to carefully scan up and down Race Street to ensure that there were no potential helpers in the area.

My abbreviated career at Goodwill ended some eighteen months after it began. Lew, my boss, would not respond to my proposals for expanding and upgrading Rehabilitation services. He did not like changes, preferring to adhere to established programs and policies.

He, along with the other managers really wanted to maintain the status quo. Then one day a guy named Jim Henderson, a retired executive from Western Electric who worked as a volunteer job placement specialist (always in trouble for actually getting people jobs), gave me some great advice. He said, "Kent, instead of bitching about your boss all the time, you either need to quit your job or go see the top man. Quit fooling around and bet the whole ball of wax. One of two things will happen: he'll listen to you and you'll be rid of your boss, or he won't, in which case you'll probably need to pack your bags and move on."

I took his advice and spent an entire Saturday (his wife even served us lunch) at the home of the executive director of the agency, laying out all my concerns but more importantly, sharing what I saw as a viable blueprint for developing a first-rate service program. I heard nothing back until the next Thursday, and the response came from Lew. While Jim's advice was still one the best and most important lessons I ever learned in the workplace, Lew's comments that day made it absolutely clear that it was time to move on. I immediately began filling out applications for Doctoral Studies in Rehabilitation, and was subsequently accepted at the Universities of Missouri, Illinois, Iowa, and Arizona; we chose Arizona and it was on to the "Old Pueblo."

Postscript:

Our brief stay in California with Carol and Frank; the dog shows, Marlys's job with the Santa Clara County Sheriff's Department, visiting the Profilets in Sacramento, and trips to the ocean were just a few remembrances that made the time there a very special period of our lives. But in recalling those days, it also brings a sense of sadness.

We spent the 1967 New Year's Eve and the next day with Bob and Karen Profilet in Sacramento. It was our last visit with Bob. He was killed in a KC-135, a refueling plane, loaded with a quarter-million gallons of fuel that failed to clear a barrier on take-off.

Then eleven years later, in 1978, the memories of those carefree, fun-filled days in California were further tarnished. Tragically for our family, and most difficult for Carol, we lost Frank to cancer in December of that year, when he was only forty-four.

Marrying Frank was one of the best moves any family member ever made. The Silva clan, headed by Juan and Leonila Silva, was a first class, storybook, up-from-the-bootstraps American success story. It was amazing to discover that a Catholic Hispanic family from tiny rural Mendota, California, had so much in common in terms of values, work ethic, integrity, and ideas of right and wrong with the Protestant German Kloepping clan of Illinois.

X. The Old Pueblo

My grandfather once told me that there are two kinds of people: Those who do the work, and those who take the credit. He told me to try to be in the first group; there was much less competition. (1)

It was the year of the "Great Flood." No, it was not the biblical epoch of Noah, nor the infamous Johnstown, Pennsylvania, disaster of 1889. The year was 1984, and it was simply upgrading the sprinkler system throughout the College of Education at the University of Arizona. The work of installing new and replacing older pipes had been completed, and one morning the system was scheduled to undergo a pressure test. Unfortunately, our unit, the Disabled Student Services Program, had not been informed that the test was taking place. At around 8:30 A.M. there was a terrific explosion that rocked our basement level offices. It was so loud, about two feet from my office wall, that we really thought a bomb had been detonated. Our secretary just down the hall began screaming hysterically, and a young man (a disabled Vietnam veteran) who was taking an early morning nap on the physical therapy mats, staggered out of the gym and exclaimed, "Jesus Christ, I thought I was back in Nam!"

Unbelievably, it was a carriage bolt that was the culprit. Actually, it wasn't the bolt that was the problem; rather, it was the individual who had failed to tighten the bolt sufficiently on the eight-inch water line of the sprinkler system. Under increasing pressure, a joint had blown apart. There was a terrific boom, followed by hundreds—no thousands—of gallons of water in the system pouring down onto the floor as all the water from the five stories above us came gushing out of the pipe. Thankfully, at 8:30 A.M. there was only one student, Hal, who was ambulatory, and a few staff on the floor.

When the water level reached a foot deep, I yelled at two ashen-faced staff members. "Hey Carol and Darlene, let's get the heck out of here!"

"Kent, how are you going to get out? We can't carry you up the steps and the elevators are flooded."

"Well, you two can carry my wheelchair up the back stairs and I'll crawl out," which I did quite rapidly.

The incident made all of the local papers, the radio-TV news, and then hit the AP news wire. The headline screamed something like, "Disabled Professor Forced to Crawl Out of Basement for Safety." The Vice President wasn't at all happy about the event, the publicity, or the ensuing barrage of editorials in the local media. Some letters suggested, others urged, and a few even demanded that the University move the Disabled Students Program out of the basement. At least that's what I assumed had made him so angry with me

"Well, goddamn it Kent! I'm sitting here wondering if the whole thing wasn't staged. Have you any idea what a mess this whole episode creates? We had it all worked out—the agreements, the space trades. Do we now have to start over?" he ranted.

I had developed a reputation on campus for not being a team player and refusing to knuckle under to the administration. Because the event couldn't have come at a better time for our program, or at a worse time for the University (with their space allocation problems) the Vice President suspected some surreptitious plot on my part. That collision of wills was just one, albeit one of the roughest, of a series of confrontations I found myself a part of with the University hierarchy. I really was innocent this time, really the beneficiary of "an act of God." On some other occasions—well, I'll just plead the Fifth.

In retrospect, it seems that beginning with our move to Tucson, Arizona, in 1967 (seventeen years prior to this encounter) for me to begin doctoral studies at the University of Arizona, and subsequently my thirty-one year career at that Institution, there was little about my years and work there that was typical or ordinary.

We left the beautiful green Santa Clara valley of central California in early June, never having been to Tucson and only vaguely aware of what the city and locale would be like. During the nine hundred mile trip from San Jose, California to Tucson over two days, the U-Haul truck that Carl and Marge Vogt (Marlys's sister and brother-in-law) were driving for us ran out of gas twice, the last time in 115-degree heat south of Needles, California, about a mile and a half north of Hades. Neither the truck nor our car had air conditioning, and on top of worrying about the dogs or us having heat stroke, Harry, our male Basenji, wouldn't take a pee.

When we finally did arrive in Tucson, there was no prearranged rental waiting for us (as promised by two friends), and we ended up in sort of a dump owned by a strange fellow named Eddie. He was, in fact, a neighbor of Joe Bonanno (the alleged boss of a New York crime family), and Eddie said he and Joe were great buddies. Bonanno, according to his doctors, couldn't travel back to New York to face a grand jury on account of heart problems. Bonanno had reportedly remarked, "I can't travel, and besides, Tucson is my town." Great, I thought, we rent a house in Tucson from a guy with Mafia connections.

We got settled, Carl and Marge left town, and Harry finally peed after two days. We awoke the second morning to a god-awful country tune and light streaming through a crack in the concrete block of our bedroom wall. Talk about feeling depressed. We had left cool, green California, two good jobs, and many friends and landed in a hot, dusty, town in a ramshackle neighborhood, renting from a guy who claimed he was a buddy of the "mob."

Well, things continued to deteriorate during the ensuing week. I went to the University to see my academic advisor, who was also going to give me the details of my part-time job as well as my schedule of classes. But he knew nothing about a part-time job, and had very little to offer concerning my beginning academic program. Frankly, I thought he was weird. He was completing his Ph.D., and I think he knew less than I did. He was a disciple of a well-known psychologist/

psychotherapist, Carl Rogers, whose therapeutic counseling forte was a technique he called Reflection of Feelings. Most simply, anything the client or patient said, old Carl "reflected" back the feelings of the words. Well, everything I said to my advisor, he repeated back to me.

I needed information about my classes, a job, start of school, etc., etc., and what I got was "You seem concerned about schedules, money, and what's next for you?" In the words of a good Minnesotan, I should have said, "By god, you got that right!" It was a terribly upsetting meeting. I finally dragged enough information out of him to register for classes, but left wondering what kind of Looney tunes program lay ahead.

Our little concrete-block house wasn't actually too bad, although we weren't in the best neighborhood in town. There was a barracks and a couple of shacks behind us, all rentals owned by our landlord Eddie. One was actually a chicken-coop, and the clientele occupying these spaces were not a very savory looking bunch. One mailbox, attached to the front wall of our house, served all of the residents in these rentals. A seedy-looking dude, who lived in back, had a habit of lingering near our front door after checking his mail. That was until Harry, our black and tan Basenji, tried to lunge through the screen door after him. After checking his mail, the guy would lean around the door jam to peek into the house. Harry leaped at him, emitting a ferocious roar, which caused the guy to stagger back and almost fall. Thereafter, he checked the mail and hustled away.

Things had started off so badly that summer that we kenneled our dogs and escaped to the Midwest for two weeks, returning somewhat reluctantly to start the fall semester. I didn't get my promised part-time job, and we lived on savings and a $180.00 a month grant. By that Thanksgiving, we had exactly $2.14 in the bank. Mom and Dad sent us five bucks. We celebrated with a chicken and a bottle of cheap wine, and hoped for things to get better.

I survived my first year of doctoral studies in the Rehabilitation Center (called Center as it administratively housed both academic and service units) and managed to put food on the table. The Center was, indeed, a rather unique University department. It was a very dynamic organization headed by Dr. David Wayne Smith, a guy in constant motion who, it seemed, daily came up with a new idea for a program or grant. He was a master at keeping the University administration frustrated and confused, especially in managing and manipulating his seemingly endless sources of revenues for the unit. He was, and remains today, a character and an "Indiana original." He might show up for work (especially on Saturday morning) attired in saddle shoes, with yellow socks, red slacks, and a checked sports coat. He wouldn't win any fashion awards, but as a grant writer and creative program developer, he had few, if any, peers at the University.

The academic faculty and service unit staff had a cadre of very bright people, but also some real screwballs. I think some of the students and staff were basically rejects from normal society who had gravitated into the field of rehabilitation to save disabled folks, as they couldn't help themselves. Also at one point, we had the wildest group of secretaries this side of the Mustang Ranch. They were dangerous.

We had a stable of really exceptional doctoral-level people, and Smith used the entire group to great advantage in grant writing, developing and running programs, and other duties. He assigned me to the Arizona Training Center for the Handicapped as a vocational counselor in 1968-1970, a thirty-hour a week job that he filled with his doctoral students. Thirty-plus years later, I still complain to my co-counselor of those days, George Lackey, that he got the office with the window in the new building. Originally, we worked in a World War II tarpaper shack with paper-thin walls. One of my fondest recollections of those days was our consulting psychiatrist who admonished me, "Kent, if you're going to become a first-rate counselor, you must be able to tell the difference between people who are mentally ill and those who are simply crazy." He was serious, and I think I have finally figured out what he meant. During that two-year period, I completed my academic coursework and began intensive study for my twelve-hour comprehensive written examination and subsequent three-hour oral exam. Assuming I passed, I would then be advanced to candidacy for the doctoral degree.

While I was playing student, my wife also made great progress as a chef. She learned how to make a world-class spaghetti sauce from a bear-sized guy who we met, when he'd stop by to kibbutz over our back fence. He lived in one of Eddie's hovels, and we got to know

Sal Pitelli well. He was a student at the University, and coming from Babylon, New York, I think he missed his family. He seemed to frequently run short of cash and would ask, "Hey, do you want me to cook for you tonight?" That really meant, "I'm broke, you buy and I'll cook." In detailing the ingredients he used, we couldn't figure out what "regort" could be. We subsequently learned that all good Italians knew it was ricotta cheese.

On one occasion we met his father, Tony, who was clearly the head of the family and his immigrant brothers. Two of the brothers had come with Tony from New York to see Sal. One of them was named Orient. I never did find out why he had that name. That evening we first met Tony he brought two or three cream pies, and we gorged on pie and coffee.

In 1969, I and two other doctoral students, George Lackey (my Texas buddy) and Norm Tully, successfully wrote a grant for $100,000 to establish a program of support services for students with disabilities at the University. July 1970 was the starting date of the $100,000 award and marked a significant departure in the direction of my then two-year course of study in Rehabilitation Counselor Education.

My original career objective in pursuing a doctoral degree program was to become a university professor training masters level folks to work with disabled individuals, and also training doctoral level people for faculty positions at the post-secondary level. There were few individuals with significant disabilities teaching at the post-secondary level; thus, a disabled person could potentially bring an entirely different perspective based on personal experience. Maybe my addition to a traditional all non-disabled faculty would be not unlike the inclusion of a person of color in a previously all-white faculty. Then the opportunity to obtain funds to establish a student services program surfaced, and I enthusiastically threw my energies into the new project.

During the initial year of the Disabled Students Program, we served about fifty students out of two offices. Norm Tully, who was completing his doctoral program that year, served as the project director and I was the program developer/coordinator. We hired a secretary who served as the interpreter for the deaf students we assisted, as well as errand girl and all around helper. She had lots of skills, but was young and had a habit of going out drinking on weeknights and then not making it to work. That in and of itself was a pain, but even worse was when she had a sudden conversion and started holding impromptu Bible study sessions during working hours.

Amazingly, during our first year of operation we encountered a significant amount of resistance from not only academic departments, but also the physical resources division (mostly due to our requests to modify physical facilities) and from what seemed like almost every organizational unit on campus. We were two decades ahead of the Americans with Disabilities Act of 1990 and there were no statutes or policies that prohibited discrimination on the basis of disability. We literally received questions from faculty such as, "Do these people really belong in a university?" And, "Do we really have to spend money on modifying facilities when it could be used for academic programs?" It was really disheartening at times.

Notwithstanding many negative attitudes, we tried hard to develop a good image across campus and put out positive publicity. But despite our best efforts, we seemed to have a penchant for disaster. We had a large student staff, and all of them worked part-time, ten-fifteen hours per week. Although they were great kids and doing fine work, at the worst possible moment there would be some monumental snafu that seemed to reverberate throughout the entire campus.

First of all there was Neil, a young man who had cerebral palsy with accompanying severe coordination problems. He struggled around campus on crutches until he finally discovered a tank-like motorized cart that he eventually convinced the State Rehabilitation Agency to purchase for him. We were concerned about his ability to drive the huge cart because of his lack of motor coordination and spasticity. Our worst fears were realized on his first trip out of our office. Neil accelerated backwards into a huge metal storage cabinet, denting it in half like a spent aluminum beer can, almost totally destroying it. We closed our eyes and hoped for the best as he roared down the hall, clipping the doorframe on his way out of the building.

Thereafter, reports began surfacing of an individual in a motorized cart leaving a woman's dormitory—not by the ramp, but down two flights of steps; a car in a residence hall parking lot discovered with a front fender collapsed (the paint smear coincidentally matched Neil's beige colored battering ram); and numerous reports of door jams being broken loose, large gashes in academic building walls, huge ruts gauged in freshly seeded lawns, and shrubbery flattened at various locations on campus. Additionally, we received numerous complaints from bicyclists and pedestrians about being run off sidewalks in their attempts to avoid a cart careening across campus. Neil didn't injure anyone or kill himself, but he also didn't do much to help the image on campus of students with disabilities.

Not to be outdone by Neil, Kathy, one of our student staff, took the occasion of a visit to campus by Ralph Nader, to stand up in the main auditorium and unmercifully attack the University for their failure to provide services for students with disabilities. She made headlines. Ralph then called the President of the University, who called our dean, who called our boss, who called us (Norm and me) into his office. He wasn't at all pleased and barked,

"Who the devil is this student. Doesn't she know about your program?"

We both gulped, and Norm stammered, "Well, yes. She works for us, Dave."

"What" he howled, "What are you guys thinking of? Don't you train these kids? You get her under control—now!"

Finally, we had a young man named Ray who was working on handicapped accessibility evaluations of campus buildings to help us develop priority lists of facilities that needed physical modifications. We were feeling a little smug since we had obtained permission for Ray to be in the Old Main Building after it was closed so he could work without interfering with normal daytime activities, including checking out the men's and women's restrooms. Ray had a severe hearing loss and also a significant visual loss, which he compensated for with hearing aids and extremely thick glasses. For some reason, rather than just turning on the lights in some areas as he was taking measurements (i.e., the width of doors, heights of mirrors and sinks), he used a flashlight to see. Such was the case when the campus policeman confronted him in the women's bathroom. The surprised and frightened Ray became inarticulate and defensive, and in the cop's estimation, downright sinister. He envisioned Ray to be an antiwar protester who was about to bomb

Old Main. They hauled him off to the police station, got the story out of him, and eventually let him go. Well, it made the papers again, and we had another item of notoriety to add to our growing list.

Modifying existing facilities to make them accessible for wheelchairs was only one of the problems we faced. Trying to ensure that new construction was accessible and usable was often an even more vexing problem. Architects, engineers, administrators, facility people and planners all seemed to have unending lists of unique reasons why new facilities could not be 100% accessible for disabled people. Their reasoning and rationale was often, in my view, ludicrous. Here is a choice example.

In the new fourteen thousand seat basketball arena, the lead architect for the project, suggested that eight wheelchair spaces would be sufficient to accommodate the large number of students on campus (probably close to one hundred) and literally hundreds more in the community. Granted, many non-disabled people could not get seats either, but the original plans initially called for sixty-four wheelchair spaces. Then the architect reduced it to thirty-two, then sixteen and finally eight. We argued and fought tooth and nail until we finally got a total of sixteen spaces. In response to my concern about the terrible inadequacy of the number, the architect replied, "Well you know Kent, things aren't always how we'd like them to be. You know, I have extra long arms and buying a suit is a real problem. So you see, we are all inconvenienced in life." My God, I thought, that's like comparing a case of uncomfortable benign hemorrhoids to colon cancer. Gene Tchida, my co-worker and a power wheelchair user, later remarked, "When he made that statement, I came close to needing to go home and change my shorts." Not only was the number of spaces woefully inadequate, the line-of-sight to the court below was obstructed when patrons in these areas stood up, which is very frequent at college basketball games.

We raised hell for years over the problem and finally got the attention of a couple of enlightened Athletic Department administrators. Bob Bockrath was the guy who really got things started, but importantly, a fellow named John Perrin was the key guy in ensuring that all athletic facilities were upgraded toward the goal of meeting the standards of reasonable accommodation.

In our continuing efforts to have residence halls modified for wheelchair access, a highly placed residence hall official seemed to sabotage our initiatives on every project we proposed. She once argued against the inclusion of disabled students in different halls, reasoning that, "What we need is a dorm to house all the 'handicapped' in one location." She cited the need to keep a close watch on these students because who could guess what calamities might occur? Maybe she really believed disabled folks needed to be closely monitored; but I'd submit that one could make a case for scrutinizing every group on campus more closely. We had dozens of battles over facilities. These examples should provide the reader a glimpse of the on-going resistance we faced. What was particularly disheartening were the many faculty members who understood what we were trying to accomplish and supported us, but simply did not have the courage to help us challenge their immediate superiors, let alone the Administration. It was very difficult trying to build coalitions with folks worrying about being labeled a non-team player.

There were many occasions when I was completely flabbergasted, outraged, and ultimately terribly discouraged by the blatant, insensitive, and openly discriminatory attitudes toward people with disabilities. It was at those low points that the students we served helped us rally and find the strength to forge ahead.

It was not only the students and their successes that were uplifting, as late in 1970, feeling flush with an annual salary of eleven thousand dollars, we bought a new house (had it built) that was completed in April of 1971. If I had a particularly tough week at the University, I could spend the weekend working off my frustrations. Our backyard was bare desert/dirt with the exception of a few creosote bushes. The first thing we did was lay concrete blocks for walkways and a kind of patio in the middle of the yard. I put down every blasted one of those 8x16 inch pavers in that yard. I got out of my chair to the ground, literally "down and dirty" to do the work.

Then we started planting trees and bushes. Frank and Carol Silva gave us a five-foot Aleppo Pine tree, today thirty-five feet tall, with massive double trunks, and an equally wide span of boughs. It dominates the backyard, and provides a marvelous barrier against the afternoon sun. Over the past thirty-five years I must have dug fifty holes for trees and shrubs, plus all the trenches for our watering systems to the plants. Some of the holes were two to three feet deep and had similar diameters.

However, I never dug one as deep as was imagined by a fellow who was walking through our back alley early one evening.

He saw me in the hole, stopped, leaned over the five-foot fence, and asked, "What are you going to plant?"

"Oh, I think a peach tree," I responded.

He paused, and stared at me intently, and asked, "My god man, how deep are you going to dig that hole? Don't you think you're deep enough already?"

Suddenly I grinned, realizing what he was seeing. He was probably sixty to seventy feet from me and it was dusk. Of course, he thought I was standing in the hole. Ground level was about at my chin, and all he could see was basically my head. He just knew my hole was five or six feet deep.

I didn't explain, just replied, "Yes, I think I'm close to being finished."

"Well I would think so," he remarked, and he walked away. He was shaking his head as he left, and probably thinking, that dummy. I'd wager he never did figure out the facts of the situation.

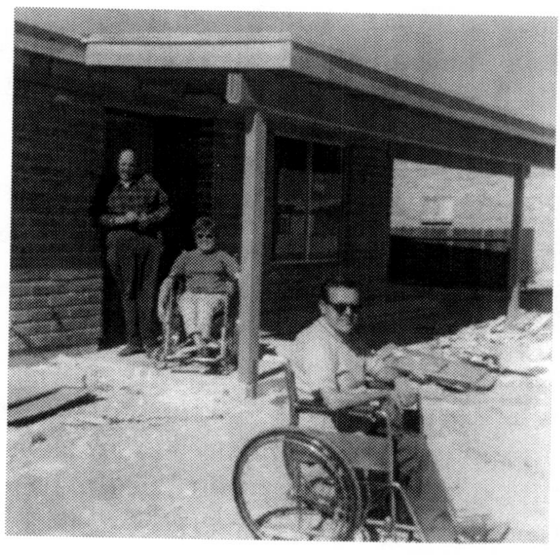

Our new home in Tucson (1972)

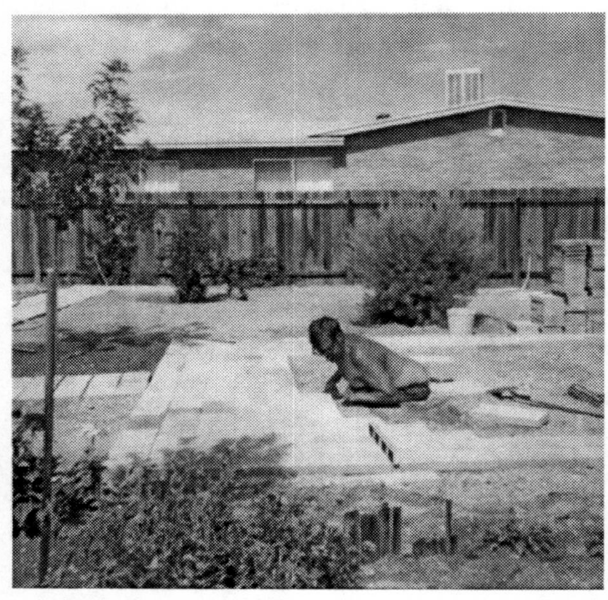

Me laying a block patio. The aleppo pine, in the center back of the picture, is today over forty feet tall. (1973)

In February 1972, I made a commitment to finish my doctoral dissertation, getting past that final hurdle and title of "ABD" (all but dissertation). I did it in five months, passing my dissertation defense in early July 1972. It was a tough five months, as in addition to my full-time position I easily averaged another forty hours a week working on the dissertation. Putting in eighty hours a week got old rather quickly.

However, little did I know at the time that those five months would dramatically change both Marlys and my life. With the completion of the degree, I became administrative head of the Disabled Students Program, which was a big deal for me. But Marlys had a bigger deal—she was pregnant! Matthew was born December 23, 1972, and as his namesake tells, he was a "gift of God." A great medical team and two doctors named Tom Foreman and Roger Perry made sure he arrived safely, and that Marlys made it through a difficult medical journey. Perry, the obstetrician, wasn't all that thrilled with the pregnancy, but Tom Foreman, not only a brilliant physician

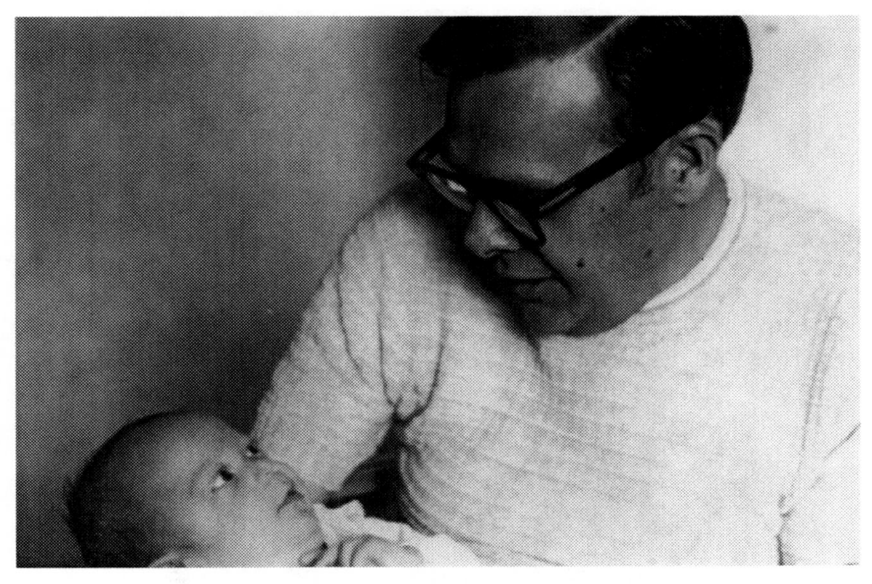

A bundle of bright-eyed joy. Matthew and me. (Spring, 1973)

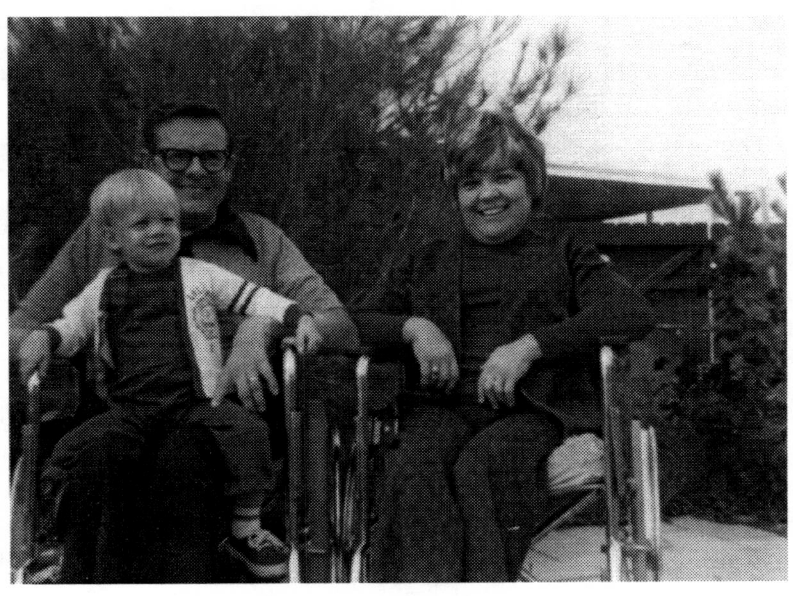

Dressed up and ready to go. Our backyard. (December, 1974)

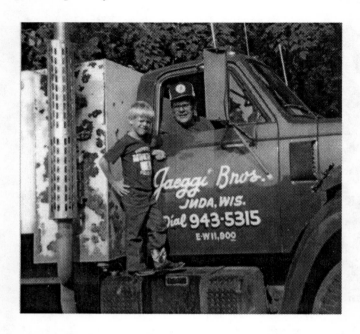

Riding with Grandpa Kloepping on his milk route one summer in Illinois (1978)

and a supportive and caring person, assured Marlys early on that, "Hey, we can do this."

There were serious and legitimate concerns about her respiratory capacity, her blood pressure problems, her kidney functioning, and the danger that the baby would not survive the pregnancy. With her post-polio paralysis, natural childbirth was problematic which meant a caesarian section was likely. However, with high blood pressure, surgery becomes a higher risk. Furthermore, her medication for the blood pressure was contraindicated for pregnancy so it had to be changed, and the new medication was not as effective. She had to be hospitalized eight weeks before the delivery date when her blood pressure began to elevate. The hope was that complete bed rest would extend the pregnancy a minimum of three weeks and if the baby came early, it would be five weeks premature. Getting past the sixth week was critical; after that time the risk of Hyaline Membrane Disease in the child was reduced. Unfortunately, her bodily functions began to deteriorate after only one week and the decision was made to deliver the baby as further delay might put Marlys in serious danger. Matthew arrived in good shape seven weeks early and after a rough twenty-four hours, Marlys began to recover. Maybe not a miracle, but with great doctors, lots of folks praying for her, and most importantly her courage to bring her baby through safely, they both made it.

In the two years after the program was established, we had at least gotten a foot in the door. But I knew that many challenges and obstacles lie ahead. One of the best decisions I ever made during my career at the University was to take time to think seriously about what I hoped to accomplish, and what strategies I needed to reach those goals. I literally spent hours ruminating over ideas and finally putting in writing what amounted to a personal philosophy about working.

I had learned as a child at the oak supper table that success was about 99% perspiration and 1% inspiration. The principle that followed was to work hard and do any job that needs to be done.

My father always said, "Accept responsibility for what you do and say," which translated to tell the truth and keep your word. I did, and it wasn't always popular, as fence riding and prevarication are highly developed art forms in universities.

A fellow student, Norman Tully, who was truly a mentor in the best sense, told me a third principle: "Don't worry about all the reasons things might fail or won't work. Concentrate on listing all the ways you can accomplish a goal."

One person can't know everything so always hire people who know more than you do about key program areas.

Have a personal philosophy and stay with it, and always be prepared to compromise on programs, but never on principles.

And finally, a sixth critical guideline, spoken by the great black abolitionist Frederick Douglas, who told a young man who had asked, "What should I do with my life?" Douglas replied, "Agitate, agitate, agitate." That fit just fine with my ideas about being persistent and insistent.

The University power structure preferred a more sanitized word than agitation—like advocacy—and wanted everyone to be team players. As one University administrator once remarked to me after I had challenged the administration on an issue, "You know, Kent, the era of confrontational politics is over (his reference to the 60's)." Alas, I think he was a poor student of history.

I carried academic rank, Assistant Professor of Rehabilitation, and also an administrative appointment as Director of Disabled Student Services. I had all the responsibilities of a full-time faculty member (except teaching), carried a large number of undergraduate advisees, served on doctoral committees, and sat on academic committees. I frequently guest lectured in our department (Rehabilitation Counselor Education) in courses such as Medical/Psychological Aspects of Disability, Principles of Rehabilitation and on specific topical areas related to disability: Marriage and Disability, Sexuality and Disability, Childrearing with a Disability and other related topics the faculty could think up. I was abreast of legislation and statutes requiring access for disabled people and as the resident gimp faculty member, was called upon frequently.

For over a year I served as Assistant Director of the Rehabilitation Center, the unit that encompassed all the academic and service programs. I was terribly busy, and worked long hours. The University got their money's worth with my tenure there.

In 1975, with the closing of the Rehabilitation Center's Medical Services Unit, we moved the Disabled Students Program from about six small offices of five hundred square feet into almost the entire first floor level of the College of Education, five thousand square feet. The first floor was below ground level (actually the basement), but space was at such a premium at the University that we elected to go below ground level, even with the limited access. We felt that the opportunity to trade this space for a comparable, ground level location would eventually materialize.

By that year, 1975, our program had gained national attention and I was invited to serve on a national planning group that led to the formation of the National Association whose membership is primarily the professionals who are the disability service providers on campuses throughout America. I obtained my license as a psychologist in the state of Arizona, #549, and the year before, I was named to the Editorial Board of the Journal of Rehabilitation, one of the primary academic journals for counselor education faculty.

In the same year, we were exceedingly fortunate to be awarded a new half-time faculty position (difficult to obtain as new academic positions were highly competitive), which was the beginning of a competitive sports program for students with disabilities. Dr. Donna Miller, a faculty member in women's physical education, was an individual highly regarded in her field and a consummate professional. She was, in reality, a visionary. After a number of discussions with Donna outlining our hopes for the future, she and I met with Dave Strack, the Director of Intercollegiate Athletics, to request the position through his department. Donna articulated our case and Dave, to my surprise committed a half-time position. Maybe I should not have been surprised, as Strack already had a record of being a forward thinker. He had hired the first African American head basketball coach at a division I school (the University of Arizona), a man named Fred Snowden. That hire of Snowden began Arizona's rise to national prominence as a basketball power, and the position he gave to us led to the wheelchair sports program at Arizona becoming a national leader today.

With an increasing visibility on campus, increasing faculty support, and a major state appropriation of funds (under the auspices of Section 504 of the 1973 Rehabilitation Act), we rapidly gained momentum and steadily raised the level of our credibility on campus. Conflicts and confrontations did increase with constituencies across campus as we pushed our agendas, and were increasingly able to justify our requests and substantiate our positions. The downside was that we not only alienated some faculty and staff, but we also made some enemies. Colleges and universities love to be labeled places of "higher learning." True in some instances, but they also have highly sophisticated, firmly entrenched bureaucracies that jealously protect the status quo. The Administration governs from the top down and distrusts anyone who is not a team player. The power groups on campus, in particular, dislike new agendas that emanate from the lower ranks of employees.

But in the process of disrupting established policies and procedures, we also found a growing cadre of allies who would become key partners in our initiatives.

About that time, I became acquainted with a guy on campus who not only became a friend, but a person I found that I could confide in and trust to keep a confidence. During tough times when I needed someone to listen to my woes, I learned that this confidant I called Guido was always available to listen, respond honestly and candidly, and offer sound advice. A university abounds with people who possess integrity, great vision, and have high levels of intelligence. Unfortunately, there also exist among the ranks a liberal number of sycophants who watch and wait silently to determine the direction of the wind before committing themselves. As much as I despised them for their deceitfulness and dishonesty in manipulating people and the system, I had an advantage because as Mark Twain said, "If you tell the truth, you don't have to remember anything."

But I did pay a heavy price for my often-frenetic pace in pursuit of work goals. In 1983, I was diagnosed with an acoustic nueroma, a benign tumor, on the 8th cranial nerve. Actually, Marlys figured it out before anyone else, including two well-known neurologists who both misdiagnosed my loss of hearing. There is, of course, no evidence to substantiate that the sudden appearance of the tumor was related to, or caused by, the daily stress and pressure of my job, but in my heart, I know it was my physical body telling my mind (literally my head) "enough already."

The eight-hour surgery was successful, but I developed a massive post-surgical infection. The infection was a virulent staphylococcus I'm sure came from the hospital. I was placed on drip antibiotics for three weeks, which killed about every bacterium in my body including the staph. Unfortunately the damage was done, and the result was permanent right side facial paralysis. The next several years were psychologically very difficult for me as I struggled with a very apparent, and to some, shocking facial asymmetry that caused children to stare and adults to pretend they didn't notice. Pictures were especially awful as they accentuated the problem.

Paul Dempsey, a great reconstructive surgeon and equally wonderful man, did cosmetic surgery on me several years later that significantly improved the symmetry of my face. I was away from work, as I recall, almost four months and wasn't sure that I could reenergize myself to once again compete successfully for space and dollars to fund staffing needs and program operations. But I did regain my stamina and most importantly, the desire and motivation to press on with our agendas.

While no institution of so-called higher learning would openly acknowledge the fact, the differing constituencies on campus jealously guard their turf, maintaining a well-defined pecking order of insiders and outsiders. Zbigniew Brzezinski, Jimmy Carter's National Security Advisor once remarked, "Collegiality is the pretense of camaraderie among highly rivalrous people." I had learned that lesson during the five years of our student services program, but had also learned about coalition building, finding money and being willing to assert myself in advocating for our program and our students. I had attained a degree of national credibility and had discovered that our staff and I had become the experts on campus in disability issues.

After fourteen (seventeen, counting the doctoral program) years working at the University, I had learned that one of the most important things people do within the institution is reorganize. Someone always has a better idea, which usually means new people have been hired and they proceed to dismantle existing policies, procedures, infrastructures and reporting lines from the president's office on down. These new organizational configurations invariably require increased staffing, more budgetary support, and, of course, more space. The groups with power on campus usually got everything they needed and more. The rest of us fought among ourselves for the leftover crumbs of dollars and facilities.

The problem for the University was that the Disabled Student Services program was rapidly expanding and gaining national credibility. Many within the Institution were also beginning to view us as an asset for the University. In effect, we were emerging as a sort of mini-power unit, and later, with the passage of the National Americans with Disabilities Act 1990, the University suddenly had to be mindful of not trampling on the rights of gimpers. We had become a legitimate protected group along with ethnic minorities, women, veterans, gays, the elderly, and many more, too numerous to mention. Notwithstanding our growing stature and attendant clout on campus, we were at a critical juncture in terms of immediate space needs and future facilities planning for the Disabled Students Program. Space was at a premium throughout the campus. And then it happened—The Great Flood of

1984, and I found myself sitting in the Vice President's office, being barraged with accusations, thinly disguised as questions.

"So you had nothing to do with this accident? Well that's probably the case. I mean, I don't suppose you physically tampered with the sprinkler system,"

"What do you call it? An act of God?"

"But the publicity—has all of that been necessary? I mean, there's an article in every damn local paper, letters to the editor, and editorials all advocating that the University 'must take immediate steps to rectify the situation.'"

"And the AP wire—how did they get the story?"

"Just how much damage was there, anyway?"

"Once the elevator is back in operation, couldn't you resume business?"

And finally, "Was that 'stunt' (crawling up the steps) you pulled necessary? You really didn't have another way out of the building?"

I had an answer for each of his questions, but I didn't think he really wanted to hear any of them.

Somehow I hadn't imagined that a university vice president would be such a garbage mouth, much less cussing me out. The accusation that I had somehow fabricated the incident really made me angry. I was so flabbergasted by his hostile remarks that I didn't know what to say. So I remained silent, listening to the guy rant and rave. He was now pacing around the office while the Senior Vice President sat quietly with a strange smirk on his face and my boss remaining completely silent. There were just the four of us to witness the tirade. It wasn't a meeting—a meeting assumes some communication between the parties. Let me assure you, this was a one-way lecture.

The Vice President continued, "How is it that this space has been perfectly fine for nine years, and suddenly it's unsafe, and you and your program simply have to move now? God damn it, Kent, you never wanted to be a team player. You're not the only program with needs. We spent a lot of money renovating those facilities."

I gulped, trying to find the courage to speak and rebut his assault, "Well," I sort of squeaked out, "I never said the basement was a good place for a program to serve students with disabilities. You know it's really..."

"Oh baloney, Kent. Now, you're raising that issue because you think it's a way out. Even if we did move your program, why do you need all the space next door—Christ —The other guys have already started to move in!"

After he, shall we say, shared his feelings, the Vice President did agree that he would move us to the ground level facility next door, displacing the College of Agriculture folks who had just moved in.

I probably should mention that I had a history with this Vice Presidential office. Several years before this confrontation, I had challenged a Senior Vice President's decision to disperse almost a quarter of a million dollars in new state funding for services to students with disabilities under mandates of section 504 of the 1973 Rehabilitation Act. I had been asked by the Vice President for Student Affairs to develop the budget for the University, as he remarked, "This is your area of expertise, and the funds will support programs in your area." When the University received the funds—the exact amount of the request to the penny—incredibly, the Vice President stated he wasn't sure how the state had arrived at that figure. He was either unbelievably forgetful or not too smart; but in fact I think he was a pretty bright fellow. His comment was made in a meeting of the President's Advisory Council for our program, and after he attempted to "blow smoke up everyone's ass," I distributed copies of the original budget request, which I had given him when the request was submitted. (In fact, he probably was the person who submitted the request). The dollar amount on each line item corresponded exactly with the amount requested. He was really pissed at me, as I had blown away his smoke screen.

But when the Administration still refused to release the money to our program, I began contacting Arizona State Legislators and writing letters regarding the matter. Probably the most blistering memo was a six-pager to the Senior Vice President, with copies to key University people and a local attorney. The day the Vice President got the memo my Dean received a phone call with a terse directive. "Tell that Kloepping guy no more memos." I did stop writing when they agreed not to distribute the funds across different campus budgets. My immediate supervisor told me later that I barely escaped being fired. I often thought it was probably my disability that saved me. It might not look good for the University to fire the Head Gimp.

Now this Associate Vice President, (the guy reviling my character) happened to work for the above referenced Senior Vice President and evidently had a long memory. He and his boss probably never could quite accept the fact that I had bested them on the budget issue. My intentions and motivation had been solely in the best interests of the University. But the powerful don't appreciate being told they are wrong, particularly by someone they view as inferior. Their pompous, elitist attitudes were infuriating to put it mildly. So I'd guess it wasn't solely the issue of space, but also a matter of some past bruised egos that would explain why the Vice President was so angry and delivered arguably the finest ass chewing of my entire career!

Our program not only physically left the College of Education (out of the Rehabilitation Department), but we were also moved organizationally to the Division of Student Services. We had officially been admitted to the ranks of Student Service Organizations, and I reported to the Dean of Students.

It didn't take long to find a couple of colleagues who weren't very good at following the company line and rules—Joshua Mihesuah, head of Native American Studies, a Comanche Indian (we called him mighty warrior), and Glen Smith, a powerfully built African American, who was an associate dean.

I liked both of them immediately. When I first met Glen, I remarked that I couldn't understand why he wasn't a finalist for the newly established position, Director of University Minority Student Affairs, as he had previously developed a similar position at another university. He gave me a Bill Cosby-like smirk and replied, "Oh, it's simple. You see, I was one shade too dark" Everyone who was involved in the screening process surely knew that an individual who was Hispanic would fill the position. But true to form, 99.9% of the politically correct types wouldn't publicly express that view. However, Glen did on the occasion of our first meeting, and I knew then he was bound to become a friend.

My other colleague, Joshua, was more reserved initially, but one morning in a serious discussion in his office I asked him why we needed specialty deans, that is, individuals ethnically representing the populations they served. He looked at me intently and in a serious tone he replied, "Well, you see, white man speak with forked tongue." I was speechless, and then he burst into laughter. The three of us became good friends, trusted colleagues, and like Guido, they became a forum for sorting out the B.S. that flowed down the chain of command.

We became a vocal minority in staff meetings and I think irked our Vice President with questions that some folks, including my supervisor, labeled troublesome. On one occasion, she advised me to carefully consider the impact of my questions on the dynamics of the meetings I attended. I guess it messed up the feelings of camaraderie and the esprit de corps. I was told that my remarks were especially distressing for that group of folks, who suffered from a malady that I called "rectal-rhinitis." It's a term reserved for individuals who have a brownish tone to their nose, and is a disorder of unknown origin. Sycophants are apparently highly susceptible. I offered to resign immediately after the Dean finished scolding me, but my offer was not accepted. As Glen Smith slyly remarked to me later, "My goodness, Kent, how would it look if the head gimp quit?"

Glen was a bright fellow, a keen observer of group dynamics and usually right on target. "You have to stay cool, Kent," he would gently remind me, "Just go with the flow."

Tragically, he developed an adult neuromuscular disorder and passed away in the early 1990's. But before he left us, he, Josh, Bill Foster, an associate dean and I took a memorable two-day fishing trip to Lake Roosevelt (April 1991) in my twenty-three foot Winnebago motor home. We were all good buddies and in many respects, the loyal opposition to all the bureaucratic crap within the University. Talk about male bonding. We all agreed on a no-holds-barred approach in getting to really know one another, learning about our racial and ethnic heritages, discussing stereotypes and myths. We'd drink a little—oh, and do some fishing. It was a hilarious two-day getaway. I kept a journal and one day I'll commit my notes to a tale worth telling. Josh and Glen were special friends and confidantes who made my time at the University better.

I'd suppose that every university has some kind of faculty senate, ostensibly to assist with institutional governance. But frankly, I really

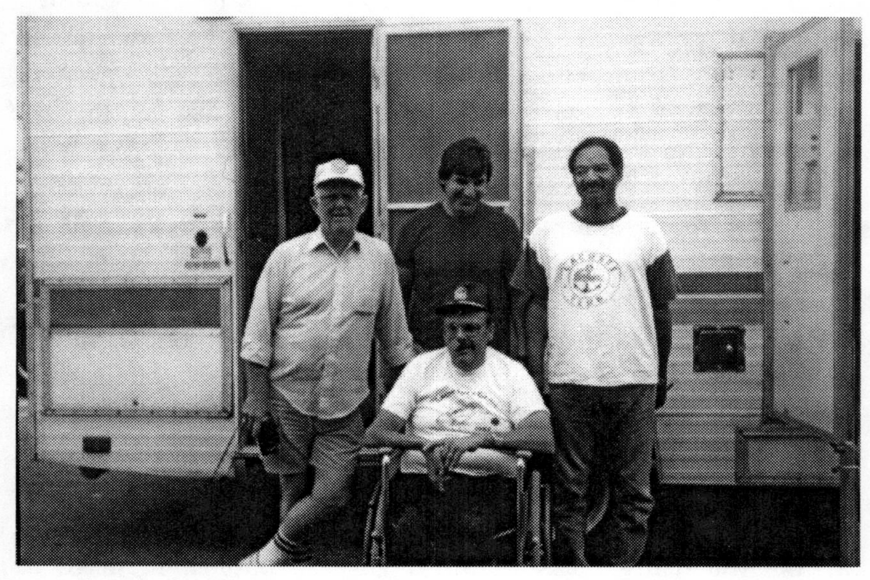

My University cohorts (L–R), Bill Foster, Josh Mihesuah, and Glen Smith, on the way to Lake Roosevelt (April, 1991)

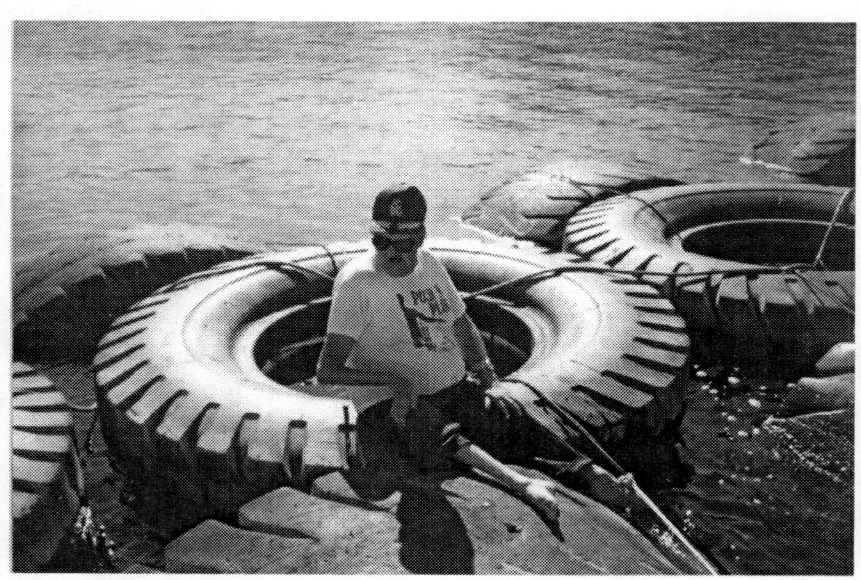

Fishing for crappies, Lake Roosevelt (April, 1991)

always believed the university administration (a small elite group) made all the important decisions. No matter. In our faculty senate there were numerous important-sounding committees covering a multitude of institutional matters. There was even a committee on committees. However, the Intercollegiate Athletic Committee (ICA) was the only one that interested me. It was a group of University and community folks who had oversight (limited) responsibilities for the workings of arguably the most powerful unit on campus. It was advisory to the director of ICA, and was highly prestigious. Each year, the faculty senate sent out ballots asking us to list the committees on which we wished to serve. One year I wrote back to the chairman of the faculty senate asking him to not send me any further ballots, as I always checked the box for the Intercollegiate Athletic Committee and nothing ever happened. I stated, "I think that election is rigged and it hurts my feelings when I receive the invitation and then my hopes are dashed." He called me and said, "We're putting your name forward for election." Well, by golly I was elected to a three-year term.

We met all the coaches; learned about their coaching philosophies; discussed athlete GPA's and graduation rates; got the inside scoop on new recruits; talked about which athlete wasn't going to make it in school; and generally acted like we were big-time operators. We got free tickets to all U of A intercollegiate games, free meals at our monthly meetings, free attendance at all the sports banquets, and even one out-of-town trip a year with a team. I flew two consecutive years to Seattle, Washington with the football Cats to watch them tangle with the Huskies. We lost 56-14 the first trip, but were ready the following year; that final score was 56-0 Washington, and they (the Huskies) went on to finish #1 in the nation. The conversations on the plane ride home that evening were quite unusual. Once those wounded warriors recovered enough to begin speaking to one another, I think I heard the "MF" word maybe a thousand times.

I served on the committee from April 1989, to May 1992, and accomplished one good thing during my term. In my final report covering the three years, I pointed out that while the racial profile of student athletes at the University probably consisted of a majority of nonwhite young folks, our committee was 100% white.

In the words of the politically correct crowd, I strongly urged them to "diversify" the group. Well, the next year two African Americans, a Dean and a Vice president appeared on the committee.

Not all of my extracurricular activities were confined to the University campus community. I also participated in meetings, think tanks, forums, committees and conferences that addressed issues of discrimination in programs for persons with disabilities. A group of community people and some University folks (including me) even staged a high-profile demonstration in the heart of campus protesting the purchase of fifty-five new buses by the City of Tucson, none of which were wheelchair accessible. We ruined the party for the University with their gleaming new buses parked on the campus mall with a huge banner announcing, "Ride with Pride." We gimpers showed up with our own banner proclaiming, "Ride with Shame." It embarrassed the City and the University, and pissed off a whole bunch of people. The local newspaper, the *Arizona Daily Star,* ran a highly critical editorial of our little protest.

"Wheelchair lifts on city buses are too costly," Saturday, May 27, 1989.

> If the city had bottomless pockets, wheelchair lifts on city buses would be a fine idea. But considering the exorbitant cost and the money already being spent on transportation for handicapped residents, the idea lost its appeal. It costs about $10,000 to equip a new bus with a wheelchair lift and another $2,000 a year to maintain it.
>
> After discovering that only five handicapped riders regularly used the 19 accessible buses, the city started pouring its money into a van service that transports 600 handicapped riders per day. Most disabled riders prefer being picked up and dropped off at their homes to waiting at bus stops. Just getting to and from the stops can be a real chore in a wheelchair. The bus vs. van controversy has been hashed and rehashed at city meetings over the years. The van system always emerges as the sensible and affordable solution.
>
> But that's never satisfied a small group of activists who insist that anything less than a full fleet of lift-equipped buses is discriminatory. This week, they blocked a ribbon cutting

heralding the arrival of 55 new city buses—sans wheelchair lifts. While the protesters had a right to demonstrate their arguments, the city can't afford to satisfy their demands. There are simply too many needs and too few dollars.

It's true that the van service has long waiting lists and punctuality isn't one of its greatest strengths. Social visits receive low priority and rides must be arranged days in advance. A lift-equipped bus would be a ticket to freedom.

But city officials must take a broader view of the purpose of mass transit. It's more than a low-cost ride service. Getting people out of their cars is a key element in the fight against air pollution. In that context, it makes more sense to buy 10 unequipped buses than five with wheelchair lifts—and serve a greater number of people.

Instead of agitating at ribbon-cuttings, handicapped people who want wheelchair lifts on buses might better spend their time raising funds for such equipment or asking city officials to place a financing measure on the ballot—perhaps along with any proposed sales tax for transportation that surfaces.

Mere insistence that taxpayers should subsidize costly wheelchair lifts doesn't sit well when taxpayers are already generously supporting subsidized transportation for handicapped residents."

I responded to their remarks several days later, labeling their editorial "Narrow Minded."

Re: May 27 editorial, "Wheelchair lifts on city buses are too costly."

The article not only demonstrates a narrow-minded bias, but additionally is very misleading.

The assertion that "most disabled riders prefer being picked up and dropped off at home," is really a response to a forced-choice circumstance of not having an option. If there is no other service, wouldn't everyone prefer that system?

As a taxpayer, I contribute toward the 55 new buses and the Para transit system that neither my wife nor I can use. Additionally, I spent $30,000 to purchase a van with a lift so my wife has transportation. Given the exorbitant costs that I personally incur for transportation, lifts have a great deal of appeal.

You admonish people with disabilities to raise funds if they want lifts. Isn't that like telling black Americans 30 years ago that if they didn't want to sit in the back of the bus, that they should go out and buy their own buses?

Taxpayers aren't "generously subsidizing transportation for citizens with disabilities." The city of Phoenix, in addition to a demand-response system, has a goal that 50 percent of the entire fleet of buses will have lifts by 1992. That's not generosity. It reflects commitment, following the law and responsible planning. About the only credible statement you made was that city officials must take a broader view of the purpose of mass transit. Now about light rail, That's a new term. I assume I will have the opportunity to help pay for it. Will I also be able to ride on it?

KENT KLOEPPING, Director
Disabled Student Services

The editor called me and apologized, saying, "We didn't want you to take the editorial as a personal attack."

"Why, hell yes I took it personally. I'm paying for a vehicle I can't ride." The city did begin to get services after our sit-in and a community group led the charge that eventually saw Tucson become a town with citywide accessible buses.

In February 1992, our program had the good fortune to be administratively moved from the Dean of Students office to the Campus Health unit. Of course the decision was made with no input or consultation from me. I was in New Zealand and one morning at 6:00 A.M. the motel clerk buzzed our room. I was groggy but finally understood that I had a phone call from America. We were in a tiny little hamlet named Twyzel, and when I got to the phone it was Murray DeArmond, who was head of Campus Health back at the

University of Arizona. I couldn't imagine why he would be calling, let alone how he knew where I was.

He said, "Kent they have administratively assigned your unit to me. Can you live with that?"

I replied, "Would it make any difference if I couldn't?"

There was a brief delay in the transmission of our remarks and then I clearly heard, "Well no."

That was essentially the substance of the call, with nothing more than a goodbye. That decision, like the journey we were on, proved to be a great move, and particularly fortuitous for our disability services program. Murray was an articulate advocate for campus health and our unit, and although I gave him a rough time on occasion, together we developed and subsequently gained approval for an outstanding new facility to house all of our operations at one location. The building was completed in early 2004.

Later that year, 1992, at the request of the University President, Dr. Manuel Pacheco, I took administrative leave from my position to coordinate the University self-study of programs and facilities for compliance with the Americans with Disabilities Act of 1990. (ADA). It was a great experience and many folks within the University community contributed great support to the effort. A serendipitous outcome of my coordinating the self-study was that my professional credibility and visibility on campus were greatly increased. I became one of the most recognizable people within the University community. At times, I felt like a small-time celebrity. I had battled so many years to ensure that our program would survive future administrations after I retired, and now the future of the program seemed assured.

I had made many friends on campus, and worked closely with many constituencies on campus. One of the nicest compliments I ever received at the University came in the form of a phone call from Dr. Jesse Hargrove, Director of the African-American Student Center. Their new facility, the Dr. Martin Luther King Jr. building, was to be dedicated that week, and Jesse asked me if I would give the keynote address.

"Me? You would like me to give the keynote? But..."

He interrupted me and said, "Yes, you. Dr. King spoke for all of us. Now you can speak on his behalf."

Our program grew dramatically over the next five to six years with increasing funding support, an influx of students, and the addition of outstanding staff. This tremendous growth spurt meant we were once again critically short of space. Despite the fact we were delivering services at eleven sites spread across campus, which was a terrible inconvenience for our students, our pleas were mostly ignored. I never ceased haranguing the administration, and eventually we were offered more space. One location was far from the main campus (across a major city street) and the second location was the basement floor beneath a basketball court. I was appalled by the offer of space so totally inappropriate for our students.

I completely blew my cork when I learned that a prime central location on campus had been given to another program, obviously as a political favor. I was extremely upset and sent a caustic letter to a senior vice-president (not the guy earlier cited), threatening to request an investigation by the U.S. Department of Justice to consider if the University had failed to provide reasonable accommodation under the ADA. Suddenly the folks responsible for space allocations (I'm sure at the urging of my Vice President) discovered that a new women's sorority house only a block away from our main building was soon to be vacated. Despite the expansion to this new site in 1996, we were still woefully short of space and continuing to provide services at eight or nine disparate locations throughout campus. But it would be our last move before we gained approval for the new facility housing all of our operations.

During the period 1996-1998, I spent many hours involved in discussions relating to implementation of the provisions of the Americans with Disabilities Act, or the ADA. That meant meetings, meetings, meetings, and hassles, hassles, hassles. I had worked for so many years advocating and fighting to ensure equal access in all University programs, had coordinated the University self-study and now, at the point of implementation, I became terribly outspoken and almost unwilling to compromise on any issue. I think the University assigned one of their attorneys, Elizabeth Buchanan, to keep tabs on me and keep me in line. Elizabeth proved to be a fair, very competent professional in assessing tough questions. She became a trusted colleague, as she was honest and candid in her views. She was a terrific resource for our program regarding disability issues. Unlike many university bureaucrats, Elizabeth actually "got it."

One day in a meeting a guy remarked, "You know, Elizabeth is the only person on campus who can tell Kent to shut up—and he does." When I got in trouble, she was my mouthpiece. By 1998, the Center for Disability Resources (new name) had become a strong, vibrant, nationally recognized program of services for individuals with disabilities at a prestigious Division One research institution. We had come a long way in twenty-eight years.

But early in 1998, after almost thirty years of doing battle with the University and many times being labeled the bad guy who wasn't a team player, I suddenly realized that I was physically, psychologically, and most disheartening, spiritually exhausted. I began to struggle with daily administrative responsibilities and had difficulty recognizing what priorities were next. The previous year I had organized a six-person management team comprised of key professional staff (including myself), each responsible for a major program component. They rapidly became an effective group and with the decision-making authority delegated to them, began to demonstrate that they were superior to me in their evaluations, planning and implementation of new programming initiatives. (That's the way it's supposed to work—hire folks smarter than you and get out of their way.) I tried to regain my motivation and energy by taking a two-month leave from February to April 1998, but upon returning, I was even less enthusiastic about going to work every day. I knew then that my job was finished.

In reflecting back on my career, I envisioned that I had been on a long, sometimes bumpy train ride, and realized that I needed to get off at the next stop. Early in June, I made the decision to retire in October at the age of sixty.

At his retirement, a friend of mine, John Perrin, the Senior Associate Athletic Director at the University and one of the really good guys, talked about what it took to achieve excellence and a great program. As he acknowledged the many individuals who had helped make the athletic department a great one at the Division I level, he finally came to the person he labeled the "Maestro." That was his boss who was the Director of Intercollegiate Athletics. Although I would in no way suggest that my job as a director could compare in magnitude to that of the athletic director, the scope of my responsibilities did encompass all the functions of the person who had overall responsibility for the unit. When I think about what I and many others achieved in the span of twenty-eight years—starting and nurturing a program, keeping the wolves at bay, and orchestrating all the players in reaching our goals—I secretly (and I suppose selfishly) hope that maybe someone also thought of me as the Maestro. But if no one remembers me or calls me by that title, I still know what I achieved, and it is a good and lasting feeling that I will carry with me.

More than once, I recall my mother admonishing us four children that one ought to think about doing something in life that might contribute to the betterment of mankind. In the spirit of her words, I hope what I did at the University was more on the positive side of the balance sheet.

Maybe, ultimately, the University did recognize and acknowledge my contributions. At the December 1997 University Commencement exercises I received the annual Alumni Achievement Award. It is the highest honor given by the association to a graduate of the University. I was truly honored and at the moment Dr. Likins presented the award to me, I had a sense that all my struggles had been validated.

The University community gave me a memorable retirement send-off in August 1998. It was a great party; groundskeepers, faculty, staff, administrators, the president, deans, family, friends, and a couple of vice-presidents (not the guy who reamed me out in 1984) all came to wish me well (or see if I really was leaving).

Saundra Taylor, the Vice-President for Student Relations said in her remarks at the party," The diversity of people here today, and the fact that they come from all walks of University life, is testimony to who Kent was, that he made no distinctions among people, he treated them all equally and fairly."

Postscript:

I didn't completely sever my ties with the University that October; I waited until January 1999, because the University had made me a great offer. They housed me in a huge office, supplied a private secretary, and paid me a nice salary for a quarter-time fund raising position. The agreement was that I could work in this capacity until at least my sixty-fifth birthday. I worked diligently for twenty-nine days in this new position and then resigned. I had a wonderful twenty-nine year career at the University, but one day short of thirty days, I discovered it was an offer I could refuse.

XI. Travels: A Brief Interlude Before the Rest of the Story

Intended to enlighten the reader of Some Snafus and Snickers of Wheelchair Travel.

In our forty-plus years of marriage and a couple of years of courtship, Marlys and I have, in spite of our wheelchairs, traveled a good deal—not only stateside, but also internationally. I made a number of business-related trips out of the country without her, and she once went to Hawaii without me. Individually or jointly, we have been to Australia, New Zealand, England (twice), Wales, Germany, Czechoslovakia, Hawaii, China, Taiwan, Indonesia, Malaysia, and closer to home, Mexico and Canada. We've been in 35 states, including all states west of the Mississippi except North Dakota. Sometimes I wonder if there really is a North Dakota. I'm not sure that we'll do much traveling in the future. It's more difficult physically, as both of our energy levels aren't what they once were. We've done OK for a couple of gimpers. Europe was always an intended destination for a prolonged visit, but maybe we should settle on an extended visit to North Dakota.

Anyone who has traveled with any frequency has more than likely been a victim, at least once, of the folks who are responsible for getting you from here to there. I'm including in this group airport workers, airline personnel, shuttle service drivers, security people, and anyone else who is supposed to ensure your trip goes smoothly. Traveling, they can lose your luggage, bump you from standby, cancel your flight on account of weather (after you have boarded the plane), lose your ticket, and even run out of rental cars. As wheelchair travelers, my wife and I face all of these potential misfortunes, but additionally there seems to be a host of other snafus reserved for disabled folks. We have endured unbelievably condescending attitudes of airline personnel, the ineptitude of people designated to assist us who have little if any training in helping passengers with disabilities, airport shuttles that are not accessible for wheelchairs, restrooms that are not accessible (particularly on airplanes), and a series of other disasters.

Traveling hasn't always been a bad experience. Some trips have been hassle-free from start to finish. But some trips have been fraught with one problem after another.

Hopefully what follows will enlighten the reader about the pitfalls of wheelchair travel, and maybe prompt a chuckle or two.

Traveling by air almost always begins with check-in at the ticket counter at your airport of departure. I was surprised, on the occasion of one of my initial work-related trips, when the ticket agent (after checking in my traveling partner) ignored me and asked, "Can he walk at all?" It was a question asked thereafter almost every time I traveled with a companion or colleague who walked. I used to travel frequently with a friend and fellow professional, Paul Leung, and the query got so ludicrous that Paul started replying, "Well, why don't you ask him?" It annoyed me, but only once did I reply, "Well, I haven't tried in a while. Should I give it a go?" The agent wasn't amused. Though I never used it, I had another smart aleck remark ready, "No, I can't walk, but you should see me crawl. Would that work?"

At most airports there are personnel who have been hired to assist travelers with disabilities. In many places both in America and overseas, they label these guys special services people. Let me tell you—most times they are very special. Worldwide, the hiring criteria for these dudes is fairly standardized: 1) limited, if any, English speaking ability; 2) no prior experience assisting persons with disabilities, especially wheelchair users; 3) usually a frayed white shirt and wrinkled tie (tattered sports coat optional); 4) to their credit, big smiles; but 5) an appalling lack of priority on personal hygiene (many of these fellows bring new meaning to the term B.O.), and in helping you, they bear hug you, lug you, and rub all over you. I mean, they really get up close and personal.

The usual method of getting a non-ambulatory passenger from the departure area to his seat is via a gurney—a narrow, L-shaped device with a seat usually wide enough for only one butt cheek, and overall, narrow enough to traverse between the airplane seats. To compensate for the fact you must balance on one cheek on the gurney, there are a series of seat belts (I have been on some gurneys with five) that fasten over your knees and shoulders and around your lower legs and belly. Frequently, my helpers (usually two) acted as if buckling the belts was their first attempt at the task. After several locks and unlocks, then re-locks, it's off to your assigned seat, bouncing, banging into seats, scraping other passengers legs, and finally arriving at your seat.

The final step in the process, getting into your seat, can be fraught with danger. None of the airline personnel seem to know how to unlock the arm rests for an easy, level slide-transfer from the gurney to the seat. No problem. I would lift myself onto the armrest and proceed to slide over and down to the seat. I once caught my privates—all of them got hung up. I literally saw stars, almost passed out and fell over into the seat. After that one excruciating painful experience, I didn't try that again. From that point forward, I leaned over on the armrest, belly first, and flopped into the seat. I'd lose shoes, pants would about come down, and glasses might flip off, but I saved the old crown jewels. Things usually got better from that point, but sometimes they got worse.

I began airline travel quite regularly in the mid 1970's, and it was mostly job-related. In the fall of 1976, I attended the National Rehabilitation Association's annual meeting in Hollywood, Florida and was to learn first hand of the many pitfalls awaiting the unsuspecting wheelchair traveler. It was October, just prior to the national election, and Bob Dole was the Vice Presidential candidate running with Gerald Ford. He dropped in at an NRA luncheon looking for a photo opportunity, and the next morning the Hollywood Newspaper front page had a picture of Dole shaking my hand with the caption, *Bob Dole meets Kent Kloepping.*

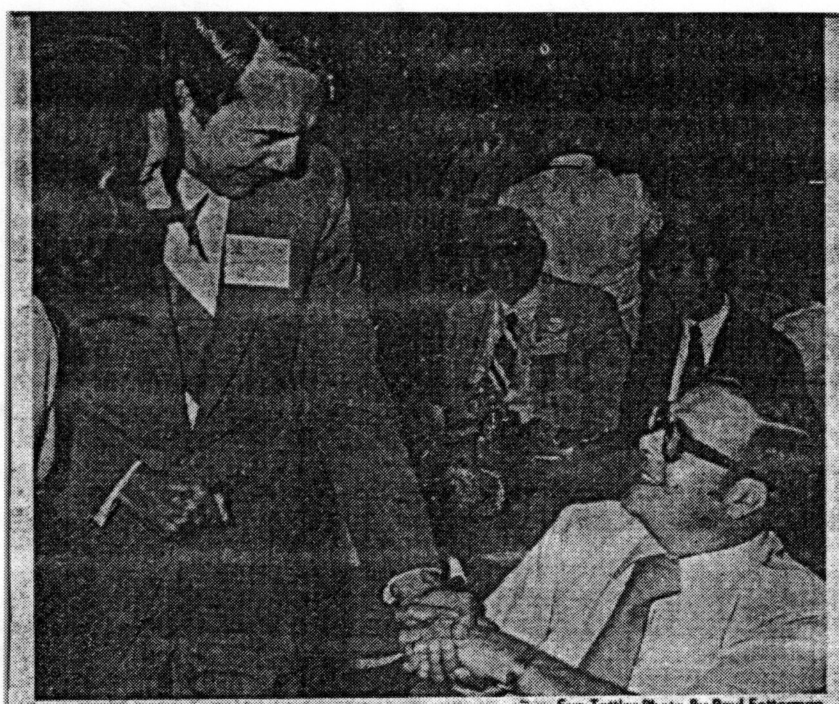

Sun-Tattler Photo By Paul Fetterman

DOLE MEETS KENT KLOEPPING, CONFINED TO WHEELCHAIR
National Rehabilitation Association Receives Dole Enthusiastically

Dole, Disabled In War, Talks To Handicapped

By EVERETT HARVEY
Sun-Tattler Staff

Some were there in wheelchairs, some on crutches, but they all had something in common with their guest speaker, Monday, Republican Vice Presidential candidate Robert Dole, a disabled war veteran.

Dole soft-pedaled politics and refrained from hurling vitriolic barbs at his Democratic opponents when he addressed approximately 1,200 delegates of the National Rehabilitation Association delegation luncheon in Regency Room of the Hotel Diplomat.

They indicated by sustained applause that they identified with the Kansas senator who was wounded in two campaigns in Italy during World War II, spent 39 months in Army

DOLE, 9A, Col. 1

A photo op for presidential candidate Bob Dole at the National Rehabilitation Association's national meeting in Hollywood, Forida (September, 1976)

Getting to Hollywood was an interesting experience. I had to change planes in Dallas, and desperately needed a restroom because I had been drinking alcohol on the flight from Tucson. There were so many wheelchair users heading for the meeting there wasn't a single airport wheelchair available for the trip to the bathroom. With loud protests from the airline, my colleague wheeled me to the nearest restroom in the airplane gurney chair.

The gurney wasn't supposed to leave the boarding area, but Tom, who was hustling me away, barked, "Hey, this is an emergency. Do you want him to pee on the floor?" I made it, and was zipping up when another colleague appeared with an airport wheelchair.

"Hurry up," he said, "We have to get out of here."

"Where did you get this chair?" I asked.

"Outside the men's restroom down the hall," he replied. "Some guy probably left it there while he went into the restroom. That means he can walk and you can't, so you need it more."

Away we raced, downstairs to the airport shuttle for the ride to another terminal. The gate to allow wheelchairs to pass was locked. Tom said, "How can we get through there?" I slipped to the floor, slithered under the gate, and my comrades lifted the chair over the railing. As I grabbed the arm rests to pull myself into the chair, I looked directly at two Catholic Sisters in full nun's regalia, staring at me with a wide-eyed look of disbelief. Although a prominent sign stated, "No strollers or wheelchairs on the shuttle," we all jumped (wheeled) on and said "Good morning Sisters." They nodded politely, but never spoke the entire ten-minute ride to the next terminal.

Another work-related trip was to an international conference on polio in St. Louis in 1985, where Albert Sabin, the fellow who developed the oral polio vaccine, spoke. I met people from all over the world and one night, at a bar, after many drinks (two of my old Southern Illinois University buddies had come over for the night), we were introducing everyone.

An Australian chap who joined our table said, "Howdy mates, I'm Hugh, a physician from Western Australia."

"Hello, what's your last name, Hugh?"

"Oh, it's Newton-John. Go ahead and ask."

"Are you?"

"Yep, Olivia is my sister;"

"Gosh, that's great."

"Oh, it's OK, don't really see her much, I guess her singing is a bit all right."

We thought it was so neat we had him call Marlys at around 2:00 A.M. back in Tucson. She didn't think it was nearly as terrific as we did.

On the topic of career related travels, I attended a 1991 conference on technology for the blind held in Prague, Czechoslovakia. Jan Halousek, a professor from Czechoslovakia, had been touring America looking at programs that served students with disabilities and was referred to our program as a model for serving visually impaired students. After he visited us in Tucson, he invited me to come to the conference the following year in Prague, a city not many years removed from the stranglehold of the Russian Communists. One could still see glimpses of the beauty and grandeur of the old city, but communism had been a disaster. It was like blight on the land, the buildings, and the people.

We (my brother Larry went along to help me) stayed in, allegedly, one of their finest new modern hotels built by the communists. It was a high-rise piece of junk, created with terrible workmanship and cheap building materials. It was absolutely colorless and dingy. The elevators banged and lurched traveling both up and down.

There was a large cast of international types attending the meeting—Russians, Germans, English, Belgians, Czechs, and Slovaks (who were already asserting their separate identity from the Republic), a few Asians, and a handful of Americans. We had the opportunity to do a good amount of sightseeing around old Prague, including visiting the famous Charles Bridge, theaters where Mozart performed, the place where the Russians smashed the Czech revolt in 1968, and many other historic buildings and places. We soon discovered that Czech beer was absolutely wonderful. We met a German guy, touring with a busload of other folks from Germany, and he readily acknowledged that a primary objective for the trip was to drink as much Czech beer as possible.

A major highlight of the conference was not on the agenda. We participated in a spontaneous international drinking bout and

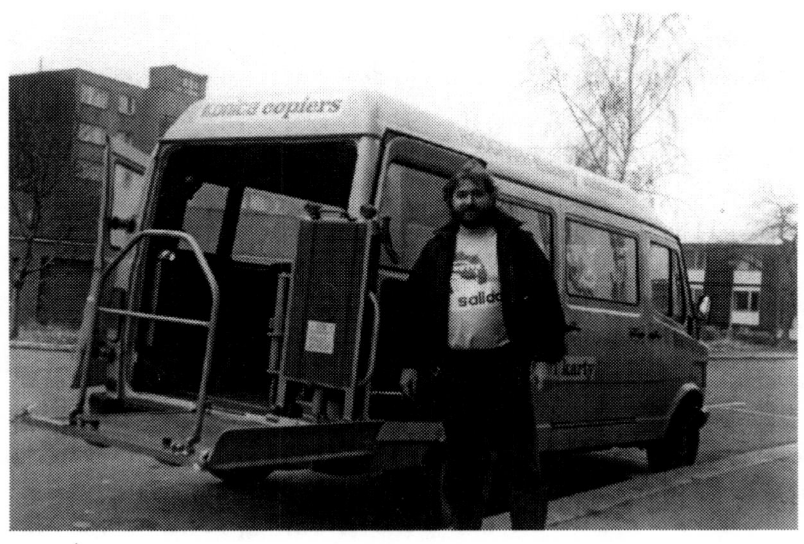

My driver in Prague, Czechoslovakia, with one of only two wheelchair-accessible vans in the city (1991)

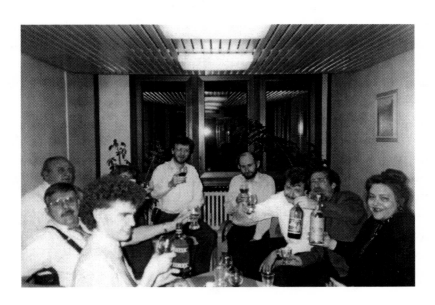

The late-night songfest at the Crystal Hotel in Prague, featuring an international cast of singers (1991)

songfest that started about midnight in the lobby area on the 10th or 11th story of the building.

It began innocently enough with an English chap, Gordon, asking, "Hey Kent, have you ever had Cragganmore Single-Malt Scotch whiskey?"

"No," I replied.

"Well, heck, why don't you come up to my floor for a little nip?"

Some Czech beer would also be good, so we bought an ample supply. We grabbed an armful of snacks and headed up the elevator. A couple of people from New Orleans joined us, toting a large bottle of brandy. After not too many drinks, as is often the case in group drinking, someone decided to sing. We thought we sounded damn good, so after finishing one tune we launched into even more melodies. Before long, a couple of German guys joined us, one an SS type (even wore a long trench coat) and the other a great fellow named Joachim Klaus. Then a big Russian dude and a couple of Russian ladies arrived with vodka. Everyone joined the swelling chorus. If they didn't know the words, they hummed or just faked it. Finally, there were two blind guys from England who came staggering down the hall yelling, "Where are you? We've come to sing." They were part of Gordon's group, The Royal National Institute for the Blind, a well-funded private organization. These fellows knew how to party, and one of them had a beautiful tenor voice. Between what must have been a god-awful crescendo when the whole group sang, we had him singing solos, really beautiful ballads.

We drank everything we had and probably around 3:00 A.M., in the final throes of inebriation, we began singing Christmas carols. Everyone loved them, especially the Germans, and we sang all of them loudly. We basically knew the tunes, and what words we forgot, we made up. It didn't matter—no one realized they weren't the right words, and furthermore didn't care. Old familiar tunes got several renditions. It was amazing that no hotel guests complained as we were terribly noisy and probably wouldn't have won any mixed choral awards.

I began to do a lot of job-related traveling, and I noticed that there were many more wheelchair users traveling, not only domestically but also internationally. I assumed seeing an individual in a

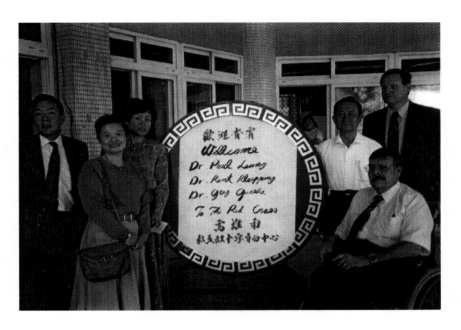

Welcoming committee, Taiwan: Paul Leung (far left), Greg Garske (far right), and me (right front). (Fall, 1993)

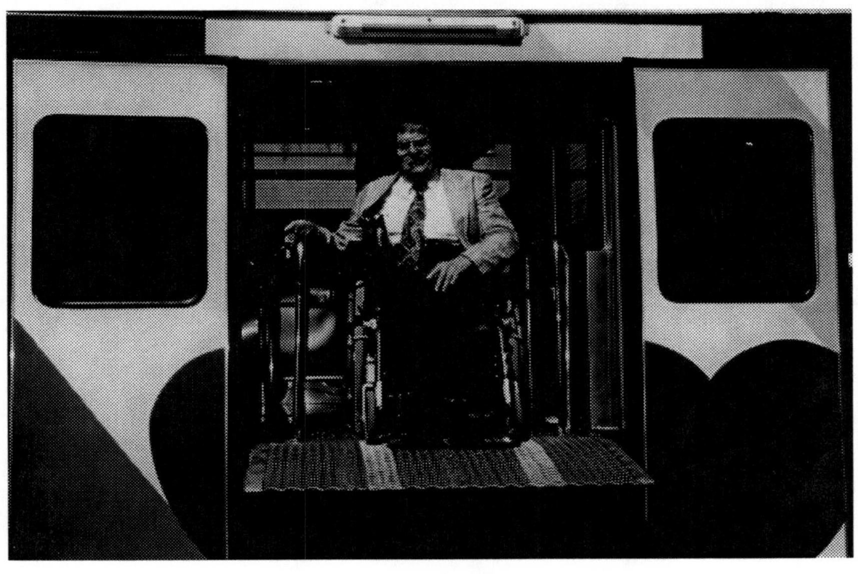

Wheelchair-accessible bus, Taiwan (1993)

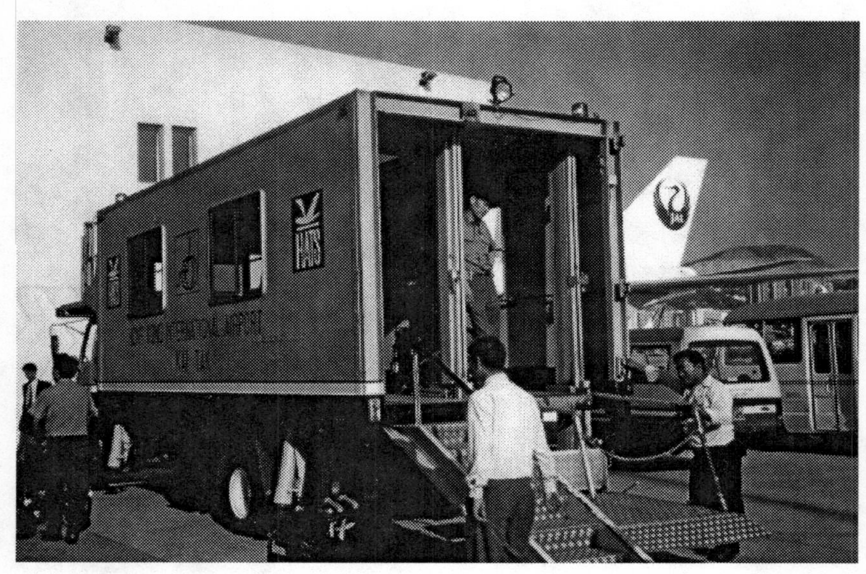

Airport transportation for me to change planes in Hong Kong (1993)

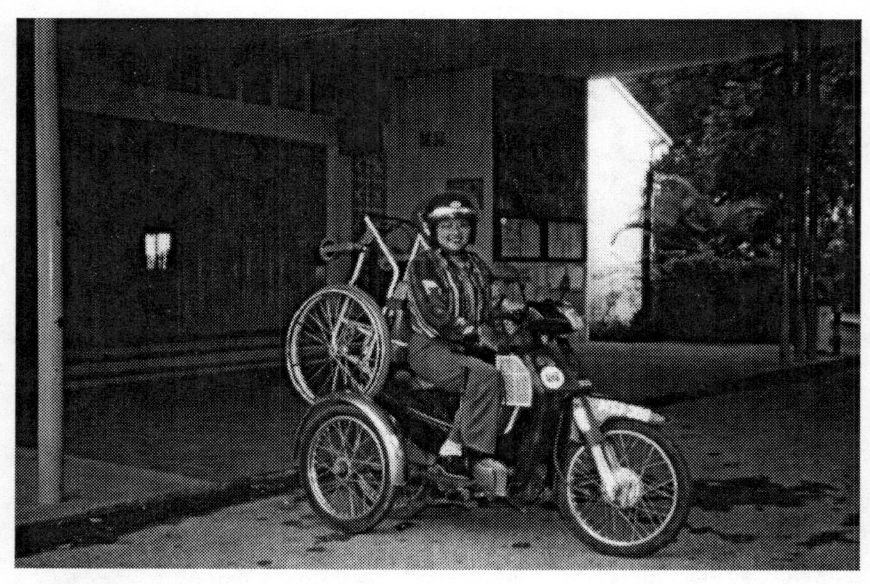

A young woman named King and her motorcycle, the only accessible transportation for her in Kuala Lumpur, Malaysia (1993)

wheelchair was a fairly common sight not only in America, but also in Europe and Asia as well. Well, that assumption was incorrect.

In 1993, Paul Leung invited me to accompany him and his faculty colleague from the University of Illinois on a three-week trip to four Asian countries.

We had landed in China's largest city, Shanghai, on the first leg of the trip. As we deplaned, I began to notice people, almost 100% of them Chinese, looking at me, some watching intently. "Oh, they'll look," said Paul, "we're somewhat of a unique threesome." Paul hailed a cab, the driver opened the door and I began the process of transferring from the wheelchair to the front seat. As I pivoted in the chair, I was stunned to see that a large crowd of people had completely ringed the cab and were silently watching every move I made. I removed the detachable footrests from the chair, which caused a minor stir in the crowd; I made the transfer, lifted the cushion from the chair, and Paul folded the collapsible lightweight chair. That brought a chorus of "oohs and aahs," and lots of jabbering among the growing throng. Paul put the chair in the trunk, and I swung my legs into the cab. Paul chuckled, "Well, you might as well get used to it." Yeah, why not, I thought. We're almost celebrities. As I reached out to close the door, I smiled at the staring, incredulous faces, and gave them a thumbs-up signal. There was a split second delay, then big smiles all around, lots of excited chatter, and a round of loud and sustained applause.

We had been scheduled to arrive in Shanghai the previous evening, but were not allowed to land and had to return to Narita Airport in Japan to spend the night. The delay caused us to miss a train trip to the interior, so we were literally shanghaied in Shanghai. While we waited to leave for Malaysia, we toured the city of Shanghai for two days, none of us prepared for the reaction of the locals. We weren't the typical threesome in the city—Greg Garske, a large Polish-German chap, Paul Leung, whose heritage is Chinese, and me in a shiny new lightweight red wheelchair. Anytime we appeared in public, people stopped in traffic (it seemed 75% or more riding bicycles) to stare at us. If we went into a souvenir shop, a crowd gathered immediately, watching every move I made. We went into a restaurant somewhere in the heart of the city, frequented mostly by Chinese, and when our lunch came, every patron stopped eating to watch us. It really got on Greg's nerves, but their curiosity was so genuine I don't recall getting annoyed. Every time I had to transfer from cab to chair or vice-versa, I tried to prolong the process a bit and accomplish my moves with flair. My exaggerations always resulted in appreciative "oohs and aahs" as the assembled crowds understood how I did it. As I recall, we saw only one other person in a wheelchair in Shanghai during our stay. No wonder they all looked. But I think it's also a cultural thing—they are curious, so they look.

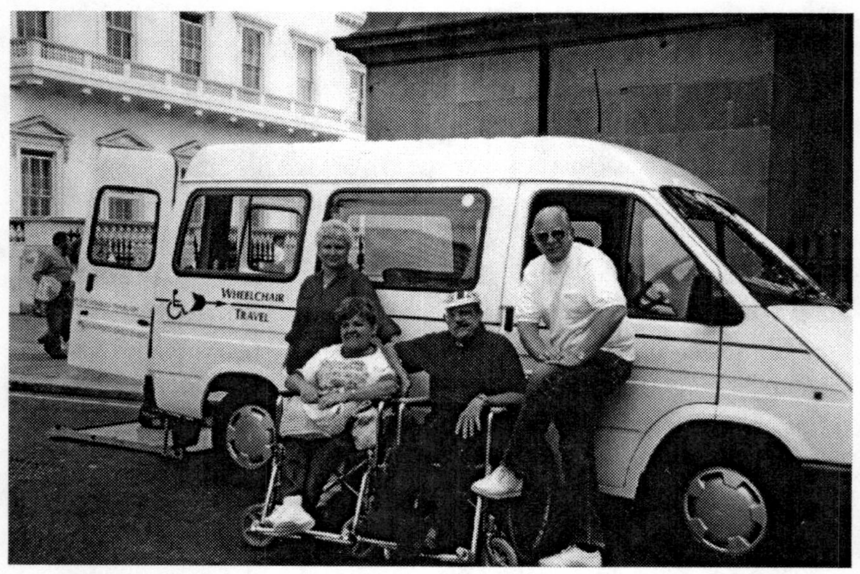

London: Our van that we traveled in throughout England and Wales. The Jensens, Marlys, and me (1990)

However, not all cultures stare, the English, by contrast, are much more discrete. They go out of their way to be polite (the traditional English, not the new immigrants) and pretend not to look. They also seem to have an innate ability to under-react and maintain a sense of normalcy, even in quite unusual circumstances.

One afternoon at Nottingham Castle, toward the end of an amazing English adventure with our neighbors, Merle and Sharon Jensen, some English fellows demonstrated that mastery of restraint. The castle, originally built by William the Conqueror, was now a museum on the original site. Oliver Cromwell had blown up the castle during the English 17th century civil war, because the area had been loyal to the Royalists. I was in dire need of a restroom after drinking good English ale with my ploughman's lunch. The men's toilet had a wheelchair accessible stall, but it was locked. Fortunately, I had the key. Throughout England, there were wheelchair accessible restrooms in a system they called RADAR (why RADAR I haven't a clue), which required a key to enter. I was in a rush and couldn't get my key to work, so one of the trusty staff marched in with his key and opened the door. The stall was very small and also had become the janitor's closet. There were two or three mops, several brooms, a mop bucket with a wringer, and an assortment of bottles (cleaning compounds, etc.) stacked in the small space.

"Wow," I sighed, "That's a problem." The English chap, quite a proper fellow, didn't seem to recognize the problem at first, so I explained that with all the supplies and the smallness of the room, I couldn't get in and close the door.

"I'll have to wait," I said.

"Well no," he chirped, "why don't we give it a go."

I backed into the stall as far as I could and the Englishman then grasped the armrests of my wheelchair and started rather vigorously trying to push me backwards further into the stall. Of course, we immediately hit the bucket and mops, but that didn't deter my determined helper. The more resistance he felt against the wheelchair, the harder he pushed. After a sustained, continuous push against the obstacles (which didn't gain much ground), he changed tactics and started using my chair like a battering ram. He pulled me forward and then lunged against the wheelchair, shoving me backwards rather violently. On about the third assault, my left foot slipped off my footrest and fell under the front wheel of my chair. By now my helper was really lathered up and didn't notice my foot as he blasted me backwards, jamming the foot between my chair and the toilet stool.

"Ow!" I howled. It really hurt.

He stopped suddenly and asked, "What's wrong?"

I gasped, "My foot, my foot is caught."

"Oh, terrible sorry, old boy, are you all right?"

I wasn't permanently damaged. I was just concerned about what further pain his next move might inflict. We—no he—managed to jam me far enough into the janitor's supplies so that the door would close. The entire affair, which had taken several minutes, had created quite a disturbance with the mop bucket, brooms, mops, and a good number of bottles and containers getting knocked about. After completing the objective of my visit, the commotion began anew.

Trying to pull up one's trousers from a sitting position is a difficult task itself, and in that cramped space, every time I moved to try and get my pants up an inch or two, I bumped the chair, which rattled mops, the bucket, and the various cans and bottles. I huffed and puffed, and swore and cursed my predicament and the smallness of that damned closet. There was no camouflaging the racket I was making, because the door had about an eight-inch section cut off of the bottom. After a ten to fifteen minute struggle, banging mops and buckets around and peppering the crashes with lots of epithets, I did finally get my pants up.

I sat trying to catch my breath and heard someone outside the door ask quietly of another individual, "I say, is everything all right in there?"

"Well, I think so. It's this handicapped chap you see...." (And his voice trailed off).

I started laughing softly as I thought about what they must have imagined was going on behind that door. When I exited, a different staff person was there.

"What a struggle," I remarked.

The fellow maintained a deadpan expression and simply said,"Oh yes. I see."

Merle told me later that two little boys had come out of the

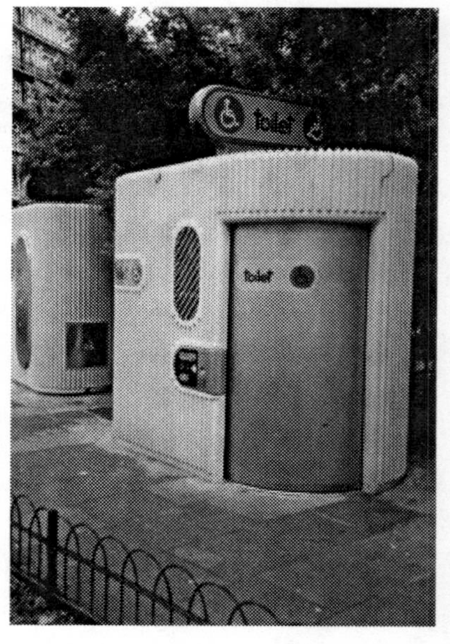

A RADAR loo in London (1990)

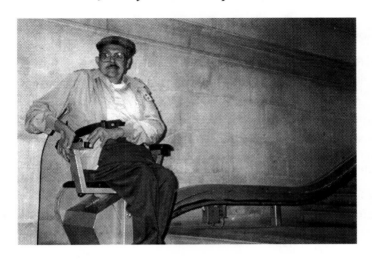

Riding to the upper floors of Castle Howard (1990)

restroom whispering that something quite unusual was going on in that loo.

The problem traveling throughout England was that I was constantly looking for a restroom. We often had two pints of beer with lunch at one of the many quaint old pubs that dot the English countryside, and then I needed to find a RADAR restroom. If all else failed, a large old oak with a girth wide enough to hide a wheelchair would have sufficed. It was really quite remarkable that we usually found an accessible restroom and not once did I have to water the countryside.

If Marlys were writing this section, she would have most assuredly included her classic experience with two of those aforementioned special services types assigned to assist disabled travelers. She encountered these two limited-English-speaking, unbathed dudes—not in a foreign land, but in her home state of Minnesota at the Minneapolis Airport. She was sitting in the aisle seat so she was the first to be helped off the plane. We could smell these two smiling young fellows the moment they came into the cabin. They were pleasant and well intentioned, but they pulled, tugged, and rearranged most of her clothes. Her bra was somewhere up close to her chin, her back brace was rotated about sixty degrees around her torso, her slacks were drooping, and her hair looked like a Janis Joplin "do!" They finally got her strapped to the gurney chair after buckling, unbuckling, and then re-buckling the straps. They tipped the gurney back slightly, and proceeded forward.

The gurney and Marlys lurched to a stop and she howled, "My gosh, those straps are terribly tight." Undeterred, the boys backed up and took another run at it, harder this time but with the same results. They both put their shoulders into the gurney, pushing, straining, and trying to get some momentum.

"Stop it!" Marlys demanded, "What the devil is going on?" They stopped and carefully rechecked the straps.

Suddenly, Marlys exclaimed, "Hey, there's the problem. Look what you did." Unbelievably, they had looped one of the seat belts from the back of the gurney, through the airplane seat, around her stomach, and buckled it securely at her navel.

They smiled apologetically, chattered excitably, and got out a rather weak" sorry."

No matter what country you go to, those blasted gurney chairs are all the same size—about the width of a 12 inch wooden plank and although padded, just as hard as a board. As uncomfortable as they are, they are preferable to having no chair available.

That was the case on the third leg of my 1993 Asian trip with Paul Leung and Greg Garske when we landed in Indonesia. There was no chair of any kind available and after exhausting all ideas and options, it came down to four guys, who weren't very enthusiastic about the idea, being told they had to carry me off the plane. I tried to communicate to them how to do a chair lift carry, with my arms around the neck of two guys, and the other two guys each supporting one leg. Had they chosen to listen to my instructions, I would've been carried out in an upright position with my weight equally distributed and in a way that was not altogether uncomfortable.

My instructions got lost in whatever language they spoke, and I ended up being carried off like a slaughtered hog or side of beef. Each of the four guys grabbed an arm or leg, but then let me droop until my ass bumped on the floor as they dragged me out of the plane. By the time we got off, it felt as if both shoulder and hip sockets were dislocated. Maybe it was because we were in a Southeast Asian country that an image of a dead Bengal tiger, all four legs tied securely to a pole being carried by four guys, flashed through my mind. It must have been some spectacle when we emerged from that plane. I could understand that a country like Indonesia might not have much experience handling people with disabilities, but I was to later learn that they hadn't totally cornered the market on that kind of incompetence.

Half a world away (and two years earlier in 1991) on a return trip to the U. S from Czechoslovakia, my brother Larry and I had to change planes in Frankfurt, Germany. We got off the plane and were met by two large Germans (storm-trooper types) who hustled us into a mini-van and proceeded to race across the tarmac at breakneck speed. They were rude, and once they realized we didn't understand German, they made it clear that we were the focus of their discussion. They laughed and yucked it up, all the while glancing back at us, snickering and not responding to any question or communication from Larry or me. They deposited us in a small room that was enclosed with wire mesh, like we were so much baggage or freight. Try as we might, we couldn't get them to respond to us and listen to our pleas that our scheduled departure was imminent. They continued to goof off long enough for us to miss our flight.

When we finally did arrive at the check-in counter, the statuesque German lady who was obviously in charge was not happy with us for showing up late. She initially began to admonish me but I quickly interrupted her, my temper rising, and made it clear that the two louts escorting us were the only reason we were late. I explained that they had caged us, refused to communicate, and had been rude and disrespectful. She then turned and began asking them a series of questions in German. Suddenly her eyes flashed and she let loose a withering barrage of verbiage, sort of a "Teutonic tirade" that actually caused them to backpedal. It was one of the most masterful performances of humiliation and degradation I had ever witnessed. Sitting behind her, looking straight at the two now-wilting krauts, I smirked like a Cheshire cat, winked at them, repeatedly covered my mouth as if to say,"Oh my!" and visibly shook my shoulders as if laughing uncontrollably throughout the entire scene. Once she banished them, she very efficiently rebooked us on another flight that left only an hour later. Missing the plane turned out to be a serendipitous happening as we flew into Cincinnati, Ohio, a much smaller and less-congested airport than New York.

Eventually I learned to mostly avoid assistance from the special services folks, and once off the plane, find my own way to the next terminal. For example, every major airport had carts conspicuously displaying the international symbol of accessibility, but they were not wheelchair accessible. They mostly transported old duffers and lots of people with large asses. On one of my last trips to Washington D.C. to read grant proposals, the Dallas Airport did have a wheelchair accessible cart. But for the previous number of years I flew back east to read for the government (I had to change plans usually in Dallas or Chicago), not one time did I get a ride or push from one terminal to the connecting flight. I usually had about sixty minutes between flights and when I deplaned, the airport personnel would call for assistance. No one would show up to push me and after waiting a half-hour, I'd tell the airline folks to call ahead to my gate of departure and tell him or her to hold the plane for me. I always made it, sometimes with no time to spare, but had I waited for those folks to arrive, most assuredly I would have missed more than one plane.

One of my strangest experiences with special service personnel occurred at Narita Airport in Japan on the final leg of the 1993 China, Malaysia, Indonesia, and Taiwan adventure with Paul Leung and Greg Garske. Paul had flown ahead to Hawaii for a scheduled meeting with folks in Honolulu, leaving Greg and me to catch a later flight to Dallas. American Airlines, our carrier, was on strike and many flights became a 50\50 probability of being canceled— including the one on which we were booked. Greg unexpectedly found a direct flight to Michigan, his home state, and without too much hemming and hawing abandoned me sitting in an ancient airport wheelchair with my personal wheelchair floating around in the bowels of Narita Airport. I was in a state of shock over his quick decision to leave, partly because he only gave me about thirty seconds to agree that I'd be fine.

The chair I was in had no push rims, so the first thing was to try to locate my own wheelchair. God, I didn't know where to start. I tried to pick out an official-looking airport person from the thousands of people milling about. I was frantically scanning the crowd when I spotted a petite, young Japanese woman walking towards me.

I thought, my gosh its Miyoshi Umeki—you know, Red Buttons wife from the movie *Sayonara.* She wasn't, of course, but she was indeed an airport official who slowly walked up to me and asked, "May I help you?" I explained that I was traveling alone and needed my wheelchair so I could find a restroom. She smiled sweetly, took a few notes (my name, arrival flight number, maybe other information), bowed slightly and said, "I will return." She did return, with my wheelchair in tow. Where she found it, I have no idea. She directed me to a snack bar and the nearest wheelchair accessible restroom, and then she was gone.

I got to the boarding area where my scheduled AA flight was to depart, and noted in bold letters my flight was on hold. I simply had to wait for notification of whether it would leave or if I'd be spending a little extra time in Japan. Suddenly, standing next to me was a stocky, very muscular Japanese fellow with a severe crew cut, wearing a suit and tie. Staring intently at me he asked, "Are you travering alone?"(Yes he said travering.) His demeanor was very stoic, almost sinister, and I thought, my god who is this guy? I was feeling a little weird and it occurred to me that maybe he was a buddy of old Tojo. No, he wasn't old enough. Yikes—maybe he was a modern day Yakuza. His shirt had a very high collar and long sleeves so I couldn't see any of the tattoos characteristic of that group of thugs. I was more than a little spooked and surprised. I did a few "well ums," and "you sees" trying to compose a rational response. It did cross my mind (in case he had seen Paul, Greg, and I arrive) to say something silly about why I was now alone, but I decided that he might not be the kind of guy who liked to be humored. Instead, I rather meekly explained my situation, trying to convey as pathetic a demeanor as I could.

He stared at me, showing no emotion and said, "You know, you may not get a flight. Then what will you do?"

"Well gee, I really don't know," was all I could muster. With that he abruptly turned and walked away. Geez, I thought, who the hell was that guy?

Suddenly and quite amazingly, AA announced that the scheduled 747 flight to Dallas was leaving in a matter of minutes. There was a limited cabin crew and only thirty or forty people on board when we left. Just before they boarded me, standing a short distance to my left stood Mr. Moto. He gazed at me, and as we passed him he said, "You were very rucky." By god, I did feel "rucky," especially not being stranded in Narita Airport with that sinister dude.

Actually, the ten or eleven hour flight was one of the most comfortable international flights I ever had. I had an entire unoccupied row of six seats for a bed, and with so few on board, it was very quiet. I slept a good part of the trip. The hostess for my section was an older gal, easily fifty plus, with lots of moxie. She quickly assessed my situation.

She asked me, "Do you have a way to use the bathroom if you need to?"

"Well, I have a urinal," I replied.

"No problem, I'll empty your jug if you need to use it." I did, and she did.

This is a nice segue into a very difficult issue. For non-ambulatory passengers on extended or international airline flights, using the restroom is difficult, if not impossible. There is no way to ever get to the airplane restroom on a domestic flight if you can't walk, as there are no on board chairs to get you there. International carriers say they have a chair, which I've seen, but it actually looked even narrower than a gurney. It did have side rails so you wouldn't fall off, but if you did manage to squeeze into it, I really seriously doubt that a person could extricate oneself from the viselike grip it would have on your ass. Women could never get a dress up, and if they got slacks down, they couldn't get them back up. It wouldn't work for a guy, as your sphincter would be pinched off so tightly you couldn't get a drip, let alone a trickle, going.

Marlys and I took a fabulous thirty-one day trip to Australia and New Zealand with our neighbors Merle and Sharon Jensen in 1992. It was really a once-in-a-lifetime adventure. The Australian leg was especially memorable as we traveled with their friends, George and Joyce Taylor. George, a world-renowned azalea breeder, was a crusty, outspoken, self-made Australian. I kept a daily journal of the trip, and anytime I glance back through it I laugh out loud recalling some of George's antics. Kangaroos of course are a main attraction in that land "down under." We saw some early in our trip in a wild animal park, but it wasn't until much later that we were mobbed by a bunch of the feisty buggers at a place called Pebbly Beach. It was amazing, birds, called lorikeets, and roos all over us.

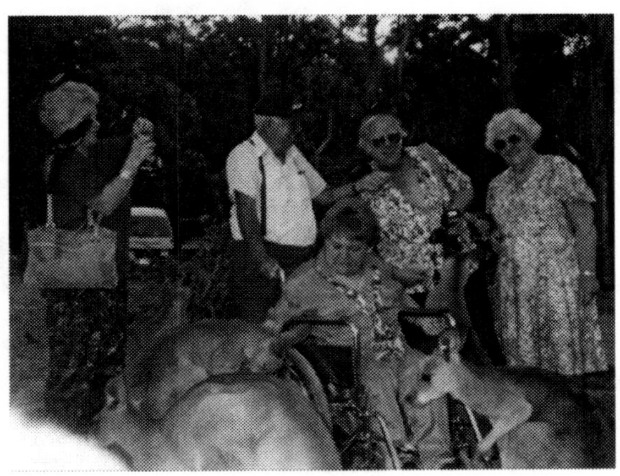

A bunch of "birds" at Pebbly Beach, Australia. (L–R) Sharon Jensen, George Taylor, Marlys, Merle Jensen, Joyce Taylor. The Taylors from Australia were friends of the Jensens. (February, 1992)

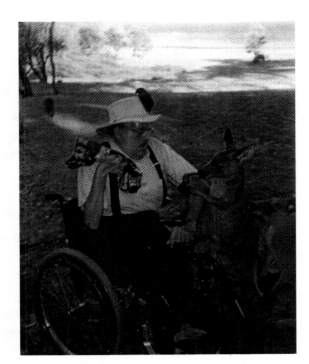

Pebbly Beach. Hey, that's my bread. (1992)

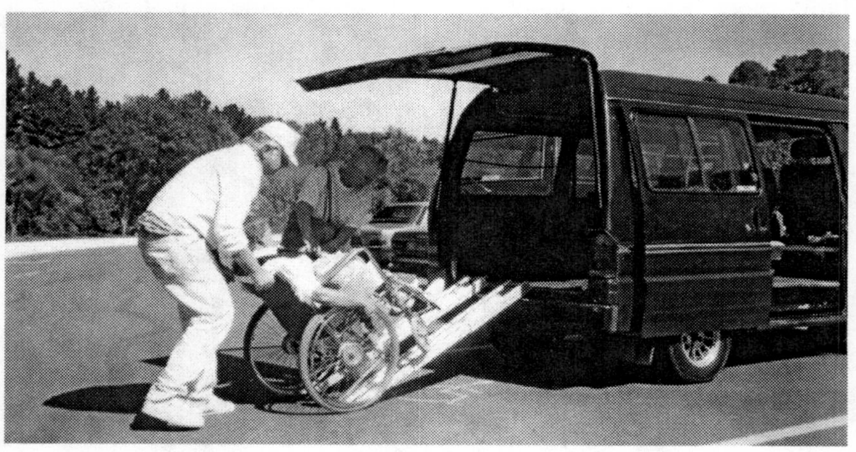

A daily routine: Merle loading Marlys (many times each day) on our thirty-one-day trip to Australia and New Zealand (1992)

Then two more weeks in New Zealand, a unique almost magical little country with people, landscapes, and cultures that will surprise and delight you. Each day we encountered unique, unexpected, and wonderful sights. The Jensen's have hauled our butts over half the globe, and on this trip we had stopped in Hawaii on the way—literally—to take a pee. Overseas flights are usually not much fun because of the unavailability of the restrooms. Outside of catherization (ouch), about the only surefire answer is to dehydrate; no liquids several hours before the flight and absolutely nothing while on board. This means that while everyone else is downing brewskies, mixed drinks, juices, and water, we're sitting there with parched throats, spitting cotton and really not feeling well.

The longest wait without using a restroom occurred on our way home to Tucson from our trip to England. Merle and Sharon had left earlier (as they had frequent flyer mileage), so Marlys and I were on our own. I was going to use the facilities at Heathrow (London) but we got into a huge flap with British Airways due to their all-female cabin crew. They had boarded Marlys and then decided they weren't going to take me. "In an emergency how would we handle you?" the head stewardess whined. I threatened them with a lawsuit, yelled, howled, and asked her how they would handle a male passenger who had just boarded, who was about 6-4 and two hundred-fifty pounds, if he had a heart attack. They finally relented, but I was so worked up that I needed a restroom as we lifted off. Some eight hours later we cleared customs in Los Angeles and were hustled outside to catch our special needs van for a short trip to U.S. Air. The van was almost an hour late, and the old codger driving it was doing about fifteen MPH. I left the curb to flag him down and hurry him up, which was against his rules; he would not stop to load us until I returned to a designated spot on the sidewalk.

We finally got loaded, and he delivered us to the U.S. Air terminal. Marlys unloaded, but the van lift was leaking hydraulic fluid so badly it would not come back up after she got out. I was frantic, desperately in need of a bathroom and terrified that we were going to miss our flight. "Yes it leaks a little," he chuckled, oblivious to my now near panic. I got out of my chair on to the dirty, greasy floor of the van, pushed my wheelchair out the door, threw my cushion on the chair, slid out into the chair and took off. . The old fellow kind of freaked out, his eyes bugging out while he repeated, "What you doin'? What you doin'?" Marlys made it to the john (I didn't) while I checked us in, and we just made our flight to Tucson. Our son picked us up, we raced home, and I got to the fritz about 6:00 P.M.—maybe fifteen hours from my last visit to a latrine.

The most maddening part of those seemingly endless hours was the old geezer and his ramshackle van (yet another of those infamous special needs guys). After all we had been through, if we had missed our plane on account of that snafu, I most likely would have arrived in Tucson in a strait jacket.

Marlys and I had lots of adventures flying here and there, but on balance, the airlines were almost always pretty good to us. We got lots of jerks and jolts getting on and off gurneys, bruised buns sliding over arm rests, and spent a good bit of time rearranging our clothes after being manhandled. On one occasion, the airlines forgot that I needed assistance getting off the plane (as I always had to deplane last), and the cleanup crew had to chase someone down to get me off the aircraft.

Believe it or not, on one trip I actually crawled to my seat from the jet way. It was an early morning flight and the agent was alone, flustered, and couldn't find an aisle chair, so I made a deal with him: Seat me in first class all the way to Washington, D.C. from Tucson, and I'd crawl the short distance from the door to first class so as not to delay boarding the other passengers. By golly, he took me up on the offer.

On another occasion, I arrived in Tucson, and as the passengers began to deplane, the cabin started to fill with smoke. Everyone, including the damn pilots, took off running and there I sat. Finally, one stewardess came back, bless her soul. As I was waiting for the explosion of flames to erupt, I told her my son Matt might be waiting for me at the top of the jet way. She disappeared and then reappeared with Matt, who carried me off. Geez, I thought if the ship or plane was in distress, the Captain was the last guy off, well so much for that myth.

Over the years, I've been carried up the steps to the plane in my wheelchair, ridden all sorts of forklifts both up and down (once it took two fork lifts to deplane from a DC-10). I've been dragged off, carried off, and even been bounced down a flight of stairs in a wheelchair; but mostly I've ridden that "one cheek pony" (gurney) on and off airliners. One of the most unique rides was on a motorized, self-propelled appliance mover. They were designed to haul refrigerators or other heavy appliances up long flights of apartment stairs, and some fool thought they'd be good to haul non-ambulatory folks up the steps. The device worked fine, but was extremely slow and had a loud thump with an accompanying jar to the derriere.

In fairness to the airlines, I must say that the problems aren't always their fault. I've also heard a number of horror stories about what some disabled folks have done and the demands they've made in the course of traveling. I know of and have witnessed unreasonable requests for accommodations that have caused a good deal of unnecessary grief for airline personnel. I once had a three hour flight to Chicago seated next to a terribly neurotic woman who had her hundred pound service dog between us on the floor. The dog was almost as bizarre as the gal; the poor thing whined, passed gas, shed its long hair all over everything, and continually jumped up on her. It was a constant agitation. The cabin crew was extremely solicitous, I think mostly because they felt sorry for the animal.

All in all, airlines do their best to be accommodating. What the industry really needs is a massive training program on how to manage and accommodate people with disabilities. Out of such training could emerge consistent, realistic, and standardized policies and procedures for serving this population of travelers. Many, if not most of those procedures would be applicable in serving elderly folks as well. Perhaps I should come out of retirement and work as a consultant for the airlines. Then again, maybe I won't.

Finally, I must share a true story about a group of disabled guys on a trip to California in 1990. I think it is one of the best anecdotes about wheelchair travel that I've ever heard. There is a wheelchair basketball team at the University of Arizona, and one spring the team was headed to San Diego for a series of games. By the time the ten, high-spirited, wisecracking wheelchair athletes boarded, settled in their seats, stowed multiple carry-ons, and secured their wheelchairs (and their multiple parts), the flight attendants were more than a little frazzled. A particularly distraught attendant began barking orders for the fellows to get their seat belts on and stop goofing off. All of them complied, including Rudy, a cherubic looking Hispanic fellow who had lost both of his legs to a land mine in Vietnam. As he was a high-level amputee (both legs gone above the knees), he could easily sit *facing* the seat, which he did, securing the seat belt at his back and quietly waiting for the attendant. In orderly fashion, she efficiently checked each athlete to ensure they were properly belted in their seat. Later reports were that when she came to Rudy, he smiled and said, "Hi." She gasped, visibly staggered, turned pale, and sat down. After she regained some composure, she made Rudy turn around and ride facing forward. The players said she never did fully recover on the trip. I wish I had been there to see that one.

I had many more misadventures, too numerous to include here. For now, it's on to the best job I ever had, RETIREMENT.

XII. Retirement

If my doctor told me I had only 6 minutes to live, I wouldn't brood. I'd type a little faster. (1)

My father passed away in January 1998. That previous August, I had flown to Illinois for my fortieth high school class reunion. It was the last time I saw my father. I asked him how he was doing and he said, "Well, you know I'm 87 and do have some problems. I'm almost blind, I can't hear very good, my left leg is shot, I have two bad ruptures, I've lost a kidney, don't sleep well, and my lungs bother me. But you know, I'm actually doing pretty good."

Now in my eighth year of retirement at the age of sixty-seven, I thought about that last face-to-face meeting with Dad and what he said. It started me thinking about my situation. To sum it up, I'm deaf in one ear, I have chronic problems with my right eye, have right-side facial paralysis, I'm overweight, have gas problems and hemorrhoids, I'm losing my hair, I can't seem to find anything, my wife says I'm paranoid, and I've become a compulsive counter. I literally have scars from my butt to the top of my head from twelve surgeries, and residuals of two hundred plus stitches in my face from a 1962 car accident. I haven't discussed the subject of my projected longevity with my doctor, but given Dad's commentary and reasoning, I must conclude I'm actually doing quite well.

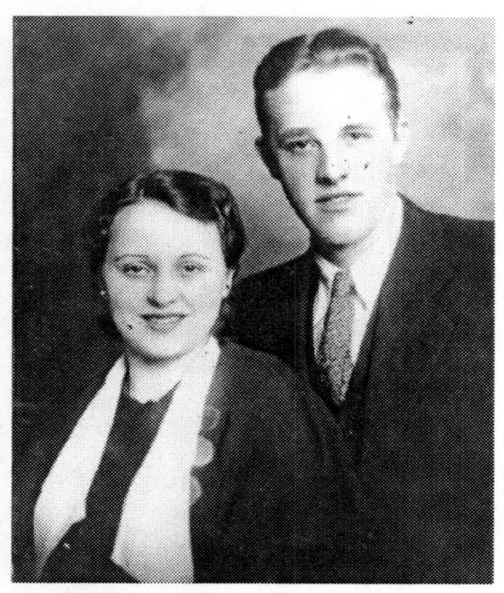

My parents, Dale and Christine Kloepping, on their wedding day (September 17, 1932)

Speaking of my father, it occurs to me that I've had little to say about either of my parents. So I think I should digress a bit.

Dale and Christine—Mom and Dad to me—were married in 1932. Dad was 6-2 and two hundred ten pounds, and Mom was a diminutive 5-2 (and that was probably in high heels). There weren't many guys around who were bigger than my father, and fortunately, he was, by nature, an easygoing individual who never used his size advantage to intimidate. He always assumed the best intentions of people. However, if others mistook his good nature for naiveté or dim-wittedness and tried to mislead or dupe him, he could quickly become a fearsome adversary. Not that he had a quick temper, mind you. He was extremely generous in his praise of others and willing to overlook almost all transgressions, but once past his tolerance level, the result was awesome. His huge, barrel

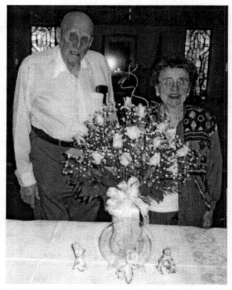

My parents on their sixty-fifth wedding anniversary (September 17, 1997)

chest seemed to expand to double its already massive girth, and I'd swear he grew two or three inches in height. His broad tanned shoulders squared from their characteristic slump; most frightening was his voice. The volume increased and was accompanied by a heightened articulateness. An older hired man who once witnessed the phenomena, remarked, "Boy, your dad is quite a talker when he gets mad."

He was at that. As we had all seen Dad in action more than once, we knew what to expect and had learned to lay low until the episode ran its course. I'd guess he was terrifying to the unsuspecting. I witnessed more than one oily tongued salesman reduced to a backpedaling twerp. While he must have appeared totally out-of-control, he was, in fact, completely in command of not only the situation, but also his emotions and behavior. Most often when the offender departed, he would chuckle over the encounter. Mom would chastise him (sort of) with a halfhearted, "Well, Dale, you don't need to get so carried away," and we kids snickered the rest of the day.

My younger sister, Jolene, reminded me of an incident that occurred in 1955 when I was seventeen years old. I included the story because I unexpectedly learned a powerful lesson about parenting from my father. There was a local drive-in theater, the Sky-Vu, at Monroe, Wisconsin, about eighteen miles from my home. It was a warm summer evening, I was bored, restless, and tried to get one of the family to take me to the show. No one would, so I pouted, sulked, and got pissed. In retrospect, I believe I was feeling left out, as I didn't drive (had no license), didn't date, couldn't play sports with my peers, and was beginning to understand that my disability did indeed impose limitations. I did a rash thing—I grabbed my wallet, crawled to the shed housing my brother's 54 Ford, got in, and drove off to the theater. I did make it, saw two of the worst films ever made, and tried quietly to skulk back home. It was 1:00 A.M. or later and the house was dark, so I crawled inside, quietly went upstairs, and got into bed.

I got up late the next morning, fearing my parents' wrath, but nothing was said. I felt pretty guilty, but it wasn't until several days later that Dad asked me to ride to town with him. I guessed that among other topics, the matter of the Sky-Vu drive-in would most likely surface. To my surprise, he spoke to me quietly, gently saying something like, "Kent, you know you hadn't ought to do things like that. It isn't your car. You could have wrecked it, hurt yourself, or worse, injured someone else. I know sometimes things don't seem fair, and they aren't, but you and I, no matter how much we want things to be different, can't change what happens to us. I think I understand why you did what you did, and I'm not angry with you, but I don't want you to do something like that again." That was it. He had reprimanded me and made it clear that it wasn't to happen again. But most importantly, he didn't embarrass or belittle me (like a child), and he didn't make me explain. He simply said that what I had done was wrong, but he understood and still loved me. He was a good Father to all his children. His thoughtful wisdom, then and frequently thereafter, helped me over many hurdles growing up. I miss him, his humor, his stories and his commentaries on everything from farming to world politics, but I especially miss him as a Dad.

He was a fair and extremely generous man, not only to all of us, but also to his neighbors. Three different older men that I interviewed for this writing used the terms "hero," "mentor," and "Father-figure" in describing their relationship with him. He was a steady, reliable helpmate for my mother, always ready to come to her aid and defend her. Mom would, at times, complain, "Well, your father rules the roost," and in the rural Midwest of the 1930's-1950's (and beyond), male dominance in marriages was the standard. But in many respects I'd suggest that my parents' marriage and relationship was very much a partnership, and differed from many other rural husband-wife relationships that I observed. Growing up, one of my most enduring recollections of their relationship was the mutual respect they had and kindness they demonstrated to one another. Both Dad and Mom genuinely liked one another, and we children saw that affection in many ways.

Now Mom, even though much smaller, wielded a good deal of clout in the relationship, despite her occasional protestations to the contrary. She was a bit quicker on the uptake than Dad. She wasn't necessarily more intelligent, but her synapses fired more rapidly than Dad's, especially in everyday conversation. I have these theories about their personalities, and consequently, their general behavioral patterns. Dad was 100% Germanic stock—thoughtful, prone to thinking through all the options before speaking.

Mom, by contrast, was much more likely to speak or act on her initial impulse or thought. Grandmother Rodenbough, who was born and raised in the Missouri hills, was like that; bright, articulate, a lady way ahead of her times, creative, a tremendously capable individual who could appraise a situation and understand the dynamics before most individuals had digested 50% of the meaning. So Mom's bloodlines were more diverse. And while she possessed great cognitive skills, she had, shall I say, a much more diverse and developed array of affective responses available to her. When Mom wanted to agitate Dad, one of her favorite barbs made reference to "slow-thinking Germans." By contrast, Dad could point to Mom's Ozark Mountain lineage and the undisciplined nature of hill folks. We kids finally figured out that people from the hills were sometimes referred to as "hillbillies." We probably only made such a reference to our Grandmother Rodenbough on one occasion. She took great exception to the label, and we carefully avoided any references thereafter. During his life, Dad read daily and regularly, mostly newspapers and farm magazines. As he got older and had more time, he read novels. I remember he especially liked James Michener, with *Centennial* his favorite.

It was, however, my mother, I think, who early on instilled in me a love of books and reading. She liked words, and any time we came upon one we didn't understand, Mom got out the dictionary. She was a prolific letter-writer, and the people to whom she wrote loved her letters. When I contracted polio, she wrote to me almost daily. I still have those letters, and the last time I read through some of them, I almost cried. They were messages of hope and encouragement. In reading them today, her grief over my situation was there between the words. Nonetheless, at the time they were terribly important for me, powerful lifelines to my family.

I hope that she feels I did a credible job in writing this book. It will be, however, awhile longer before I know what she thinks. She passed away on Mothers Day, May 14, 2006.

But that is a far subject from retirement. As to the term retirement, it is, I think, a misnomer, as I'm not sure what it means. Most people probably think it's the time when one no longer gets up early

Monday through Friday, heads to a designated work site, reports to a boss, and in return, gets a paycheck every two weeks (mostly a statement of deductions) which is automatically deposited in your bank. Retirement is, I think, just a different job, and frankly, it is the best one I've ever had. Finding things to do isn't a problem (a common fear of people facing retirement). In fact, the longer I'm retired, the more there seems to be a growing inverse relationship between time available and things that I must do.

One fact that has become crystal clear since I left my job is that retirement is a great equalizer. Things we thought important like titles, awards and accolades, social status, money, or having been an important person isn't very relevant as we begin the twilight years of our lives. I borrowed that expression, twilight years, from Ronald Reagan, who used that phrase in his farewell to America speech, as he left public life. I always thought it was a classic remark, so perfect to describe this time of our journey in life. Now, twilight doesn't imply a dimming; it's simply a point in our later life chronology. In fact, twilight is a time for illumination and enlightenment, for uncovering truths, to understand our mortality, attending to important things like family and friends, and discovering our real inner self. But if that's too burdensome of a responsibility, do something a whole lot simpler and much more enjoyable—like hanging out in a mall and ogling the gals with big hooters.

I know much has been written about how to ensure that our golden years are satisfying, and I've tried to read a few of those self-help guides for oldies, but they always turn me off. However, I once heard a simple, yet profound commentary on how we might live our life each day. It was the 1993 ESPY Awards speech by Jimmy Valvano, former North Carolina State basketball coach, just two weeks from death from the ravages of cancer. He said that to truly have a life of fulfillment, *each day,* we must do three things: 1) Laugh, 2) take time to think seriously about important issues of the day, and 3) be in touch with our emotions. It was a simple, yet powerful prescription for living, whatever our individual circumstances.

Growing up, I recall lively, humor-filled discussions during supper around the old round oak kitchen table. "Philosophizing," we called it. Maybe it was early training for developing a process to identify and resolve life's values and how to live successfully. Then again, maybe it was just we four kids trying to one-up each other. Whatever the case, (and I think it was a bit of both) they were meaningful interactions, and we children learned much about life's issues those nights.

So what should I say about retirement? Talk about what I should do, or what I think I should do, and what I actually do? Probably recounting what I actually do is the easiest topic. Every one of us, throughout our lives, has good intentions about getting things done, doing things, or going places. Because we simply don't have the time to accomplish everything we want to during our working years, we tell ourselves big fibs that we will do it when we retire. Major life goals like going to Europe, or Hawaii, or driving the Alcan Highway to Alaska in a motor home, or writing a novel or growing the best roses in town are all things we plan to do when we're no longer working.

Maybe it's just doing jobs of a more mundane nature, like clearing out the garage so we can actually park our cars in the space; painting the outbuildings on the farm; cleaning out and rearranging closets; keeping the house tidy; refinishing furniture; keeping the address book up-to-date; getting rid of no longer used stuff; and getting more involved in community affairs. It doesn't matter what activities you identify that you think you will finally accomplish with all that free time in retirement, because it mostly doesn't happen. The most frequent comment I hear from other retirees is, "How the devil did I have time to work?" Having been released from the curse of the leisure class (aka work), I can't seem to find time to get anything done. It is indeed a mystery how all the things we have to do multiplies, almost exponentially, to fill the time available to do them. Like this memoir, I keep putting things off because I have so many other things to do.

My latest cholesterol count (March 2006) was one ninety-five, and my doctor said, "That's a little elevated." I am overweight and ought to lose some pounds to ease the load on the old ticker. So I have to start eating more healthy stuff to lower the cholesterol and I also have to lose some weight. I'll do that very soon. Matt and Marlys are really quite good about their diets. Low fat this and that, brown bread, few—if any—cookies or doughnuts, fat free milk, less meat, no beef, and more soy and vegetables. They now try to ration my cookie fixes to a weekly schedule. I discovered a meatless sausage called Morning Star that's delicious. I now eat it on an almost daily basis. Matt, who is very health conscious, worries that I might be overdoing this essentially soy product (it could lower my testosterone level). He implies that in a T-shirt I look like I'm about a B cup size. Really? I told my wife that I was going to get a large-sized "Tom Jones helper" and one morning come into the kitchen wearing only my under shorts with Tom's phony tally-wacker strategically positioned. He'll surely notice. That will give me an opening for revealing my sudden unexpected surge in my testosterone level.

There are actually a number of routines that I have been able to implement that give me a subliminal sense of security and make me feel that I'm really being productive. Things like keeping two bird feeders full; winding our seven-day chiming clock; paying bills daily; balancing the checkbook monthly; keeping the freezer, refrigerator and pantry fully stocked; actually reading completely through the daily and Sunday newspapers; and weekly picking up doggie "fertilizer" all contribute to my sense of fulfillment. Ah yes, life in order and order in life!

Speaking of routines, one of my favorite things to do is attend the weekly meeting of the "Monday Morning Irregulars." Four guys—Roger, Ron, Gordon, and myself—constitute the core group of irregulars who meet weekly at Bruegger's Bagelry. We review the past week's world news and events, discuss politics (I wonder if I'm really the only conservative), and keep abreast of the world of sports—particularly the University of Arizona Wildcats. During the basketball season, Lute Olson and his usual group of bluebloods are a favorite topic. We also discuss books, a bit of history, the stock market, computers, (several guys are nerds and really know their stuff), religion, issues of morality, movies, and tell lots of jokes. One fellow, Jerry, who occasionally drops in, is an expert in Southwestern art and textiles (Indian blankets.) Other folks stop by, adding a bit of diversity; Bill, who became a regular Irregular for a while, suddenly departed. He was a newlywed in his early seventies, and had added a new wrinkle to the group by bringing along his cribbage board. His new wife was quite a bit younger, and I hope his absence isn't related to problems of too much physical exertion. That can happen, as we get older.

I need to clarify that meetings of the Monday Morning Irregulars are in Tucson, our *winter* home; because I really did do something in retirement that I had planned to do years before, and that is to also have a *summer* home. Now, before the reader concludes that that we must have a lot of money, I must tell you that the total purchase price of both homes was only 1/3 or even 1/4 of the cost of a mid-range home in Tucson today.

In October 2003, we bought a cute little bungalow in Truman, Minnesota, Marlys's home territory, just a block and a half from her sister Marge and brother-in-law Carl. It has two bedrooms, no basement, my first real garage (instead of a carport) it's air-conditioned, and a perfect place for us. We have two great neighbors—guys who mow our lawn and keep an eye on the place. Carl only charges $75.00 an hour for house-calls for things like changing light bulbs, putting in a screw, attaching a hose, or lighting a pilot light. I mean, how can you beat that? Most of Marlys's family lives within a maximum of twenty-five miles, so we have a built-in social group, who are always ready to go places and do things.

But unlike the weekly forum with the fellows in Tucson, I meet daily with the local guys at the Truman Cafe. Liars dice is the glue that holds the group together. There are from five to seven, sometimes even more guys who show up for the daily ritual of coffee, sometimes breakfast, gossip, and always the hotly contested games of liars dice. We always play four games at $.25 an ante, which means you could lose a whole dollar every morning. These fellows are mostly quite conservative, with a few "We'd-vote-Democrat-even-if-the-candidate-was-the-devil" folks thrown in. So now May or June to September, it's Minnesota at the Truman Cafe, with the Truman Mafia (that's my private nickname for them) guys for liars dice; and September to May or June it's Tucson, Arizona, at Bruegger's with the Irregulars, cussing and discussing and maybe learning cribbage.

Actually, Marlys and I first spent the entire summer in Minnesota in 1999, the year after I retired. We had an apartment at the Booz Baptist Apartments, a facility (twenty units) for mostly retired elderly locals, many in their seventies, eighties and even nineties. We loved the place and those dear folks who lived there (some still do). I kept journals of our time there, and one day I'll get the notes into readable form. We had much fun, laughter, and good times with those honest, straight-talking Minnesotans.

In1998, during one of our annual treks to Minnesota, my brother-in-law, Roland Stradtman asked me if I wanted to go to a country auction. I did and I bought a small mixing bowl called a beater jar. It was not just any old bowl—it was Red Wing Stoneware. Yes, Red Wing Stoneware, an almost hallowed word in the upper Midwest. There are crocks, jugs, pitchers, bowls, plates, water coolers, churns, all made of clay, fired in kilns, and essentially our earliest earthen Tupperware. Made in Red Wing, Minnesota, until 1967, it has become quite collectible, with some of the more rare and unique pieces appraising quite high. I took that small beater jar home and the more I fondled it, the more I became mesmerized. So I began going to more sales and buying more Red Wing Stoneware. Country auctions, many times at the farm-site of the individuals having the sale, feature hayrack wagons piled high with everything the family had accumulated for sometimes over a hundred years, are excellent sites to find Red Wing Stoneware. There is always a lunch stand hosted by a church group, hundreds of locals, and antique dealers from far-flung places in a noisy, fair-like atmosphere. Everyone is looking for that great bargain and the bidding is spirited. I think I developed a craving for Red Wing like some folks crave chocolate or coffee or sex. I'd go to a sale every day if I could find one (if my wife would agree and it didn't interfere with a family gathering, of course).

By 2005, I had accumulated a horde (my son's words) of over one hundred-fifty items of Red Wing stoneware, from chamber pots to a thirty-gallon crock. Just weeks before completing this initial final draft in November 2005, I got a fifty-gallon behemoth in Tucson.

I told the guy, "My wife will kill me."

"Ok then, tell her it's your coffin," he replied. By golly, I think it would hold me! There are thousands of Red Wing pieces out there, and I used to fantasize about cornering the market in Red Wing. I don't know. I'm sixty-seven and have limited expendable income, so I may not get it all before I die

My wife sometimes admonishes me for wanting to acquire all those material things.

"But I love them." I protest.

"How can you love an inanimate object that can't return the love?" she asks. Well, maybe love is not the word, but I do like to fondle the various pieces. I'll bet I'm not alone in discovering that as we get older, we spend less time fondling our wives, mostly because they don't like it as much. So there is, I'm sure, an inverse correlation between time spent fondling our wives and time spent fondling other things. For me, the Red Wing seems pretty innocuous and keeps me from looking elsewhere.

Now with two houses, one in Arizona and one in Minnesota, I have two locations to stash my stoneware. This stoneware does have real utilitarian value besides being a nice hobby—the thirty-gallon crock in Minnesota serves as our TV stand. It really looks nice, too. A fifteen-gallon beauty served as the base for our 2004 Yule tree; two to five gallon crocks can be used as waste containers or storage, but some (the more expensive ones) are just to look at and enjoy. A final serendipitous result of the Red Wing obsession was our "crock house." We enclosed (with wrought iron and screen) a portion of our back patio in Tucson, which resulted in a bug-free, lovely out-of-doors eating-lounging area. It's really quite nice. Best of all, when you're in the room, you are surrounded by all manner of stoneware, crocks, jugs, churns, and coolers. I tell Marlys it's kind of a religious experience for me.

Stoneware isn't my only retirement avocation. Back in Minnesota, Neal, who's married to my wife's niece and frequently takes me fishing (we've got thirteen thousand lakes to choose from) sent me an e-mail the fall of 2004, jokingly suggesting we buy a home on a local lake that listed for a mere quarter-million. My reply was to suggest that what I really needed was a boat, a pontoon boat, so my wife and I could just roll from the dock onto the boat.

Well, the stars lined up. The guy had one and was in a hurry to sell. The boat was a real bargain, but after much discussion, I agreed with Marlys that we probably shouldn't buy it. Notwithstanding, one phone call later from Neal and the guy and presto, I had an 8x16 foot silver and blue Palm Beach pontoon boat, outfitted with a forty HP Mercury Marine outboard with a new water pump. It also has a trolling motor, a great travel trailer, and probably other features unknown to me as I bought it over the phone without having seen it. But what a deal—a terrific buy, Neal assured me.

How could I not buy that boat? As I explained to Marlys after she recovered from the shock of my having done a 180-degree about-face: This is not simply a fishing boat. It, like the Red Wing Stoneware, has much practical, utilitarian value. Now we can take whole families fishing—eight or ten people, maybe more. Just think of the bonding that can happen on family excursions. We can have guy's only trips, or ladies day or outings just for the kids. Neal will have nightmares envisioning multiple lines entangled, broken lines, snags, lost rods and reels, baiting hooks, and taking off fish.

Hmmm, maybe I should have given this a little more thought. Nah. We can take beverages, food, our grill (for burgers, dogs, and brats), pillows, blankets, cots if we need them, and a port-a-pot. God, what luxury. The thought crossed my mind that if I antagonized my wife, I might one night need a place to sleep over. Can you imagine how serene it would be to fall asleep being gently rocked by the waves? Yes, this pontoon boat is a good thing.

Well, here I am, rambling on for some time and not sure if I've even begun to address the topic of retirement. Before I reached this state of affairs (pre-retired), I thought one had to have hobbies. The word always conjures up images of things like coin or stamp collecting, photography, making scrapbooks, putting puzzles together—sedentary types of things. But a hobby can be almost anything, can't it? Enjoyment of the activity seems key to me. It could be reading, watching TV, playing cards—all the sedentary things I mentioned—even washing dishes, doing laundry, hiking, watching girls, chasing grizzlies, maybe even sleeping. I had thought that a better word for hobby might be pastime. But one of my Monday morning irregular buddies—Ron, I think—said no, we should call it "real time, like now, not pastime." I think he's right. So what we do after our work careers end is begin to do real time stuff. I have a lot of these real time activities on my plate. Gardening is really one of my big-time avocations; growing vegetables; flowers; doing some propagating; some in ground and a lot of potted plants. I do a pretty good job. I have a winter garden and flowers in Arizona, and a summer garden in Minnesota.

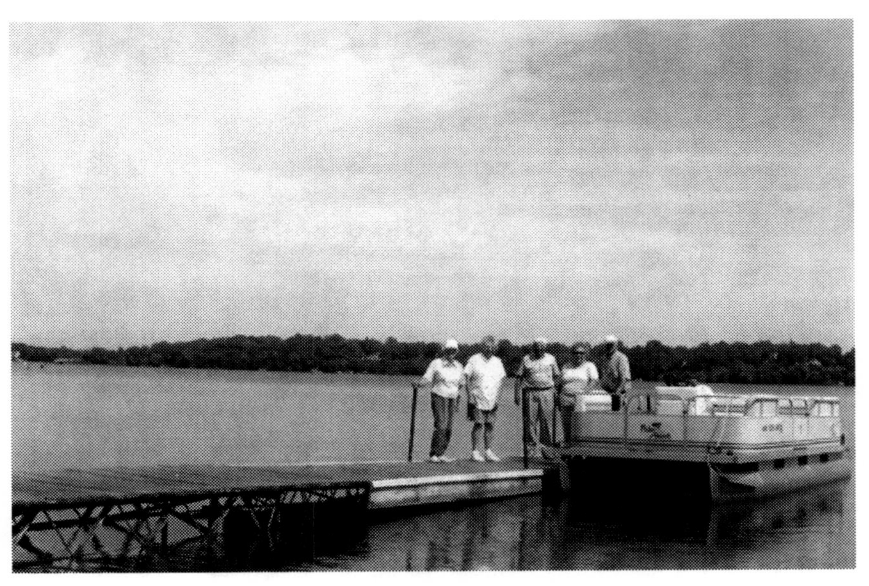

My pontoon boat, the Mary Lilly, *at Fairmont, Minnesota (summer, 2005)*

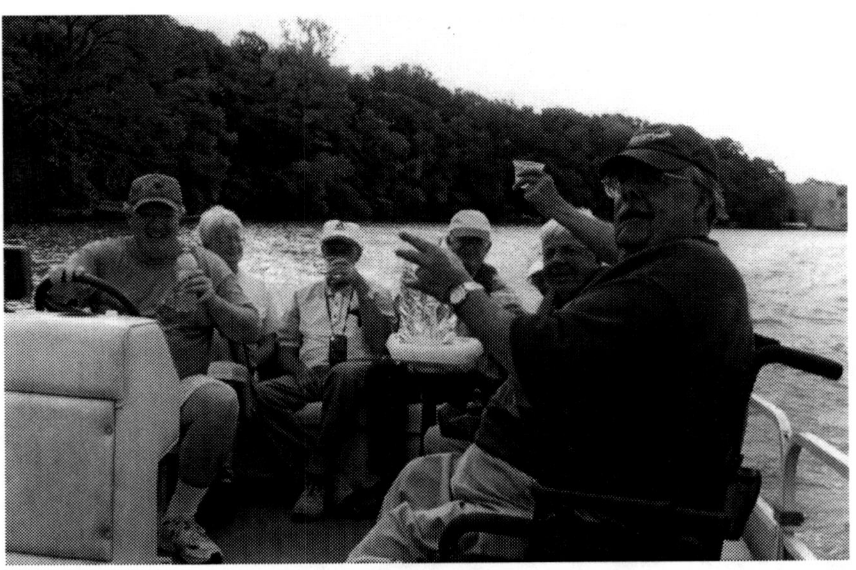

A party on board! (L–R) Neal and Debbie Belgard (Marlys's niece and her husband), brothers-in-law, Hank Kohn, Roland Stradtman, Carl Vogt, and me. Marlys and sisters behind us. (Summer, 2005)

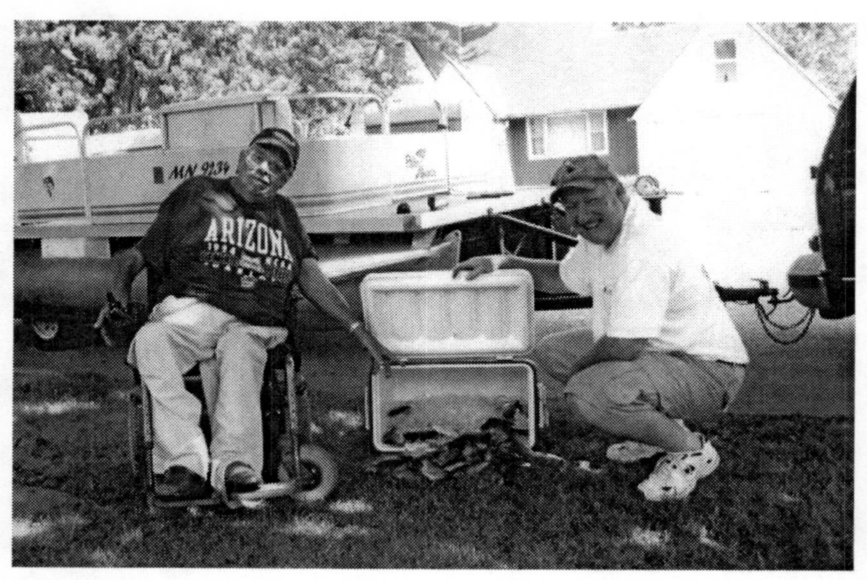

Neal and me with a nice catch of crappies. Truman, Minnesota. (Summer, 2005)

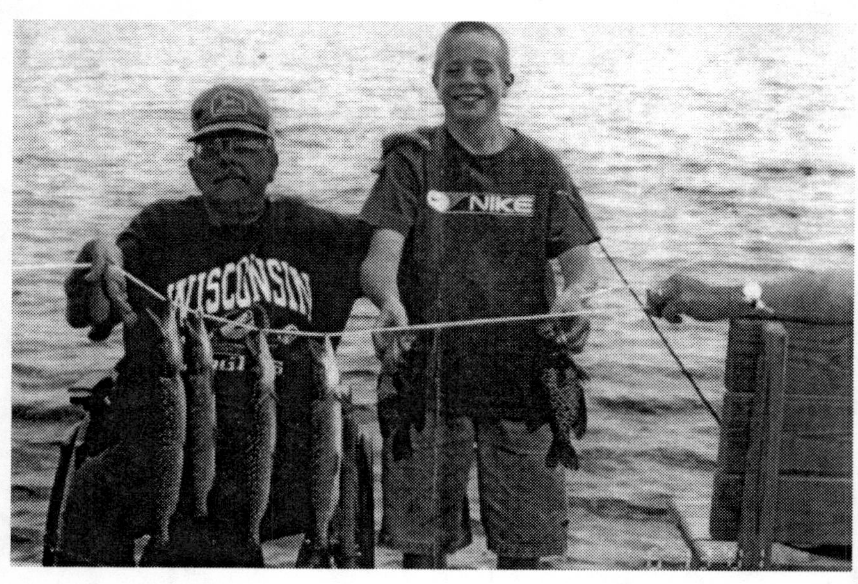

A stringer of northern pike. Small, but fun to catch. Great-nephew Jordan Viland and I. Lake Pemush, Minnesota. (Summer, 2001)

I'm not sophisticated enough to have gone through the University's program and acquire the somewhat grandiose (at least for me) title of Master Gardener. I'm more the dirt-farmer type. I think one big difference between the two types is that many master-gardener types may wear gloves to keep their hands and nails clean. We dirt-farmer types actually like the feel of soil; it connects one more closely to earth. It means that one handles composted manure, soil amendments, and fertilizers with bare hands.

Time with friends, going to movies, the theater, antique fairs, and eating out are good retirement real-time activities. Jerry Bobs restaurant in Tucson is one of my favorite places. Breakfast (with no meat) of eggs, toast, potatoes (I usually have grits), and coffee is $1.99, and a nice hamburger with fries for lunch is also $1.99 (recently raised to a sky-high$2.39.) It's one of those places where America eats. It isn't fancy, but Mr. Kim keeps his overhead low, and the place is always full of regulars. It's not only the blue-collar crowd who eats there, I know a seven million dollar lottery winner who likes the atmosphere and the prices.

Minnesota also has those hometown places, like the Home Town buffet in St. James, and the Cottage Cafe in another small town close-by, and of course, the Truman Café. For a change of pace, I can also go to St. James for coffee at McDonald's (seventeen cent coffee) instead of doing liars dice in Truman. The boys in St. James are mostly Democrats, so I get a different take on the news—plus cheap coffee.

Coffee-time is usually around 8:30 or 9:00 A.M., (some guys go earlier) which means I can get in several early morning hours of fishing from the pier at St. James lake. Hank Kohn, another brother-in-law, joins me and we often get a nice bunch of pan fish, crappies, bluegills, sunfish, some bass and also occasionally a walleye or a northern. Hank and I have done a lot of fishing together in the past, and we've had some memorable times. As I think about all my past fishing expeditions, and there were hundreds, maybe I should put them together in another book.

Maybe activities and interests in my real-time retirement appear mundane to the reader; I suppose deep-sea diving, mountain climbing, an African safari, or running with the bulls in Pamplona, might actually be more exciting. But I don't think it's either the magnitude or the uniqueness of what we do, rather it's the quality of each undertaking that we glean from the experience. For example, I'd suggest that one could travel the world and in fact observe and understand little of the meaning of where they were and what they saw.

Ah, now is not the time to get philosophical; and besides, every now and then I do try something a bit more adventurous; like taking a spin in Carl Vogt's fully restored (even to the Army colors) 1941 PT-13 Steirman bi-plane. Getting into the plane took some old fashioned ingenuity, as well as a durable block and tackle from the Truman fire rescue squad. Carl was legitimately concerned that I could wreck the fabric on the fuselage if they tried to hoist me up over the lower wing into the seat. The solution, (see photo) wasn't pretty, but it worked. My pilot, Tim Steier, did a few rolls and dives, enough to unclog my adrenaline valves for several years. Now for my next big thrill, let me think; I wonder if gimpers can skydive?

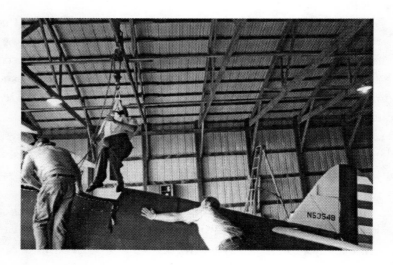

How I got in the 1941 Steirman that was restored by brother-in-law Carl Vogt. Up to the rafters and then down! Blue Earth, Minnesota. (Summer, 1999 or 2000)

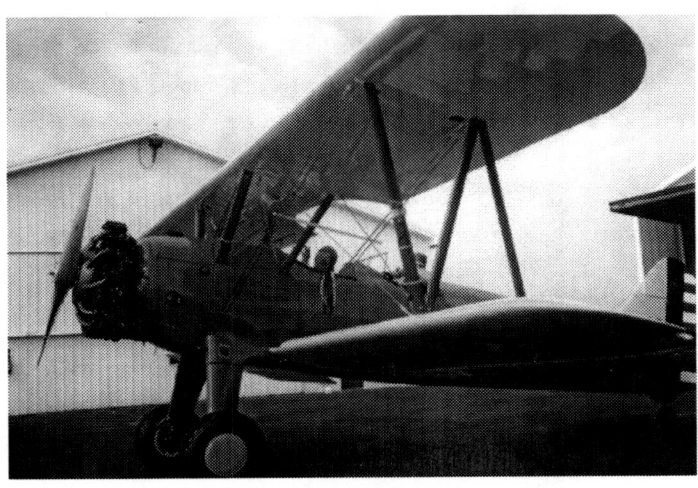

Ready to roll. I'm in front with the Red Baron-type scarf. Blue Earth, Minnesota. (Summer, 1999 or 2000)

The reader will recall Jimmy Valvano's second axiom of his 1993 ESPY Awards speech was that we take time to think about and ponder important issues in life. I do some of that in these real-time years. I try to think seriously about important local, national and even international matters. I think about questions of morality, my values, where our country is heading on these issues (seemingly rushing to the left). I haven't figured out much of anything yet, but I think the important thing is to keep an open mind, remain inquisitive, stay informed, and continue to search for answers.

However, I must tell you that this dedication to finding truths sometimes does pay off. A matter on which I had spent considerable time pondering did become clear to me. Having been born and reared in the Midwest, I had become accustomed to the regular summer activity of people mowing lawns. It seemed that someone was always mowing—early mornings, midday, evenings, and on into the night. I left the Midwest more or less permanently almost forty years ago, but now with our home in Minnesota and spending summers there, I'm always surprised, actually quite amazed, at all of the mowing that goes on. It's not only lawns that get mowed. They mow road ditches, highway medians, vacant lots, and anyplace that grass grows. Young and old, men and women, and kids too are involved in mowing acres and acres of turf. I observed that continually riding those mowers (or walking behind a self-propelled machine) seemed almost obsessive. I began to give serious thought to the matter, trying to understand the meaning of this behavior. Well, by golly, relaxing in our summer apartment in the Booz Home several years back, the answer came to me. Yes, it was "The Truth of It." And the revelation follows:

THE TRUTH OF IT

Now Carl Jung was a very smart man
Born over a hundred years ago in Switzerland.
He had these theories few thought true,
That we can inherit behavior, you know, what we do.
His teacher was Freud, that wild old guy,
But behavior thru the genes, hey, that's pie-in-the-sky.
Then, eureka! Like a bolt from the blue,
I discovered that what Jung said was probably true.
Reflecting in the solitude of a Midwest dawn
I realized there is a gene for mowing lawn!
For years I had asked sometimes quite brash,
"Why is everyone always mowing grass?"
In swirling dusk, its 95, and storms men should fear,
They'll still be out there on a Snapper or Deere.
Yes, life was good, the grass was green,
Nonstop mowing, what an idyllic scene.
But, alas and alack, the winds turned dry,
No rain fell from that aluminum sky.
The grass turned brown from lack of rain.
Mowers were silent, there was genuine pain.
People were listless, they lost their spunk,
Holy cow, the whole county was in a funk!
For mowing lawns and acres more
Is not an option, it's deep in our core.
As air and water are essential to grow
So life has no quality if we can't mow.
Many prayed, and the good Lord sent rain

And mowing at a frenetic pace began again.
When I was young and not so wise
I thought mowing an obsession in disguise.
Shaving lawns and roadsides too
Was simply, "what one ought to do."
But truth, as for all, has set me free
So; I'm getting a 4-foot Wheel horse and going on a spree.
Remember my friends, if you've got the blahs and are feeling low,
Take heart, crank up that engine, you need to mow!

So now you know writing silly ditties is a real time hobby of mine. Not everyone may think my new understanding of why people mow is important, but it is to me. One of life's mysteries finally solved.

Frivolities aside, I sometimes wonder if during our lifetimes we really figure out much about anything. At one time in my life I thought I knew most all of the *answers*, today I mostly just have all the *questions*. Maybe that's the point—we're here to try and work out the details. Maybe it's the process, and working on it in real time is the thing that matters. At a minimum, I hope I can stick around a few more years enjoying my real time—retirement.

XIII. Finis

"I shall tell you a great secret my friend. Do not wait for the last judgment, it takes place every day." (1)

Webster's Third New International Dictionary, unabridged, and Seven Language Dictionary has several definitions for the word memoir. I used this particular reference book, as it was part of the Great Books series that I thought was a must for anyone who deemed themselves (or aspired to be) intellectual. Impulsively, I bought them in 1966, and over forty years later, I am still not an intellect. Notwithstanding, I am still trying to justify the purchase by demonstrating that I am using them. Memoir: 1) "An account of something regarded as noteworthy;" 2) "An autobiographical account, often anecdotal or intimate in tone, whose focus is usually on the persons, events or times known to the writer;" 3) "The record of the proceedings of a learned society."

Clearly, this manuscript doesn't fit the definition of number three; it's also highly unlikely that anyone would suggest it approaches the substance embodied in number one; which leaves us with Webster's second definition as the likely—if not only—choice. In fact, it does fit with what I attempted to accomplish. It is not a Kloepping family history or even a recounting of what I did or could remember throughout my life.

This memoir is simply about experiences I had during my life that collectively provide a sort of sense for how I got where I am today, and why I think as I do. It has been a very therapeutic process reaching back to my recollections and memories of my mother, relatives, siblings, friends, co-workers, wife, and into my own sometimes-dark recesses. Reminiscing about past good times and tough times has not only been satisfying, but also enlightening. In so many ways, I was lucky to have the family I had, the great friends in my early years and in high school, and the many great folks I have met along the way.

Writing about my career and the struggles as a disability rights advocate was very cathartic. In actuality, I was a pioneer in my field (and who doesn't want to be a pioneer?); not the earliest, certainly, but during the early days of my career there were few guidelines to follow. What my contemporaries and I accomplished was to establish foundations and set standards for those who followed. A memoir can help one relive the best of times. I hope the reader recognizes my sense of fulfillment and understands that I would do it the same way again.

How does one end a memoir? Literally, it could continue until one dies. One day you are writing and the next day, "pffft," you are gone. Therefore, when to stop is an arbitrary date. I originally decided to stop on July 18, 2003, as I had just turned sixty-five. I would use the occasion of my just past sixty-fifth birthday, June 6, as the end date. However, I had much more to write. I procrastinated, and suddenly it was December 2004. I made a commitment to complete the text by the end of Spring 2005. I didn't make that deadline, but now it's May 2006, and I have finished. But before I end, I have one more serious topic to discuss. Then, of course, I can't help myself from ending with a little frivolity.

The serious thoughts that I had concern the two most important people in my life, Marlys and Matthew, my wife and my son. They are my most intimate family, each of them bright individuals, at times my strongest supporters, and also at times, my most articulate critics. They are both private, modest people who don't need and want to be the center of attention. So I need to tread lightly.

Matthew, an attorney now licensed in two states, inherited among other qualities my father-in-law's problem solving skills. He is a talented fellow, unaware, in a number of respects, of the depths of his abilities. He's a thoughtful individual who is able to grasp and synthesize information, reaching logical, rational conclusions. He didn't get that from me. I think he ought to be a writer. He's great with words and has a rapier wit. He is, as are Marlys and I, politically conservative and keeps abreast of national and world issues. His humor has given me many great one-liners, e.g., "Ted Kennedy is living proof that spam floats;" he also coined the term "wedding tackle" in a discussion we were having on weddings; he also calls himself a Native American (which he, Marlys, and I are); we belong to the "Hon-Kee" tribe. I could write much more about my son, and I'd like to. However, given his nature and understanding his wishes, I'll leave any further matters of his notoriety to his own designs (besides, he's a lot bigger than I am).

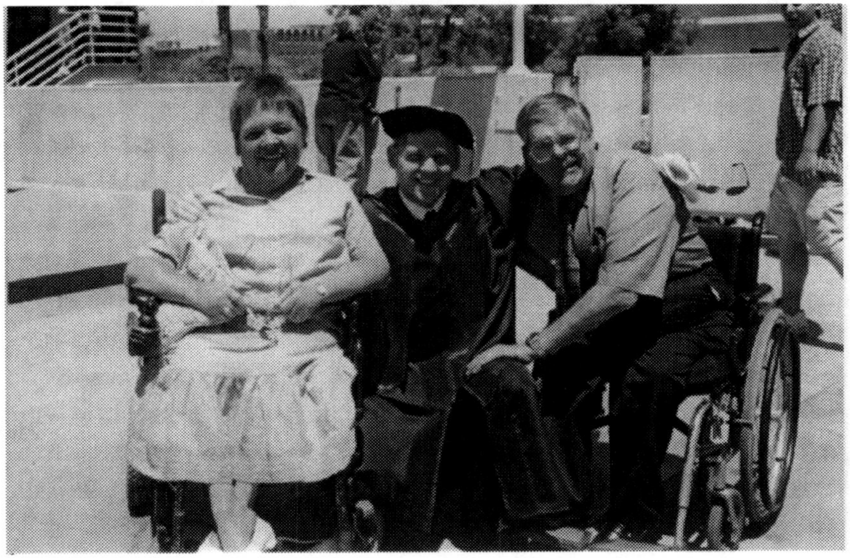

The law school graduate and proud parents. James Rogers College of Law, University of Arizona. (Summer, 2000)

Marlys is, likewise, one who doesn't need or want the limelight. But in her case she is smaller than I am and since I don't think she'd physically assault me, I feel safer revealing a bit more about her. She has put up with me for over forty years, and that fact alone is testimony to the strength of her personal resolve.

Marlys contracted polio in 1948 when she was ten years old and living in rural southern Minnesota. As noted earlier, she came from good German stock and like my family, her parents, three sisters and extended family were a tremendous support. She had significant loss of respiratory function as a result of polio. In spite of that rather severe limitation (30% remaining lung capacity), she developed a truly amazing ability to accomplish whatever she decided to do. Not only has she successfully managed our household for over forty years, she had time to work as a speech pathologist in the local school systems for seventeen years and took time out to give birth to our son, a medically very difficult event for her.

All during Matthew's early years, while I was busy with career-related activities, she was the primary cook, parent, chauffeur for scouts, soccer, 4-H, the fair, etc., etc. We also entertained small and large groups of friends and colleagues on a fairly regular basis, and most times she prepared all of the food for the party. Oh, I'd open the wine and mix drinks and probably helped with clean up, but mostly it was her effort. She sewed many of her clothes, and was always a great bargain-hunter when shopping for groceries and consumer goods.

She had great parents and sisters. They taught her to be strong and secure in her beliefs and she has often told me, "I'm comfortable with what I believe, and furthermore, I rather enjoy spending time with just myself." She has been a steadying, levelheaded partner in our marriage. Oh, she ain't perfect, but among other attributes she has three really admirable qualities: honesty, trustworthiness, and a keen sense of fairness. They are rare in people today, and folks she calls friend, are indeed fortunate.

Yes, what you see is what you get with Mary Lily. That's the old French name for Marlys. And like my pontoon boat, christened *The Mary Lily,* she keeps our marriage and life on a pretty even keel, even though there are, at times, turbulent waters.

Although I've done fairly well here, I'm most often reluctant to outwardly express my feelings about them, especially when I think seriously about what they truly mean to me, Invariably my father comes to mind. He deeply loved his family, but was not one to make public displays or verbalizations of affection. It wasn't his style, and maybe I have embraced that legacy. Or maybe I'm chicken, afraid of intimacy. Maybe it's sufficient to say marrying Marlys was undoubtedly the best decision I ever made, and Matthew is undoubtedly the best thing that will ever happen to Marlys and me.

And finally a last silly story related to the occasion of my sixty-fifth birthday, which was the original target date to end this memoir. Marlys had asked me what I wanted for my official passage into old guy status. I couldn't come up with anything too exciting, so she suggested two options, a trip to Las Vegas or attendance at two antique auctions in Minnesota .She wanted to stay home with our great little schnauzer, Mina who was very ill; Marlys didn't want her to die in a kennel. She said, "I'll pay for either trip, all expenses, within reason." If I went to Minnesota, I would attend two Red Wing Stoneware auctions with some really great pieces on sale. Option two would be a trip to Vegas to gamble, carouse, and do whatever else I wanted (she just requested I not tell her about it).

In considering the Las Vegas trip, a story came to mind: Two grandsons of a ninety year old fellow decided to give him a special gift in honor of his ninth decade. The family had lodged him in the finest hotel, had a sumptuous banquet brought to him, served him fine wine and applauded his vigor. It was a truly magnificent tribute. Later that evening, the two boys hired a gorgeous young woman to spend the night with the old gentleman.

When he opened the door to the exquisite beauty, she said alluringly, "I'm here to give you super sex."

He paused a moment, thinking to himself, "Soup or sex…" He replied, "I think I'll have the soup."

The decision on which trip to take was an easy one for me. I love those Minnesota auctions and the opportunity to fondle those crocks and jugs (stoneware, of course). So how did that choice of the two trips (Vegas or Minnesota) influence the end date for my memoir? Well, if I had chosen the Las Vegas trip, I would have had to write about it.

XIV. Epilogue: On Being A Gimp: Differently Abled.

I often use the word "gimp" in describing a person with a disability. Some folks think the word is offensive—if not derogatory—but it isn't. Laura Tieke, a severely disabled young woman who frequently refers to herself using the term, told me, "Kent, gimp is a wonderful word. It means God Improved Me Personally."

Disability throughout history, across cultures, and for the individual, has differing meanings. This manuscript is a reflection of my experiences and views as a person with a disability. Thus, it is inherently biased, as it reflects my worldview. My observations and what I have written may be completely valid, or then again maybe not. In an attempt to provide a balanced view of disability and disability issues, (writings, research, and other viewpoints) the following is a very brief overview of this complex topic, presenting some differing perspectives and interpretations of the subject.

This past summer I was wheeling into Park Mall here in Tucson. As I approached the automatic sliding entrance door, a fortyish, pleasantly plump gal gave me a sweet smile and remarked,

"How are you doing honey?"

"Oh, fine," I replied, "How are you?"

"Great Hon."

It was a friendly greeting, but her words and manner communicated more. Her salutation, although probably used commonly, is not one you might expect stranger to stranger. However, I am frequently addressed as "hon," "sweetie," "honey," or "babe" by (mostly female) individuals I don't know. I'm not really pick-up material—I'm quite porky, not a flashy dresser, and often don't shave before going out in public. In fact, I have pretty much gone to seed. Despite my appearance, I am repeatedly greeted with one of these rather intimate salutations. I usually don't get offended (unless it's a guy), because I don't think the intent is malicious or demeaning. I do believe, however, these comments are predicated on the other individual seeing me as different from most sixty-seven year-old males. It is my disability, I think, that elicits the response. Whether it is a reflection of compassion, sympathy, empathy, or some combination of all, it is a more gentle and solicitous greeting than one would expect if one were a "Tab," a temporarily able-bodied person.

After living with a disability for over sixty years, and having learned how to adapt and accommodate for the limitations, I think of myself as a normal person. I don't ever remember waking up and exclaiming, "Oh my god, I'm a gimper!" But the well-meaning lady at the Mall once again reminded me that in her paradigm of normal people, I didn't quite fit. It's not a question of disability paranoia. After six decades and countless encounters with people who respond first to my disability, my gimper radar readily picks up on the disability/discomfort signals. Visible physical disability is often a conundrum for many people. However, responding to the disability rather than the person, whether positive or negative, has the effect of introducing an element of artificiality or disingenuousness into the situation, and that is very apparent to me. I am rarely offended by these behaviors or remarks that reflect obvious discomfort, but they do serve to reinforce and communicate that I am, at best, different, or at worst, deviant. In either case, I am not viewed as a "whole" person. Adults are usually subtler (or think they are) because often they will not verbalize their feelings of discomfort. Children, on the other hand, are more often quite direct and will want to ask questions about what they observe.

Most times, the questions are simply based on a desire to understand and seem quite innocuous. Then again, I must admit to wanting to backhand some snot-nosed types who screech, "Hey mister, what's wrong with you?"

I vividly recall my first soul-jarring experience of being seen as different and feeling that something was terribly wrong with me. It wasn't long after I had returned home from my initial hospitalization with polio. One Sunday afternoon, my family and a group of extended relatives (who we didn't see on a regular basis), gathered for sort of a mini-reunion at Grandmother Kloepping's home in the small village of Rock Grove, Illinois. One of the clans, whom I had never met, had four or five boys who were very energetic and kind of rough-tough kids. It wasn't long after their arrival that they noted I was crawling on the front lawn rather than walking, as a normal eight-year-old would do. I think they were initially puzzled, but they weren't bashful fellows, and shortly they confronted me, taunting me to get up and stop crawling. I was intimidated by their brashness, and rather meekly tried to explain that I couldn't walk. They didn't buy that and several of them grabbed me and physically tried to force me to get up. I was probably like a limp rag—a stance that they interpreted as resistance—so they began an all-out assault. Some of my siblings and other cousins came to my rescue and reported the incident to the adults. I remember their parents then taking them aside and speaking to them at length. Whatever was said, the boys avoided me for the duration of the day, like I had the plague. Throughout the afternoon, I'd notice them staring at me suspiciously from a distance, or whispering among themselves. That didn't feel very good.

Based on a good many years of empirical observations of people and countless interactions with them, it seems clear to me that humans have a keen capacity for detecting differences among individuals and responding to the dissonance they perceive. In my University days, lecturing to students on issues of disability in America, we'd discuss the general concept of "perceived difference" and how it fit within the normal response continuum of people. I liked to use the example of Dolly Parton (maybe in a bikini) walking into a room of average women, suggesting that we would all most likely notice that she was quite different. Similarly, a young Paul Newman or Robert Redford in a group of average-looking guys would surely be seen as significantly different from the rest of the fellows. In both situations, these three folks would appear to be clearly outside the norm. While people readily recognize these differences, equally relevant or even more to the point is that the individual who doesn't fit the norm also clearly feels or experiences that they are being seen as different. Most times those vibes don't bother me, as there are positive as well as negative aspects. But the fact remains that I am different, most cogently because I'm viewed as belonging to a distinct class of people—people with disabilities.

I recall when growing up that a common expression was "Oh, that's all in their/your head." But it isn't only my own empirical observations that support this hypothesis of being seen as different as a disabled person. Contemporary researchers and writers have investigated the matter of attitudes toward persons with disabilities. Beatrice Wright (1), an early writer/researcher on the subject, found high correlations in attitudes held toward disabled individuals and those towards minority groups. The findings can be understood as deriving from a more basic ethno-cultural attitude toward out-group members in general. The following are a few additional concepts relating to the perception of disability.

Stigma: As man became more adept at controlling his environment through his abstracting abilities, he developed a more complex society. Because of this complexity, he needed to learn to control his environment, so he learned to classify events, circumstances, and people, and to label them. Those who did not fit the "norm," were labeled as "other"—deviant and not normal. The label became negative and is the barb of stigmatizing words-ideas-beliefs-practices: "crippled," "gimp," and "bad legs," a "useless limb," "idiot," "deaf and dumb." Those who were not understood or were seen as deviant had a label—a stigma. Words such as "retardo","schizo", "spastic", "hunchback" can all evoke images of beings who are abnormal.

Tamara Dembo and Tane-Baskin (2) talked about the concept of *Spread Effect.* This is the power of a single characteristic to evoke inferences about an individual. Disability is often viewed as more severe than it really is; research findings suggest that given a single characteristic, people feel able to rate groups with whom they have had no contact. Thus, if the salient characteristic of the person is disability, not only may specific characteristics of the person be inferred, but also sometimes the person as a whole is evaluated. This issue is especially harmful when global devaluation takes place so that the individual is seen as less worthy, less valuable, and less desirable. Individuals with severe cerebral palsy, with accompanying involuntary movement, often-unintelligible speech, drooling, and difficulty in eating are frequently assumed to also have low intelligence. Obvious disfigurement, of birth or traumatic origin, can also cause people to generalize about the lack of abilities in the individual. Conversely, in our society we often assume or ascribe qualities of intellect if the person is handsome, or tall and physically well proportioned—particularly if said individual is an Anglo male.

I believe it's relevant to relate two examples of what I perceive as blatant acts of discrimination based on our disabilities that Marlys and I encountered. It was, I believe, the concept of "the spread effect" in operation.

The year before we arrived in Tucson, Marlys had worked for the Santa Clara County Sheriff's Office in San Jose, California, and came with a highly complimentary work and personal recommendation. After we had moved to Tucson, she took a civil service examination for the city and received the highest score out of all the applicants; but when she went in for her first interview, the man she was to meet saw her wheelchair, turned his back, closed his door, and sent his secretary to tell her that she would not be able to handle the job.

Similarly, several years after moving to Tucson, another fellow who was a wheelchair user and I answered the call of the Big Brothers agency to serve as Big Brothers for young boys from broken or difficult home situations where male role models were needed. Our interest and enthusiasm resulted in a phone call informing both of us that the agency felt it would not be in the best interests of these boys to have an individual in a wheelchair serve as a Big Brother. The other fellow pursued the agency for an explanation with no satisfaction; I was too humiliated to do anything further.

Marlys didn't get that job with the city of Tucson, but instead, she applied for and received a very lucrative U.S. Public Health Service grant, which paid for her master's degree program in Speech Pathology. She then had a terrible time getting an opportunity to practice her profession (speech and language specialist) in the elementary classroom, as traditional school administrators feared that a person in a wheelchair would be unable to handle a classroom emergency. Most likely of greater concern (but not verbalized) were their views concerning the impact of a teacher with a disability on the children. Kids, however, are often more perceptive than adults, because at a young age they have not had their thinking polluted by adults regarding matters of race, religion, disability, or any of the myriad myths that adults hold to separate us, one from another. These are the roots of suspicion, alienation, fear and ultimately, hate. Marlys got an opportunity one spring semester when the incumbent specialist took pregnancy leave. Well, the kids loved Marlys. About one session on the details of her wheelchair, how she drove, got dressed, cooked, and why she was in the wheelchair, and her disability and related questions rarely ever resurfaced.

Disability is often seen as a state of deviance from the "norm"—an abnormality if you will. The extent/degree to which a person with a disability is seen as different/deviant goes a long way in determining comfort level, development of a relationship, and ultimately the degree to which that individual is included or excluded in the dynamics of the situation. Beatrice Wright (3) said it well with, "to be different is to be set apart" which, in the language of interpersonal relationships, may signify rejection. Research demonstrates that we tend to like and agree more with persons we see as similar.

Since the early work of Wright, there have been a multitude of studies dealing with the topic of attitudes toward persons with disabilities. Harold Yuker has been a major theoretician, writer and researcher in the past several decades, and the book *Attitudes Toward Persons With Disabilities* (4) is a comprehensive look into the topic. A short abstract of the book described the contents: "explores attitudes toward persons with disabilities in five sections: basic issues, sources of attitudes, measurement of attitudes, attitudes of and toward specific groups, and attitude change. It includes teacher attitudes, attitudes of health-care personnel, self-help groups and attitudes that affect employment opportunities for persons with disabilities." Frankly, after reading (skimming) through the book, I began to develop some really bad attitudes toward the topic. There is so much research and attention given to the topic in academia, which is a good thing, but it doesn't make (for me at least) the most exciting bedtime reading in my post-academic career.

But aside from my facetiousness, it is instructive and maybe important also to look back at historical thinking about disability. How do we explain, or begin to understand, modern-era research regarding the perceptions of people with disabilities and how the disabled are viewed? And what about my own empirical observations and personal experiences? What are the origins, the antecedents if you will, that might provide some insights into the place of persons with disabilities in contemporary society? We need, I believe, to look back some two thousand years, possibly even more, to help enlighten us.

Colin Barnes states ".... I will suggest that contemporary attitudes toward people with perceived impairments have their roots in the ancient worlds of the Greeks and Romans.... p2." (5) There is evidence of consistent cultural bias against people with disabilities in the antecedents of what we termed western society long before the emergence of industrial capitalism. Examples of this bias can be found in Greek culture, Judean/Christian religion, and European drama and art. The Greeks who pursued physical and mental perfection had no room for any form of flaw, and infanticide in the form of exposure to the elements for the disabled child was widely practiced. The Romans, too, were enthusiastic advocates of infanticide for "sickly or weak" children, drowning them in the Tiber River. Years before the Greeks and Romans, at the dawn of history, in ancient Egypt, Akenathon, husband of the beautiful Nefertiti was notable as the first historical person to establish monotheism. Some scholars believe that the later Hebrew prophets' (seven hundred-fifty years later) concept of a universal God was partially derived from his belief system. Interestingly, Akenathon was severely disabled. Images in temple and tomb paintings depict him with a curved distorted body, a misshapen stomach, and an elongated head. His successor Tutankhamen tried to destroy all of Akenathon's images, as he believed he was a curse on Egypt for his monotheism. I wonder what, if any, of Akenathon's impairments played a role in the view that he was a curse on Egypt?

Bob Mauro writes: "Religion can create symbols, images and stereotypes – both negative and positive. Many of the world's religions have done just that." America was founded as a nation of Christians who believed the Bible was the path to salvation—the document that governed not only our morality, but also influenced how we viewed the world. It was written during the time when early society was heavily influenced by the Greek world. And today, many acknowledge that those ancient Greeks laid the foundations of western civilization. (6)

In the Bible there are one hundred eighty incidences of disability according to Charles Kokaska's *Disabled People in the Bible* (7). Mauro continues, "The Bible portrays those with disabilities often as castaways and as people shunned by society. This can be seen in Samuel-2, 5-8; wherefore they said the blind and the lame shall not come into this house." The Bible has over forty instances in which the "cripple" is connected to sin and sinners. In Luke 5:20 a paralyzed man is brought to Jesus, who says, "man your sins are forgiven." There is the classic question in John 9 1:2 (which I heard when I first contracted polio) "Rabbi who sinned, this man or his parents that he was born blind?" Christ challenged this belief, but generations of Christians mostly recall the question and not Jesus' answer.

Our Western literary traditions are replete with negative themes concerning disability. During the dark ages, men, women, and children with disabilities were viewed as curses of the devil, possessed by demons or their impairments as punishment from God. St Augustine, sixth century, claimed that impairment was a " punishment for the fall of Adam and other sins."(8) Martin Luther, the protestant reformer, (1485-1546), said that he saw the devil in disabled children and recommended killing them. (9)

Shakespeare gives us an infamous disabled demon, Richard III. He is portrayed as an angry, vindictive cripple and also maybe a murderer. In speaking of the meaning of the disability of Richard III, Leonard Kreigel (10) states "...Shakespeare provides us with two fundamental images of what cripples are accorded in western literature. The cripple is threat, and also recipient of compassion, both to be damned as he is to be pitied." (11) Akin to Kreigel's idea and theme, we find other demonic cripples in literature:

Captain Hook in *Peter Pan,* Long John Silver in *Treasure Island,*

and Captain Ahab in *Moby Dick*; there are also the "charity cripples" like Tiny Tim in *Christmas Story*.

Throughout history, people with disabilities have been the target of violence and abuse. We know the Greeks killed imperfect infants, and the Romans liked to throw disabled children under horse's hooves in the coliseum. Disability and witchcraft were linked in the middle ages and led to burnings at the stake. During Hitler's time in the third Reich, one of his initial targets in ridding the country of "useless eaters" and "race polluters" were the physically and mentally disabled. Probably two hundred-forty thousand disabled men, women and children were gassed under his T-4 extermination program. The German church and locals living near the crematoriums raised an outcry, and Hitler did stop killing the disabled. Tragically, he used the knowledge gained in exterminating the handicapped for what he termed his "final solution" of the Jews.

Historically, if the disabled weren't killed, public ridicule was an accepted practice. During the Middle Ages, as was true in the ancient world, the disabled were a welcome source of public amusement. Children and adults with physical abnormalities were often put on display at village fairs. Visits to Bedlam, where the developmentally disabled, paralyzed, hearing and visually impaired were housed in filthy, diseased, hell-holes, was a common source of amusement for the populace; keeping "idiots" as objects of entertainment was prevalent among the wealthy (12)

Contemporary society has not rid itself of the negative images of disability. For example, the list of films connecting impairment to wickedness and villainy is seemingly endless. In addition to guys like Captains Hook and Ahab, we have Peter Sellers as the demented multiply disabled Dr. Strangelove. Dr. Jekyll is hunched and ugly, while Mr. Hyde is handsome and whole. Then there is the procession of disabled villains in the James Bond movies (James the virile good guy), and the amputee in the *Fugitive* and on and on.

While I have focused on tracing historical antecedents in our Western culture, Eastern thought has also contributed negative images of disability. The Hindu concept of Dharma explains one's condition as the consequences of past behavior; there is no sympathy for the disabled—they're responsible for their individual circumstances.

Considering the roughly two thousand years plus of our Western culture and the negative images of disabled people from the Greeks, through the Bible, in literature, in social policy, and into modern society (the twentieth century), I would submit that persons with disabilities have a powerful and pervasive negative legacy to overcome.

In the year 2005, what can we say about attitudes toward persons with disabilities in our society? In the introduction to the Library of Congress National Library Service for the Blind and Physically Handicapped, the author states, "… however the emphasis in the literature on disability (since 1984) has been shifting from a focus on differentness and limitation to a focus on abilities and potential."(13)

The passage of the Americans with Disabilities Act, ADA in July 1990, which mandated non-discrimination in employment, public services, education, public accommodations, transportation services, and other areas of everyday life, provided a major impetus for redefining the place of disabled individuals in American society. Disability is " out of the closet." Today, the media celebrates the achievements of super-crips in heroic terms. Persons with all manner of impairments (i.e. paraplegics and blind individuals) climb mountains, ski, scuba dive, wheel across America supporting a particular cause, participate in track, push their wheelchairs in marathons and have even carved out a niche in the every-four-years Olympic games. Disabled comedians have emerged (no superstars to date) and writers like John Hockenberry, John Callahan, Irving Zola, Leonard Kreigel, Dr. Nancy Mairs and Frank Bowe (to name only a few) have become notable on the national scene. Society has evolved a whole new set of jargon, all quite politically correct, to describe folks with disabilities; "Handica pable,""differently abled," "otherwise abled," and the ever-popular, "physically challenged."

So, too, have many colleges and universities risen to the challenge to rethink, redefine, and redo the image of disabled folks. Similar to their immediate predecessors, Black Studies and Women's Studies, now Disability Studies curriculums are appearing in institutions of higher education. Many of these programs focus on socio/cultural aspects of disability and seek to develop new conceptual models of disability. They attempt to avoid traditional medical models and instead seek to redefine disability as a sociological construct. I think that means more like a minority group and less like gimpers.

The Disability Rights movement of the 70's, 80's, and into the 90's resulted in greatly increased visibility of disability issues and disabled people, and resulted in many program, policy and legislative changes that benefited people with disabilities. This, ultimately, led to the passage of the ADA, the national civil rights law for disabled people.

The next step in the evolution of disability into the mainstream of society was a systematic search by the disability community and their advocates to identify heroes and persons of note who had disabilities. Depending on who compiled the list, there is no shortage of well-known people who have been identified/labeled. To head the list, how about one of my heroes, Julius Caesar (reputed to be epileptic)? Or perhaps Claudius the Roman emperor (polio); Beethoven (deaf); Toulouse-Lautrec (short stature); Helen Keller (deaf/blind); Kent Kloepping (ha, just checking to see if you're paying attention here); a group of folks alleged to be learning disabled (although the term wasn't coined until the mid- twentieth century) including: Churchill, Einstein, Edison, and Alexander G. Bell. Entertainers, Ray Charles, Marlee Martin, Christopher Reeve, Roy Orbison, Itzak Perlman, Politicians Bob Dole, Max Cleland, and of course, F.D.R., Jim Abbott (a major league pitcher with only one hand). Today people want to include Muhammed Ali; and if so, then folks like Roy Campanella (the great Dodger catcher), and the also great jockey Bill Shoemaker would be on the list.

So can we assume that today everyone or almost everyone loves gimpers? Probably not, but it is true that attitudes are much enlightened and opportunities abound for disabled individuals (in America) to lead productive, meaningful lives. Discrimination against people with disabilities will likely never completely vanish, but that is also the case for individuals based on race, gender, age, culture or any other categorization we can contrive for people. I don't believe life will ever be equitable across any dimension one might measure.

After taking this brief tour of some historical views and practices related to disability, we have brought the topic forward to contemporary times. I'd like to rather abruptly change gears here, well sort of, and discuss a matter that is at least tangentially related to the subject at hand. I haven't spent much time, if any, on the matter of my personal spirituality, or religion, if you prefer. I've always had sort of a schizophrenic relationship with organized religion. I don't have any doubts about a Creator, but have struggled throughout my life with how one stays in touch with the Almighty (some people would say prayer).

But anytime I think I'm about to get it straight, there seems to be a new twist, like one fine morning in April of 1999. Since our marriage in 1963, we had attended church on sort of an irregular basis. Then in the early 1970's we became very active members of an Evangelical Lutheran Church of America, ELCA, congregation here in Tucson. We attended church regularly, both served on committees, and at one point, I was elected congregational president for a two-year term.

Over the years, I had grown weary of university politics, and with my retirement in 1998, I had essentially also retired/retreated from formal committee activities in the church, as there were many of the same organizational dynamics in both institutions. However, with the onset of the Lenten Season, we decided to take steps towards personal spiritual renewal. We signed up early for an all-day church sponsored retreat at a local resort. The total number in the group to be led by our senior pastor was probably close to twenty people. I knew many, if not most, of the people who arrived that morning at La Mariposa resort for the special day. When we entered, a tall, smiling lady, who had a puzzled/pained expression, greeted us.

"Good morning," I chirped quite piously, "Are you staff?"

"No, I'm your substitute pastor's wife, and I've handled all the arrangements."

"Good, nice to meet you. I'm Kent Kloepping and this is my wife, Marlys. Where's the seminar room?"

She hesitated as if collecting her thoughts and said, "Well, it's upstairs."

"Oh. Where's the elevator?"

Again she paused, and I had a sinking feeling that I wasn't going to like her answer.

"Well, you see there isn't one," she said. I felt the wind go out of me. I felt deflated. My enthusiasm and upbeat mood evaporated like a punctured tire.

I sighed and asked," Well, how do you propose that we get up there to attend the retreat?"

"Well," she became quite animated and said excitedly "Let's just get three or four fellows, grab those big power chairs and whisk you up those stairs."

I sagged even more in my chair and asked, "Ma'am, are you serious?"

"Why sure," she answered enthusiastically.

" But these chairs weigh close to four hundred pounds with us in them, and they really have no designated freight carrying handles. What's more, have you noticed that the stairway is only about three feet wide with a 90 degree turn and switchback at about stair #10?" I asked.

"Oh dear, it does appear to be a bit of a problem," she replied, her brow knit in thought.

"Problem, problem, you say, I was thinking of something of a little greater magnitude, like more along the lines of a catastrophe!"

Her demeanor changed, to something akin to a little cottontail looking down the barrel of a 12-gauge shotgun.

"How could you do this to us," I asked, "We signed up early to avoid any problems like this. My gosh, how many people in wheelchairs named Kloepping are currently attending that Lutheran church?" The poor lady stared at me as if her mind had turned to jelly.

Before she could respond, (although I'm not sure she would have) I barked to Marlys, "Come on, let's just get out of here." We pushed open the front doors and exited out into the cool overcast morning. She followed us out, muttering and wringing her hands.

"Oh dear", she exclaimed," Well, at least let me give you a hug."

"Hug? Did you say hug?" I howled, "What do you think is happening here, the end of a Special Olympics event?"

As we left the building, I noticed the senior pastor rapidly hustling up the stairs. As he and the church council had been the target of my comments regarding seating for black folks to complement the wheelchair seating in the back of the church, he wasn't about to address this "snafu." We left, called good friends, went to breakfast and fumed for most of the day. But that wasn't the end of the saga. Upon our return home some four hours later (we had gone to the casino as they are always accessible), our son informed us that a note had been left on our front door that stated, "Don't make plans for dinner. We're bringing you food from the retreat." I wish the note had said (or even better, that the group had called) they were moving the retreat to an accessible location.

Maybe the food was seen as a substitute for us not being able to attend the event. You know, like bringing food to "shut-ins." Concerning the note that was left, it was ironically taped to the top of our wrought iron doorframe. That's about eighty inches up. "Holy cow" (or maybe something stronger) I exclaimed to Marlys, "Who hasn't noticed that we are both in wheelchairs?"

I had finally cooled off, having reached a kind of adrenaline withdrawal stupor, when the phone rang. It was the cheerful voice of the pastor's wife.

"Oh hello, did you get our note? We have the food ready to deliver." She continued, "We had a wonderful retreat and I'd like to share some highlights with you and your wife." I took a deep breath and sat shaking my head in disbelief. I decided the course of least resistance was simply to lie.

So I said, "Well, we didn't get home very early and we already ate, so don't bother to bring any food." But I couldn't let the offer to share retreat highlights go without a parting shot. "Furthermore, I don't want to hear any highlights or any thing else about the retreat. Could you try to see it from our perspective? We were excluded from the event because of a really ludicrous oversight, and then when it became clear we could not get upstairs, there was no consideration given to moving to an accessible location. Now, listening to you describe the day would be like rubbing salt in an open wound." I explained.

"Well, well maybe I should come over and we can talk about it," she stammered.

"No, no", I replied," I don't want to talk about this day anymore."

"Oh," she said quietly.

Then silence.

"Would you like to speak to my wife?" I asked.

There was a barely audible, "OK."

Marlys did speak with her for some time, and what they discussed I never did ask, but we didn't get any leftovers or a report of the day's activities.

That ended the La Mariposa fiasco and probably my retreat days. Several Sundays later, I happened to notice the pastor's wife staring at me with a quizzical look on her face. Her expression made me think she might be wondering if I had some type of chronic psychosis. She didn't speak to me, and I'm sure she had little awareness of the frustration I experienced that day.

Should the reader feel that my recounting of the Mariposa affair was overblown, I'd suggest they consider the incident as akin to, say, a black person who'd arrived at a café with a sign that said "no colored people served here." Some would suggest the two situations are different, as the former was unintentional and the latter deliberate. But the situations really are quite similar. They both result in exclusion, and both reflect a lack of understanding and sensitivity to the issue. Whatever view one might have on the matter, as a recipient, I can tell you it doesn't feel very good. It stays with you awhile and it leaves a nick in your dignity.

The lesson for me (and also my suggestion for anyone who has suffered unfairness at the hands of society) would be to work constructively to change/improve what we can, but ultimately just GET OVER IT! I think Marlys and I have mostly passed that hurdle.

I began this chapter with a short anecdote about *being seen* as a person with a disability: This last story is about *being* a disabled person. Oddly, the difficulty for me is I don't feel like a disabled person. I think that I am "normal." I've led a pretty typical middle-class kind of lifestyle. I had a good career, have a reasonable retirement income, live in a nice neighborhood, have two homes, two cars, a boat, some antiques, and lots of other stuff. I'm losing hair from my head, growing more in my ears and nose, I'm going gray, I forget to shave, have problems with gas, and now and then catch myself picking my nose.

Doesn't that sound fairly normal for a guy my age? My wife

tells me that I often don't face reality. Maybe she means that I have delusions about what is or is not real. I have already admitted that I have a schitzy kind of relationship with my religion, but maybe the malady is more pervasive. Perhaps it's at the center of who I am. Several elements central to the definition of schizophrenia are, loss of contact with one's environment" and "retreat into a fantasy world." Nah, that's not me. I'm just "Differently Abled."

XV. Notes And Sources.

1. Acknowledgements.

(1) Mark Twain, letter to George Bainton, 1888. March 25, 2005. <http://www. Twain Quotes.com>

11. Chilldhood-Changes

(1) *Chickory Chick*. Leo's Lyrics. March 2005. <http:/ leoslyrics.com/ list

lyrics.php?sid>

2.Interview: Christine Kloepping. November 19,2001. Rock Grove, Illinois

3.Interview: Christine Kloepping. November 2001. Rock Grove, Illinois.

4 Ibid. July 12,2002. Monroe, Wisconsin.

5. Interview: Frederick "Fritz" Kolb. July 9,2002. Blanchardville, Wisconsin.

6. Interview: Esther (Andereck) Grenzow. July 2002. Juda, Wisconsin.

7. Interview: Larry Kloepping. February 24, 2003. Tucson, Arizona.

8. Interview: Carol (Kloepping) Silva. May 2004. Tucson, Arizona.

III. Polio: The Short Story.

(1) Carlin. George. *Napalm and Silly Putty*. Hyperion, 77 W. 66th St. New York, New York. (P.51)

(2) Bruno, Richard L. *The Polio Paradox.* New York: Warner Books, 2002 (p.34)

(3) Ibid. (p. 58)

(4) *Winnebago County Chapter, National Foundation For Infantile Paralysis.* Rockford, Illinois, 1945.

(5) "Poliomyelitis: 4th Century B.C. Egypt. *Polio Epic Newsletter.* January-February 2003. Tucson, Arizona.

(6) Bruno, Richard L. *The Polio Paradox.* New York: Warner Books. 2002 (p.39)

(7) Business Week Online. *A Summer Plague, Polio and its Survivors.* Tony Gould. Yale University Press. (Book Excerpt) July 23, 2003. < http:// www. Businessweek. Com/ chapter/gould/htm. >

(8) Jane Smith, *Patenting the Sun. Polio and the Salk Vaccine* (New York William Morrow and Co, Inc. 1990.) pp.126-127. (Cited at) In Fear of Polio in the 1950's. (Beth Sokol) July 23, 2003. <http: // www. Inform. Umd. Edu/honr269J/. www/ Projects/ Sokol. Html>

(9) Horstman, Dorothy. *Three Landmark Articles About Poliomyelitis. Medicine.* September 1992 (pp. 320-325)

(10) *Poliomyelitis.* August 1,2003. <http: // www. Cdc.gov/ncp/ Publications/ Pink/Polio. Pdf>

(11) *UNICEF-Immunization plus – Eradicating polio.* http://www.
unicef.org/immunization/index_polio.htm

(12) Corbett, Barry: Alan Toy: The Voice Of Polio Past and Future. *New Mobility.* March 1996. (Pp. 42-48)

(13) *History of Polio.* July 23, 2003. http:// oror. Essortmeent. Com. History of polio_rkgd.htm>

(14) Poliomyelitis-*Medical Dictionary of Popular Medical Terms to Help You*

Better Understand. July 23.2003. <http:// www. Medterns. Com/ Script/

Maim/ art. Asp? Article Key=4974>

(15) Thomas H. Weller-Biography. August 20,2003. <http:// www. *Nobel. se/*

*Medicine/Laureates/ 1954/*Weller-bio. Html>

(16) Jon F. Enders-Biography. August 20,2003. < http:// www. *Nobel se/ Medicine/laureates/ 1954/*enders-bio. Html>

ADDENDUM A *A History of Polio:* A Hypertext Timeline. http:/ www. Cloudnet .com/~ edrbsass/ poliotimeline.htm.

IV. Dusty Lane Days.

1. What my father said to me in 1947 when I complained about not being able to do things other children could.

2.Interview: Christine Kloepping. November 19, 2001. Rock Grove, Illinois.

3.Interview: Jolene (Kloepping) Brudi.November 20, 2001. Rock Grove, Illinois.

4.Interview: Linda Scheider (fellow patient at Deaconess Hospital Freeport, Illinois in1948. November 21, 2001. Rock

Grove, Illinois.

5.Interview: Esther (Andereck) Grenzow. November 2001, Monroe, Wisconsin.

6. Interview: Kenneth Nott (longtime family friend and neighbor during this period). November 2001. Rock Grove, Illinois.

7. Jackie Robinson story (game day and statistics). April 10,2005. <http:// www. *Baseballlibrary/teams/*1951//cubs.stm>

V. High School.

1.Interview: Carol (Kloepping) Silva. May 2004. Tucson, Arizona.

2.Interview: Richard Rockey (childhood and current friend). November 2001. Rock Grove, Illinois.

VI. Illinois Research: A Summer in Chicago.

1.Interview: Christine Kloepping. July 12, 2002. Monroe, Wisconsin.

2.Interview: Carol (Kloepping) Silva. May 2004. Tucson, Arizona.

V11. University of Illinois: A Brief Visit Across The River Styx.

(1) Mickey Rooney. March 20, 2005. <http:// www. Quotations page. Com/quotes/ Mickey Rooney_Rooney/>

2. Interview: Marlys Kloepping. January 2005. Tucson, Arizona.

VIII Southern Illinois University: Redemption in Little Egypt.

1.Interview: Marlys (Sternberg) Kloepping. April 2004. Tucson, Arizona.

2.Interview: Sue (Hackley) Poppaw. April 2004. Green Valley, Arizona.

IX. The Road West: To Find a Job.

(1) Thomas Edison. March 21,2005. <http:// www. Quotations page. Com. Quotes. Php3 author= Thomas+A+Edison. >

2. Interview: Marlys (Sternberg) Kloepping. April 2004. Tucson, Arizona.

X. The Old Pueblo.

(1) Indira Ghandi. March 28, 2005. <http. www. Saidwhat. Co uk/ quotes/i/ indira-ghandi-279 php>

XI1.Travels: A Brief Interlude Before The Rest of The Story

1. Interview: Paul Leung. February 2004. Tucson, Arizona.

2. Interview: Marlys (Sternberg) Kloepping. February 2004. Tucson, Arizona.

3.Gallego Anecdote. As related to me by David Herr-Cardillo, Director Adapted Athletics, University of Arizona. April 23, 2002.

X1I. Retirement.

(1) Isaac Asimov. April 6, 2005. http:// braineyquote. Com/ quotes/i/ isaacasimov/ 46215. html>

2.Jimmy Valvano. 1993 ESPY Awards Acceptance Speech. April 6, 2005. http:// Jimmy Org/ remembering Jim/ espy.efm>

XIII Finis.

1. Calmus, Albert. April 5, 2005. <http:// braineyquote. Com/ quotes/ authors/ Albert Calmus_html>

XIV. EPILOUGE: On Being a Gimp; Differently Abled.

(1) Wright, Beatrice A. (1960) *Physical Disability a Psychological Approach.* Harper and Row, New York.

(2) Dembo, Tamara and Tane-Baskin, E. (1955) The Noticeability of the cosmetic Glove. *Artificial Limb, 2. 47-56.*

(3) Wright, Beatrice A. (1960) Ibid.

(4) Yuker, Harold E., ed. *Attitudes Toward Persons With Disabilities.* New York: Springer, 1988 336p.

(5) A legacy Of Oppression*: A History of Disability in Western Culture.* Colin Barnes. January 19, 2005. <http:// www. Leeds. ac. uk/ disability-studies/ archive uk/ Barnes/ chap 1 pdf.

(6) The Writings of Bob Mauro: *130,000 years of Disability Images from the Stone Age to Beyond Today.* January 18, 2005. <http:// www. Geocites. Com/ ram 87200Newimage.Htm>

(7) Kokasko, Charles. Et al. "Disabled People in The Bible." *Rehabilitation Literature* 45, no. 1-2 1984 (20-21)

(8) *A Legacy of Oppression: A history of Disability in Western Culture.* Colin Barnes. January 19, 2005. Ibid

(9) Haffter, C. (1968) "The Changeling: History and Psychodynamics of Attitudes to Handicapped Children in European Folklore" *Journal of History Behavioural Science*s no 4, pp. 55-61. (Cited in, A Legacy Of Oppression: A History of Disability in Western Culture. Colin Barnes)

(10) Kriegel, L. (1987) The Cripple in Literature, in A. Gartner and T. Joe (Eds*) Images of the Disabled, Disabling Images* (New York, Praege)

(11) Nicholli, O. 1990. *Sex and Gender unhistorical Perspective,* Baltimore John Hopkins University Press. (Cited at: <http: // www. Leeds. ac.uk/disability studies/ Archive uk /Barnes/ chap 1 .pdf>

(12) Ryan, J and Thomas 1987. *The Politics of Mental Handicap* (Revised Edition) London, Free Association Books. (Cited at <http: //. www. Leeds. ac uk/ disability-studies/archiveuk/Branes/ chap. 1. pdf>

(13) *Bibliography on Disability Awareness and Changing Attitudes.* February 8, 2005. <http: // www. rit. edu / ~ easi/pubs/ezbib2. htm>

Other Sources.

(14) The Holy Bible. Authorized King James Version. Edited by Rev. C. I. Schofeild D.D. New York Oxford University Press.

XV. Notes and Sources.

Printed in the United States
77307LV00003B/22-36

9 781587 366413